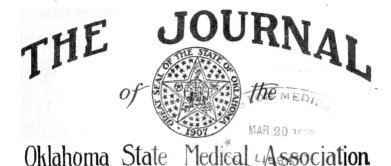

THE JOURNAL

of the

Oklahoma State Medical Association

VOLUME XI   MUSKOGEE, OKLA., JANUARY, 1918   NUMBER 1

GONORRHEA IN THE FEMALE.*

By L. M. SACKETT, M. D., Oklahoma City, Okla.

So surely and regularly does gonorrhea in the female from time to time present its sub-acute manifestations before the practitioner, so does the subject sub-acute itself with the same regular precision before the medical societies of the country.

I know this often discussed condition becomes very burdensome to many of us, yet it does to the female also, and herein lies the purport of this paper,—to impress upon your minds and review with you the real necessity of its early recognition—the endeavor to prevent energetic, persistent and patient treatment of this very serious infection. This same infection which has caused so much unhappiness, suffering and destruction to so many individuals and homes.

This subject is too large to disclose all the different phases or to itemize all that is in the history of gonorrheal infection in women. Just a few important features to mention briefly, and not burden you with the regular routine remarks on what gonorrhea is, where it goes, and what it does.

Accordingly, I hope it will do to pay some attention to the important necessity of pathological recognition of the various stages of its cycle in gonorrheal infection. You will agree and appreciate as the treatment is applied to the understanding of its different stages, so may the results in treatment depend. To mind that without this knowledge and observation can we ever expect results of treatment in any stage. Taking, for instance, the acute stage; if we would recognize and abort by careful appropriate treatment, we might limit the process and prevent the later advance or complications with chronicity, which so inevitably follow.

Therefore, we should know that in the average case, the organism plants himself in the beginning in the Skenes glands, soon attacking the urethra and glands of Bartholin. The glandular structures become swollen, hyperemic and tender, thus disclosing their indentity. The gonococcus imbedded in the gland element. Should we attempt to abort, strong applications are applied to these parts, not intending to seal up infection, but severe enough not only to destroy the organism, but the cellular gland tissue which contains the infection. The severe reaction following brings greater blood supply, bearing greater numbers of leucocytes to assist in repelling the attack. Many times this is possible; occasionally, however, the vulvo-vaginal gland gives trouble.. Abscesses develop, because the infection travels the duct and follows one or all of its branches as they diverge into

*Read at Lawton-Medicine Park, Okla., May 9, 1917.

this gland structure, which is of the racemose type. Often in opening and draining and curetting this gland, we fail to cure for the reason that we do not reach all of the cells making up the gland and the infection reaches here through a different branch than the route we chose, hence it is necessary to remove this vulvo-vaginal gland in its entirety, before permanent result is obtained.

Should we be unsuccessful in the abortive attempt, the folds of mucous membrane at the introitus become bathed and hide quantities of pus which finds its way into the vagina.

Normally, the vagina offers a natural resistance from the fact that it is paved with stratified epithelial cells and offers great resistance to infection, and it is a fact that we do not have gonorrhea existing in the vagina proper, although the walls are hyperemic and tender from the irritating exudate. Regardless of the cleansing douche, the folds of mucous membrane store this infection and allow for plenty of resource for the infection, by continuity and contiguity to invade the cervix.

The cervix, once attacked, becomes a very troublesome presistent office. Here the stratified epithelium is converted into the columnar type containing numerous mucous glands. With this change in structure, the susceptibility is greatly increased. Popular impression has been that the organism enters these cells proper and the greatest activity results from this source, but it is the glandular element, the individual gland infections that represent the difficulty and affords the fortification for future action.

The glands are swollen, their cell lining hypertrophied and eroded, occlusion follows and the drainage obstructed; a sealing in process results only to break out at different intervals, resisting our active, patient treatment. The erosions, the cysts, the chronic leucorrhea persists.

To me the endometrium presents an interesting role with its relation to gonorrheal infection. Here again, theories have changed rapidly; for instance, gonorrheal endometritis is rather rare, at least not the rule, in the list of complications. Now, undoubtedly, while gonorrheal endometritis does exist, it is a great deal more uncommon than is ordinarily supposed. The endometrium acts merely as a side-walk for the gonococcus to pass over to the tubes. The infection may sojourn here for a while, but with little or no pathological significance. The endometrium seemingly has a strong natural immunity to invasion, much stronger than the cervix, whether or not due to a papular arrangement, a lower grade columnar epithelium, utricular gland structure or their secretions, yet it is noted that if the stratified epithelium is thicker and extends further up in the cervical canal, there is greater resistance to infection. Following menstruation, however, there is always a greater susceptibility, as the underlying cell glands are swollen and as the superficial layers are cast off, the port-holes are widened more open and permit of easier infection.

If gonorrheal endometritis does exist, it is either but for a short time, as resolution is very rapid, or the symptoms are more manifest from the constant irritation of leaky tubes.

This theory is well proven by scraping and post-mortem evidence with the use of the microscope. At this point then, it will be well to mention by word of caution and condemn the reckless use of a curette. After local treatments are failing, which, by the way, should never extend beyond the cervical canal for the same following reasons—the curette is to be used.

Now the curette should not be carried beyond the cervical district, for the great danger of carrying infectious material into the uterus, which either subsequently involves the tubes surely or light up their former activities. This, I am sure, is an error in practice. In our knowing of gonorrheal infection in the history and in our desire to stop this troublesome leucorrhea, etc., we curette the entire organ. This is unnecessary, superfluous and dangerous in the majority of the average cases. We not only lessen the normal immunity but are apt to carry in the mixed type of infections, start up old tubal trouble, which can and does set up the local peritoneal symptoms and possibly general peritonitis.

. Next in order the Fallopian tubes are attacked with such unfortunate frequency. In by far the greatest number of cases, both tubes are involved nearly simultaneously; rarely one alone, although in one tube the process may be arrested, early resolution, and the fact escape our notice.

The infection is carried to these structures by the continuity of mucous membrane, the blood and lymph streams, most often by the first route. The mucous membrane is thickened, swollen, the muscular coats congested, their fibers elongated, the whole tube red and angry looking and enlarged, the ostium closes. Pus may form rapidly and in a few days be in great quantity.

Most usually the process is slower, the columnar epithelium is highly inflamed, thickened and swollen; the celia are lost. The rugae or folds of mucous membrane ulcerate and become glued together in different areas of the tube. Termination of this pathological process—the gradual accumulation of pus distending, distorting the tube with its many already formed adhesions from exuded lymph, either ruptures and drains back into the uterus or ruptures into the pelvic cavity or becomes sealed up. The activity lessens and disappears for a time only to flare up again under some exciting, irritating influence. Repeating these menacing performances until it is necessary for surgery to put an end to the condition.

Some cases are more fortunate; the process, active for a time, may subside with resolution and absorption and the patency of the tube restored. It is these changing pathological conditions that afford the opportunity for tubal pregnancies. The ovum traveling down the duct is stopped by minute strictures or adhesions which have followed in the wake of inflammation. In times gone by, it was declared that with gonorrheal pus tubes women were rendered sterile—that is not true, because we all can recall instances with a gonorrheal history prior to confinement. She had gonorrheal tubes but with good resolution. Here again should great conservatism be exercised in surgical treatment. Especially, in young women anxious to become mothers—better many times to amputate a portion of the tube and build a new ostium and draw closer to the ovary. Conserve, save, do all that you can to help her, then if necessary do a secondary operation later.

The last and very vital consideration is the ovary. Infection reaches this delicate organ by way of contiguity, continuity, blood and lymph supply. It often happens that an ovary is infected without the infection ever reaching the tubes. How? By the lymph channels draining the endocervical and endometrial regions through the broad ligaments and lateral structures.

Curiously in the descriptive type, only the surface of the ovary is first involved, often no further extension. An excessive amount of lymph is produced around it, responsible for the extensive adhesions which from in this vicinity. Much swollen and extemely edematous. Should the process extend, infiltration occurs into the deep stroma. Here small islands of pus develop, sooner or later there can be a general coalescing and a true ovarian abscess will result, followed by sterility.

Should the opposite condition occur, viz., resolution, we note that the small foci of infection are isolated or absorbed. The attending connective tissue intergrowth with its tendency to contract and retract results in a cirrhotic condition— a cirrhotic ovary.

Sterility is apt to follow here also. Why? Because of the infection or destruction of the viable follicles or on account of the dense thickened stroma of inflammatory connective tissue, cirrhotic stroma, making it impossible for a mature rupturing Graffian follicle to force its way through such a resisting network of fibrous tissue. Consequently, the ovum never reaches the surface.

The adhesions which are associated with gonorrheal infection in the female pelvis are worth mentioning. It is in this condition that they are more rapidly and more securely developed than in any other type of pelvic inflammation. Another instance of how quickly nature assists in grave dangers. The adhesions formed from extravasated lymph in any style, from threadlike bands to solid masses, are the strongest and the safest of all the different types. Instead of disappearing by traction and absorption as they do for instance, in a per cent. in septic peritonitis or tubercular peritonitis, not a trace remaining years afterwards in many cases, these *gonorrheal* monuments remain only to grow harder and firmer, binding together structures, immobilizing the uterus and its appendages, limiting functions of anything and everything that inhabits the pelvic cavity. Troublesome in the extreme.

From the obstetrical standpoint, many are of our unexplained, long-drawn-out, tedious labor cases due to inertia, as we say—but what has caused the inertia? Earlier gonorrheal infection is unquestionably responsible in a per cent. When the uterus is involved in infection, the parenchyma, especially the inner layer of muscle fibers, are attacked. · The resulting connective tissue formation with its characteristic non-elastic qualities, resisting muscular activity, and they fail to respond to the nerve stimulus of the pregnant uterus, and hence the inertia. Later poor absorption of fatty degeneration on account of connective interstital tissue leaving varying degrees of sub-involution.

Little will be said on treatment as it has not changed much from the ideas which we all have; only mentioned to caution against things not to be done.

If one is attempting to abort gonorrhea, necessarily he must use strong caustic application. If he fails or sees the case after abortion is out of the question, the treatment is to be mild at first—rest in bed, very light, low, bland douches. Avoid the dangers of driving infection upward with the douche stream or by the nozzle itself. External douches are frequently the better of the two. Constant local application to the endocervix only, and not beyond.

Various tamponades for relief of local irritation and support are advisable when the infection has attacked the upper structures. Later on thorough curettage of just the endocervix brings good results if thoroughly done. I have seen with good results the endocervix and the endometrium cauterized with pure phenol following curettage—to be sure to get all the infection or destroy all of the infected glands. Yet there is a danger towards an atresia of some degree following too long and too strong cauterization.

Lastly, surgery, conservative surgery, is resorted to for permanent relief and protection from the frequent, troublesome, sub-acute attacks which allows the patient so little comfort or good health mentally and physically between cycles.

This now is the real appeal of this paper—to regard more, study more, learn more of the true condition in gonorrheal inflammation. Be able to decide from the pathological findings the best course to pursue in your treatment. When to conserve or when to sacrifice tissue for the best benefit of your patient.

Learn by the touch what the pathology is, what it means, what structures are involved and how applied to the various symptoms, especially in the neurotic types.

Summary: I am very glad that this paper has brought criticism; that it may stimulate us all to be more observant in future cases. In criticism we are all made better. To me a paper should not be given to represent a man's own personal experience nor observation—we have all had that—but to hunt up and quote the experiences, the findings and the proofs of men whose opportunities and training have been greater than ours. Whose results have been accepted by the majority of the profession as standard for authority. Among those whom I consulted are Graves, Norris, Ashton, Bandler, Boldt, Taylor, Kelley and Noble.

CHRONIC VESICULITIS.

Physiology, Symptoms and Treatment.

By WILLIAM J. WALLACE, Ph. G., M. D., Associate Professor Genito-Urinary
Diseases, and Syphilis, University of Oklahoma.

The seminal vesicles were first noted by the anatomists Berendi de Carpi, in 1523, and again by Fallopius in 1562, but were not discovered from a pathological standpoint till 1815 by Baillie of London. Among the urologists of recent years who have devoted special attention to the diseases of these glands, may be mentioned, Fuller, Belfield, Guiteras, Young, Squier and Keyes.

We know at this time, and recognize that obscure joint, neuralgic or neurologic-nephritic, vesical and cardiac diseases are to be found in remote organs or foci. Comparatively recently the tonsils, teeth, nasal cavity and throat have been regarded as the most frequent site of such infections. The genito-urinary tract, which to my experience is to blame in a great number of cases, has not been appreciated as a causative factor. It has long been recognized that gonorrhea, both acute and chronic, is responsible for many general infections, but the seminal vesicles, up to the present time, have received but very little attention. In this article I shall confine my discussion to the role of the seminal vesicles in their chronic state, the toxemias and remote symptoms.

Physiology.

The function of the seminal vesicles is to act as a storage reservoir for the seminal fluid, and to contribute a secretion, which acts as a nourishment or fertilizer, and which also has the faculty of preserving the vitality, and activity of the spermotozoa. It is also possessed of a peristalsis similar to that of other parts of the body. With the physiological stimulus the peristalic wave begins and empties contents.

Pathology.

The most frequent cause of chronic vesiculitis is a result of an extensive posterior gonorrheal, urethritis, or prostatitis. If the case is of long standing, which is always true of the chronic, a mixed infection will usually be found present in the vesicles, namely: streptococci, staphylococci, and the colon and proteus bacillus, etc., which resist all ordinary measures of treatment available to the average physician. There are three stages of chronic vesiculitis to deal with from a pathological standpoint: 1st, the hypertrophic. 2nd, the atrophic, which are the result of an extension of a specific disease, (namely gonorrhea). 3rd, the atonic, a condition of the vesicle which is non-specific, and brought about by abnormal abuses, etc.

First, in the hypertrophic form, we have a general septic inflammatory condition with infiltration, and with inflammation of the mucosa, sub-mucosa and the muscular structure and peri-inflammatory condition of the entire seminal vesicle, which is considerably enlarged and presses up under the bladder in the region of the trigone, and upon the ureters near their entrance in the bladder. The result of this inflamed condition of the vesicles, consists of an altered secretion of the parts, together with the products of an exudative or separative inflammation, in this condition the peritoneum frequently extends well down the vesicle and is attached to them, hence the frequent peritoneal symptoms.

Second. The atrophic is the result of the hypertrophic, and is characterized first, by an overgrowth of tissue, which if untreated, results in the mucosa being deprived of its normal blood supply and function, then the vesicles become atrophied either in part, or completely, destroying the entire vesicles. Sometimes we have calcareous deposits in the diverticulum of the vesicle which is bound down by numerous fibrous bands.

Third. This form, atonic, or non-specific, is the result very frequently of abnormal abuses, lack of indulgence, or over-indulgence. In this the entire vesicles have become relaxed with no strength of power to stimulate the peristalsis, so it can empty itself of its contents, hence they are soft, mushy and putty-like. The pathology of these three forms is mentioned because each calls for a separate and distinct treatment.

Symptoms.

Chronic seminal vesiculitis is nearly always a continuation of a previous acute vesiculitis which was uncured. At least 70 per cent of the acute cases become chronic. The close association of the symptoms of the chronic vesiculitis with sexual irritability give the appearance of neuresthenia, and mental affections. In the hands of the majority of physicians these cases are often treated for neurasthenia, without the real underlying cause being recognized.

Pain: Felt deep in the perineum, sometimes it is described as a gnawing pain radiating from the groin, frequently accompanied by a sense of weariness and often assumes the form of itching or tickling. Pain interferes with rest and sleep, which hastens the onset of the classical symptoms of neurasthenia. When the bladder is full, the pain is in the supra-pubic region and also is felt in the loin over the kidneys, the latter being caused by counter-pressure by the distended bladder above, against an inflamed vesicle underneath, which extends up and into the ureteral entrance into the bladder. With this pressure we get a direct reflex pain to the kidneys. In the terminal act of urination pain is also felt in the perineum and supra-pubic region and there is also a sensation of fullness in the bladder as though it had not been thoroughly emptied—all due to the inflamed and diseased vesicles which lie underneath the trigonum.

Urinary: The disturbances of micturition are very common. Burning along the urethral canal during micturition or the same sensation may be confined to the prostatic urethra, or to the head of the glans penis. Frequent urination is not such an annoying symptom in chronic vesiculitis as it would be in the acute form, but the desire to urinate is more than it would be in a normal bladder on account of the inability of the bladder to distend, as over-distention presses on the vesicles.

Sexual erethism: Sexual erethism is evident only in the hypertrophic form of seminal vesiculitis. It is characterized by priapism, or frequent erections, due to the congestion of the vesicles, or the pressure of their contents with secretory edema. The erections may be so frequent as to prevent the patient from sleeping at night. The desire is stimulated, and the ejaculation may be painful. Nocturnal emissions accompanied by lascivious dreams are present at first; later, the emissions occur without dreams, and without sensation, or apparent cause, due to the passing from the hypertrophic into the atrophic form.

Impotency: This is due to two pathological conditions of the seminal vesicles, the atrophic and atonic. First, the atrophic form, which is a direct result of the hypertrophic, is the result of a cicatricial contraction, occulsion and destruction of the vesicles. The vesicles are thickened, hard and sclerosed, and calculi are frequently formed. The normal secretion is no longer present to dilute and activate the spermatozoa, hence incurable impotency.

Next, in the atonic form the vesicles have no strength, no power to empty their contents, no circulation and no tone—hence a physiological impotency which is curable.

Spermatorrhea: Spermatorrhea, or gleet, is a very frequent symptom, and most annoying to the patient. The ever present "morning drop" calls up all manner of dire forebodings in the patient's mind, and causes him to consult a physician for relief. If there be only the spermatorrhea present, the discharge is clear and watery; if a mixed infection has occurred, the discharge will be more purulent, containing pus together with epithelial cells and occasionally a few blood corpuscles.

Arthritis: The role of seminal vesiculitis in producing arthritis has been recognized only recently. This systemic effect is due to the absorption of toxins and bacteria, especially gonorrhea, from the vesicular infection. The symptoms are pain in the lumbar region, severe pain in the coccyx, stiffness of the muscles attached to the tuberosity of the ischium, causing a stiffness when the patient sets down or stands up. Arthritis is often manifested in the form of tender heels, inflammation of the joints, periarthritis and periostitis. Sometimes it is impossible to locate the source of the infection, but if the vesicles are enlarged, it is safe to say that drainage of them will cure the arthritis.

Abdominal: These are usually intestinal in character. Peritoneal symptoms are not uncommon. Attacks of pain, with the concomitant signs and symptoms, have frequently been mistaken for appendicitis, and Schmidt reports numerous cases in which operations have been performed. The peritoneum is frequently attached to inflamed vesicles.

Rectal: There is a feeling of fullness, sometimes pain, sensation of feeling a lump or some obstruction—no power to expel the contents. Anal irritation and eczema are not uncommon.

Ureters: Young reports ten cases in which there was operation for renal calculus, the symptoms of which were typical—intermittent, colicky pains radiating to the groins, simulating ureteral calculi.

Neurasthenia: Nervous symptoms play a prominent part in chronic vesiculitis and are among the most difficult to overcome. These neurotic patients are usually deeply depressed, because of the long standing of their symptoms, and are favorable subjects for melancholia. They brood over their condition, and the prospect of early sterility, together with the fear of insanity, occasionally leads them to commit suicide. If an occlusion of the ejaculatory ducts occurs as a result of the vesicular infection, there is no emission. This causes a severe deep perineal pain with profound nervous shock and depression. Mental lassitude, occipital headache, loss of sleep, aggravated by sexual excitement, are usual symptoms. The feet, hands and back may feel cold and numb; anesthesia and paresthesia may be present in certain parts of the body. Sensation of numbness and atrophy of genitals; flushing of face, indigestion and constipation are common. There is a lack of desire to work and inability to concentrate the mind on any particular task.

Differential Diagnosis:

The normal healthy vesicles are not palpable to the touch, and if the physician is certain that he feels them, there is reason to believe they are diseased. Seminal vesiculitis is most frequently mistaken for chronic prostatitis, posterior urethritis, stricture and varicocele.

Prostatitis: Chronic prostatitis very closely resembles seminal vesiculitis, and the fact that both may be present in the same patient makes it extremely difficult to decide which one predominates. A microscopical examination of the fluid in prostatitis shows the presence of Boettcher's crystals and amyloid corpuscles, which in vesiculitis spermin and spermatozoa are present. Prostatic discharge is more frequent after defecation in prostatitis than it is in the chronic vesiculitis. Rectal examination will show the prostate enlarged, soft and flabby or irregular; while in vesiculitis it is normal and the vesicles are palpable, irregular, tortuous and swollen. Chronic vesiculitis often follows chronic prostatitis. The urine after massage in prostatitis is turbid and contains pus and inflammatory products; while in the vesiculitis it contains only globulin and shreds of membrane.

Chronic Urethritis: Because of the urethral discharge, chronic urethritis is often mistaken for chronic vesiculitis. In vesiculitis, the discharge is clear, and contains spermatozoa; while in posterior urethritis it contains pus, gonococci, and spermatozoa are absent. In urethritis the urine shows shreds; in vesiculitis it is clear until the last, when there is some detritus consisting of membrane, shreds and globulin. Rectal examination shows vesiculitis. Endoscopic examination in posterior urethritis shows granular patches and areas of ulceration.

Stricture: Stricture should never be confused with chronic vesiculitis. The passage of sounds and palpation of the vesicles is all that is necessary to differentiate.

Varicocele: Varicocele is likewise confused with vesiculitis only by the physician who neglects to examine the vesicles. The pain in the groin and testes is common in both diseases.

Treatment:

The treatment consists of constitutional, local and in one form, surgical. The first step is to classify the pathology of the case to be treated, that is, whether atonic, atrophic or hypertrophic.

Atonic: The first form to be considered is the atonic. This is usually non-specific and generally found in neurotic individuals who never had a specific disease, and in many instances have never even exposed themselves, but have suffered from self-abuse and as a result we find them in a nervous, anemic and weakened condition, mentally, physically and psychologically.

The first of this class in our line of treatment will be constitutional, hygienic and suggestive—advice as to patient's mode of living and suggestions as to exercise and general physical development—definite instructions as to the regulation of sexual habits. It is very necessary to impress upon these patients that the case is serious, but curable, and they must follow instructions implicitly and work in cooperation with the physician as the treatment will extend a considerable length of time.

The local treatment is begun in a systematic way, as follows:

Massage: First, massage the vesicles jointly with the prostate gland, and let me say here that it is very necessary to understand how to give the massage. Patient must lean forward with hands grasping legs, as near ankle as possible, legs widely separated, and straight with no bending of the knee and toes turned in. Introduce the index finger in rectum very carefully, as the latter is frequently very sensitive, carrying the finger over the prostate gland up to the bladder to the back of the seminal vesicles, 2 1-2 to 4 inches from the anus. Begin with a very gentle light stroke back and forth movement, slow and steady, as hard rapid pressure will not empty the vesicles as well as the former method. This should be done slowly several times ascertaining from the patient if anything is passing from the meatus. The time required is usually about three minutes over each vesicle. The prostate is then massaged with very much more force to empty the contents of it as well as the vesicles, as the prostate is usually enlarged too.

Meatotomy: A meatotomy should be performed if a small meatus exists, then introduce a sound into the bladder, the larger the better, preferably size 30 French, allowing this to remain in the bladder for 5 minutes. After withdrawal of sound give deep instillation, both into the prostatic urethra and into the bladder of a stimulating antiseptic. This treatment is given every second or third day. Once a week this instillation consists of 1-2 of 1 per cent of nitrate of silver solution as something is needed to stimulate and build up the part. This treatment systematically used with the cooperation and confidence of the patient, together with the advice of marriage and well regulated sexual hygiene, will cure the patient of vesicular symptoms.

Atrophic: The atrophic is a result of a previous hypertrophic condition causing a destruction, contraction and occlusion of the vesicles. In this we have no vesicular action, merely scar tissue and adhesions, frequently calcareous deposits and nerve pressure, hence reflex symptoms—incurable impotency, and general mental depression. The prognosis in this case is very bad, but can be benefitted by the following treatment.

First treatment is constitutional, as described in the atonic. Locally the treatment will be centered upon an effort to stimulate a circulation through the scar tissue and to liberate and break down the adhesions around and through the vesicles.

First, introduce a sound clear into the bladder, size 30 to 32 F., the patient in same position as previously described, finger introduced into rectum upon the vesicles and a similar massage given against the counter-pressure of the sound. In this way we can break down some of the adhesions and stimulate a new circulation. This treatment every third day for a period of several months will bring very happy results.

Hypertrophic: In the hypertrophic condition, the treatment is somewhat different from those previously described, as here we have an infiltrated and inflamed, suppurative and circumscribed vesicular abscess, with all the resultant constitutional, neurotic, and local symptoms, with an adhesion or obstruction to normal drainage. So the treatment must be to liberate the contents by drainage. This should be done by local and operative methods.

Local: In the local treatment introduce a sound as previously described, which must remain for 5 minutes—carefully withdraw. Then massage vesicles, each one for three minutes—repeating every day with the object in view of liberating the suppurative contents. The massage must be gentle and slow and should be given each day until the condition is thoroughly cleared and symptoms relieved. This may take from three weeks to three months. Use the sound not oftener than every third day, following with a deep instillation of some antiseptic. If this treatment is carried out it will establish a cure in 95 per cent of the cases.

The remaining uncured cases, which have not yielded to the above treatment, have resolved themselves into circumscribed vesicular abscesses, which must be drained, as these are the foci from which remote constitutional symptoms will arise. Hence a perineal, vesiculotomy is necessary to effect a cure.

Technic For Operation: The patient is placed in the extreme lithotomy position. The skin incision should be either the semilunar, or the inverted V incision, extending from tuberosity to tuberosity. The median tendon is exposed and divided. The urethral-rectal muscle is located by blunt dissection and divided, thus permitting the exposure of the vesicles, which are hidden beneath the fascia of Denon Villier. A Young's prostatic retractor, at this point in the operation will be found useful in bringing the vesicles down into view. Squier passes a needle threaded with heavy silk on each side at the juncture of the bladder and prostate, using this as a tractor; while Schmidt uses tenaculum forceps applied at this point. The fascia is dissected first from one vesicle, and then from the other; the vesicles are opened and a drainage tube of small calibre is fastened into each one by catgut sutures, through the adjoining fascia and tube. The drain is left in place from ten to fifteen days.

References:
1. Schmidt, J. A. M. A., Jan. 15, 1916.
2. Anderson, J. Tenn. S. M. A., April, 1916.
3. Shropshire, Southern Medical Journal, Oct., 1916.
4. Bremmermann, Interstate Medical Journal, August, 1916.
5. Jacobsohn, Munich, Med. Wchnchr., Sept. 9, 1916.

SPOROTRICHOSIS.

To the total number of cases of sporotrichosis observed in this country, amounting to less than a hundred, another is added by E. H. McLean, Omaha (*Journal A. M. A.*, Nov. 24, 1917). Though discovered in America the disease has been more thoroughly studied in France where there is an extensive literature on the subject. In the case reported, a clinical diagnosis of glanders was made but cultures revealed the sporothrix. The case adds another from the Missouri Valley, from which section of the country have come the largest number of reports of the disease.

A RELATION OF FOCAL INFECTION TO SKIN DISEASES.*

By EVERETT S. LAIN, M. D.,

Associate Professor and Head of Department of Dermatology, University of Oklahoma,
School of Medicine, Oklahoma City, Okla.

Progressive medicine has always made its advances through diligent pursuits along a particular line until said line of thought or suggestion has been fully developed. Advancement in dermatology, one of the specialties in medicine, has been no exception to this rule. It has been unfortunate, indeed, that for a long period of time practically the only lines of original research or advancement were made along the line of histo-pathology, diagnosis, and in more recent years nomenclature of diseases.

Until recently few men had given serious or diligent thought to the etiology of that large class of dermatological lesions which have been classified as "unknown," "idiopathic," or "trophoneurotic."

After experimental work done and announcements to the world which came from the laboratory of Billings and Rosenow, in the years of 1912 and 1913, wherein they had positively proven a relation of focal infections to rheumatism and a number of other systemic or constitutional diseases, quite a few of our dermatologists, as well as men in other branches of medicine, were awakened to the possible etiologies and soon began investigations of focal infections and what relation the same might have to certain diseases. We soon had announcements from Galloway upon the observation of a number of erythematous eruptions which were accompanied by and associated with rheumatism with a focal infection. Immediately following this, Gerber made observations and studies in ten cases of erythema nodosum, declaring that he had found present in the cutaneous veins, cocci which were similar to those also found in the tonsils, or apical abscesses of the same patient. Soon thereafter, or about November, 1915, Rosenow again announced his proven theory of elective localization of streptococci. Also in the same studies he was able to produce, experimentally, herpes zoster in rabbits which had been innoculated with an emulsion from tonsils or teeth of patients suffering from the same disease.

After hearing and reading of these almost startling discoveries, the author was inspired to examine briefly, and later more carefully, both the tonsils and teeth of every patient who came under his observation suffering with a skin disease whose etiology was not already known. The studies were begun early in the year 1914 and have lasted until the present day. The usual routine consisted of inspection and perhaps palpation of the tonsils in an effort to ascertain whether there might be lacunae filled with pus, also an inspection of the teeth with reference to pyorrhoeal infection or probable apical abscesses.

In the early months of our studies we merely inspected the teeth and made no radiographs unless a tooth presented clear evidence of death of its pulp or nerve. We soon learned, however, that no method other than a complete X-ray picture or radiograph would reveal the true condition presented at the apex of a tooth. Therefore, we do not finally accept any tooth as sound or that there exists no focus of infection until a clear picture is taken which proves same.

Our studies have been largely of such diseases as erythema multiforma, and nodosum, psoriasis, herpes zoster, lupus erythematosis, eczemas, ptyriasis, urticaria, acne and lichen planus. To date we have carefully examined several hundred cases. Within this number we have had quite a few successive cases of each of the above named diseases. Therefore, we feel justified in presenting some of our observations for whatever value they may give to others and trust for a further investigation to reveal the truth or fallacies of our conclusions.

*Read at Lawton-Medicine Park, Okla., May 9, 1917.

The length of this paper will not permit of a discussion of each of these diseases as regards the relation or lack of relation of a local foci of infection to their etiology. Therefore, we shall only mention a few of said diseases which have offered most encouragement for our studies or in which there have been almost constantly associated either apical abscesses or diseased tonsils.

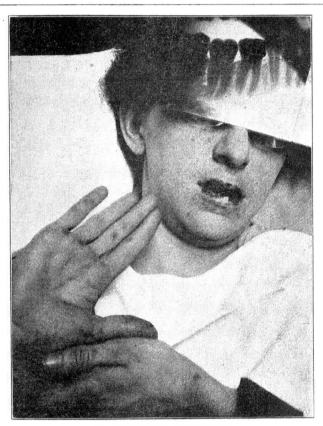

NO. 1. ERYTHEMA MULTIFORMA.
Recurrence of Erythema Multiforma involving hands, also large area of mucous surface of mouth and lips. Apical abscesses under first molar.

The well known disease of psoriasis has furnished us a large number of cases for investigation and we have been able to note either an infected tonsil or apical abscesses in a large percentage of the cases examined. In a few cases, perhaps ten per cent, we have not been able to locate a probable focus either within the tonsils or under the teeth. However, when we are reminded by Rosenow and others that a stomach ulcer, diseased appendix, or an infection of the genito urinary tract and other organs are not infrequent sources for the etiology of diseases which may have a special localization for other than their tissues, we still feel encouraged to prosecute the study of psoriasis for a longer period.

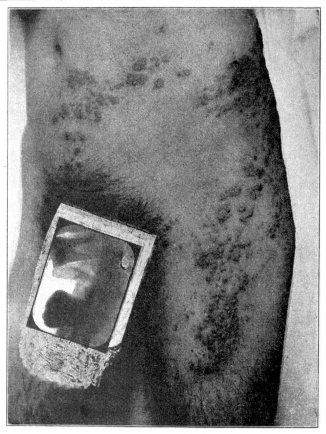

NO. 2. HERPES ZOSTER.
Extensive Herpes Zoster, with necrosing fragments of teeth.

Erythema multiforma has in our recent investigations been almost constantly associated with apical abscesses or diseased tonsils. In a recent case of extreme type, in which the mucous surfaces of the mouth and lips were extensively involved, we found teeth and tonsils apparently good, though a radiograph of the teeth disclosed a large apical abscess under a molar of which the patient was unconscious. The present eruption was only one of a number of preceding attacks during the past three years. The first having occurred some four or six months after a dentist had attempted to kill the nerve and fill the canal of said affected first molar.

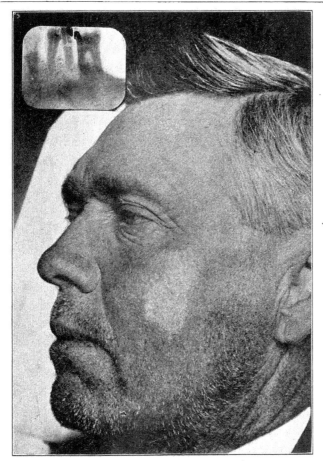

NO. 3. LUPUS ERYTHEMATOSIS.
Two or more sharply defined apical abscesses.

Lupus erythematosis is also offering a very favorable field for study. We did not begin the study of this disease until the past year. Therefore, have not a sufficient number of cases from which to draw conclusions. Of the few cases we have so far examined, we found the tonsils were affected in a large number, in most of said cases even to a degree of marked hypertrophy. In one case a man, age about 50, retained roots and two or more distinct apical abscesses were dis-

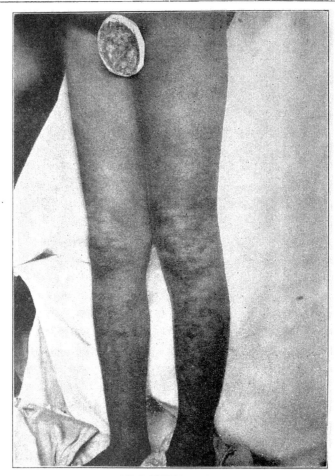

NO. 4. LICHEN PLANUS.
Large pus filled tonsils. After removal of same, a complete recovery within three weeks.

closed by the X-ray. The lesion had dated from a period immediately following a toothache with an attempt at extraction.

Two diseases in our studies have from the beginning been constantly associated with a focal infection, namely: lichen planus and herpes zoster. We have examined quite a number of each during the past two and one-half years, and in every case of lichen planus we have been able to discover either one or more apical abscesses, or abscessing fragments of teeth. Or as in most cases in which the patient was under twenty-five years of age, clearly defined hypertrophied pus infected tonsils.

The etiology of herpes zoster can no longer be doubted, since Rosenow's declarations of November, 1915, wherein he related a number of experimental cases produced by innoculations from apical abscesses or infected tonsils. Zoster was one of the first diseases studied by the author and his associate, Dr. M. M. Roland, who has worked side by side with the author from the first to the last case studied. In our studies of herpes zoster, approximately 100 per cent have given evidence of a focal infection.

It now appears almost like a stupidity of our minds that we were not able at an earlier date to classify both rheumatism and zoster, also some of the neuralgias, as a focal infection, for they have always been closely associated with diseased tonsils or pus infected teeth.

Every general practitioner can recall such cases wherein their patients affected with zoster had been affected with repeated attacks of tonsillitis or possessed a foul smelling mouth, wherein there rested fragments of decayed teeth or a constant pyorrhoeal discharge.

In conclusion we are convinced that quite a few dermatological lesions shall soon be classified as focal infections. Some two or four of said diseases we feel confident now shall be among this group, namely: herpes zoster, lichen planus and erythema nodosum, with a probable addition of erythema multiforma and lupus erythematosis. No doubt others may also be classified as those which in rare instances may be caused from a localized foci.

However, it behooves us to study carefully and not jump at conclusions or make wild declarations as some are prone, which are exemplified in a few articles appearing in some of our journals. Let us study carefully and prove all the ground for our conclusions both by microscope, cultures, and the X-ray as well as by clinical findings.

CHRONIC NEPHRITIS.

William Ophuls, San Francisco (*Journal A. M. A.*, Oct. 13, 1917), reports a study of diffuse glomerulonephritis, a term which he prefers for cases in which the renal tissue shows diffuse hematogenous inflammatory lesion. Excluding all focal lesions of lesser importance, the term includes the various types of nephritis in which the lesions of the glomeruli play an important part. The author notices some of the prominent contributions on the bacteriology of these cases, and reports the results of experimental intravenous injection in animals. These results seem to support his former suggestion that the glomeruli lesions are probably embolic and due to the rapid lysis of the bacteria within the vascular loops of the glomeruli. He also describes the course of the three types, acute, subacute, and chronic, and summarizes as follows: "1. There is a well defined disease of the kidneys caused by general sepsis arising from some infected focus and often made progressive by the persistence of such a focus. 2. Since the glomeruli in this disease show the most characteristic and constant lesions, we may speak of it as glomerulonephritis, and as the lesions are so distinctly of an inflammatory character, as true nephritis. 3. The disease occurs in three forms—the acute, the subacute and the chronic type. 4. The characteristic glomerular lesions may be reproduced in animals by injection of bacteria into the blood stream. 5. The majority of cases in man are due to streptococci, but other bacteria may cause similar lesions in the kidneys and elsewhere. 6. Many of the chronic cases seem to be caused by a peculiar form of chronic suppurative tonsillitis due to diplostreptococcic infection."

DIAGNOSIS OF GASTRO-INTESTINAL LESIONS BY X-RAY.*

By J. T. MARTIN, M. D., Oklahoma City, Okla.

Accuracy in diagnosis is the goal of present day progress. In the different fields of pathologic physiology and anatomy of the abdominal organs the radio-scope and radiograph is establishing itself. This field is truly modern, and the memory of each one of us vividly pictures the hopes and dreams of its dawning.

I shall endeavor to give briefly the present value as derived from current literature and our experiences at the X-ray laboratory of St. Anthony's hospital in Oklahoma City.

There are two methods in vogue. The one, direct, or American, as Leonard and George call it, and the other the indirect,' or continental method. Both are based upon giving an opaque substance in a given menstra and the study of the subsequent shadow. The Ridel meal, more used in the continental schools, consists of 40 gms. of bismuth in 300 cc. of porridge. The usual American meal is 100 gms. to 150 gms. of bismuth in a fluid menstra as buttermilk. The observations with the different meals are not comparable either as to time motility factor of filling power. The fluid meals are more rapid moving and fill both normal and abnormal recesses better than the porridge meals.

The indirect or continental method is chiefly fluoroscopic. It is called the indirect method because the diagnosis is derived by symptom complex, e. g., diagnosis of gastric ulcer by interruption of peristalic wave and rapid emptying.

The direct method attempts to and does demonstrate the lesion on a series of permanent records. The direct method, besides demonstrating the actual lesion at the time, gives an opportunity to study the findings at your leisure and in con-junction with the other evidence in the case. The fluorscopic method leaves no permanent evidence except the record of personal interruption. The wonderful work of Cole, of New York, demonstrates the highest type of the plate method. A judicious combination of the two methods is now the more popular.

The patients presenting themselves for roentgenologic examination of the abdomen should preferably have a gentle cathartic the previous night. Breakfast is prohibited, but water and coffee are allowed. It is wise to take the first view before an opaque meal is given. Fluoroscopy of parts suspected, i. e., at time the opaque meal is in the suspected parts and recording of any abnormality by permanent picture is advised. This should not interfere with, or supersede set plate records of areas as pylorus, caput, ileocaecal, the colonic flexures taken at definite times as on ingestion, the one hour, 3, 6, 9, 12 and 24 hour.

Stomach: Roentgenologic study of the stomach has changed our ideas as to location and shape. The stomach is a collapsible bag hanging in the abdominal cavity. The cardiac orifice is attached to the diaphragm. The pyloric orifice is attached to the slightly movable duodenum. The lesser curvature is less movable than the greater curvature on account of peritoneal attachments. The normal position of the stomach varies, these loose attachments being considered, accord-ing to size, general individual development, tone of muscle walls and irritability. The greater curvature may normally be 3 or 4 finger breadths above the umbilicus to the same distance below. The umbilicus, which is often used as a localizing point, is a very movable affair; hence it is better to locate the stomach by the vertebra or the bony pelvis. We may have the stomach above the second lumbar vertebra or to the pelvic brim and yet be normal to that individual.

Ulcer of the stomach can be demonstrated because of the induration and erosion of the stomach wall making an irregularity in the contour of the shadow. The fluoroscope can demonstrate interruption and change in the peristaltic wave and changes in the motility. By plates filling defects an actual outline of the

*Read at Lawton-Medicine Park, Okla., May 9, 1917.

ulcer can be shown. Plates should be made immediately after ingestion of opaque meal after 1-2, 3, 6 and 12 hours. In case of ulcer should show: 1. Projection of shadow in wall. 2. Defect in shadow due to infiltration of ulcer wall. 3. Contraction—permanent hour glass. 4. Retention—pylorospasm.

1st: Projection of shadow in gastric wall is due to denuded surfaces on lesser and greater curvatures. This is pathognomic of ulcer. If the ulcer has perforated the gastric wall, the shadow is punched outside the stomach wall.

2nd: Defect in the shadow due to infiltration of the stomach wall. This is shown by filling defect and interruption of peristaltic waves over a definite local rigid area. Fluoroscopy is here valuable.

3rd: Temporary and permanent hour glass stomach are most often ulcer accompaniments. The former is found in both acute and chronic ulcer; the latter is chronic scars of adhesions.

4th: Retention due to pyloric obstruction may be spasm, benign cicatrix, adhesions, outside pressure or new growth. The first three conditions suggest ulcer. Besides definite spasm deep indentations of the incisura is suspicious of ulcer.

Malignancy: The value of the roentgenologic study in malignancy of the stomach is of great importance because it is the most definite of the early evidences we have upon which to base an early diagnosis. The gastric cancer picture is a filling defect, usually near the pylorus, annular in shape and permanent in character. Leonard and George claim the pyloric annular filling defect that has an irregular bitten out appearance is diagnostic of cancer. Advanced cancer has a similar shadow. The annular character may become so marked as to make the lumen appear as a canal; dilitation may follow and atony and retention be the picture presented.

Duodenum: Lewis G. Cole's wonderful work has demonstrated that: 1. Duodenal cap can always be demonstrated in the normal. 2. Defect in its smooth outlines indicates ulcer, adhesions or outside pressure.

It may be very difficult to demonstrate the cap, and many different views may be required. Any abdominal pathology may so turn the duodenum and require lateral and oblique views to demonstrate it. Mesenteric fat also adds greatly to the difficulties in some individuals. Dr. Cole advises that next to the posterior anterior view the left to right oblique is most satisfactory.

Leonard and George say: "In simple adhesions, no matter how extensive, the deformity of the bismuth is greater at the beginning of the examination, gradually lessening as the stomach empties and while the stomach, when first filled, will be found in the sub-hepatic region, it will be found in successive plates to have moved back to the median line as the stomach empties. When the degree of deformity remains the same from the beginning of the examination until the stomach has almost emptied itself, it is the more characteristic of ulcer. A constant deformity of the duodenum is peculiar to ulcer and to no other lesion."

Dr. Carmen of the Mayo clinic emphasizes gastric hyper-peristalsis and six hour residue and classifies hyper-motility and hyper-peristalsis of stomach, and lagging of bismuth in the duodenum as minor points.

Small Intestine: The passage of the opaque meal through the small intestines is rapid and the appearance of the shadow is foam like. Displacing pressure from without, kinks, adhesions and ileal stasis are the chief findings. Condition of stasis is shown when the bismuth meal becomes markedly massed and the massed appearance continues for some time.

Appendix: Acute appendices have definite signs and are usually clearly diagnosed without the use of the X-ray. Chronic appendices that are hard to diagnose and by X-ray are often readily determined.

By using the buttermilk bismuth (or barium) meal the six hour or the twenty-four hour plate will usually show the appendix. All normal appendices can be shown on plate, unusual positions may make it difficult to bring the organ into view. An appendix that cannot be shown is diseased.

The fluorscope has its greatest field in clearing up the diagnoses of this pirate of the abdomen. Palpatation with the roentgenscope will reveal appendix tender point, movability of the organ and perhaps concretions. All of these findings indicate appendicitis. Thus the X-ray is added to the forces that are daily bringing more offenses home to the right illiac region.

Colon: The technique of colon examination includes the bismuth enema. The picture of the colon following enema is much different from that of the colon filled from above. It is an exaggerated picture and must be carefully studied. It is most useful in malignancy and organic diseases.

Dr. Arthur Hertz' studies of constipation by X-ray are an interesting contribution to the literature of the last decade. The many findings of interest he outlined cannot be even briefly touched in a general paper like this one.

New growth of the colon is a filling defect that usually shows in twelve or twenty-four hour picture. Obstruction, of course, can be shown if present. Opaque enema are more apt to show the obstructive tendencies than the meal; this is on account of the growing mass accommodation for the usual passage of the stream and not for the unusual.

Mal-position and mal-formation, as Hirschprung's disease, are easily shown and easily interrupted. Adhesions can be demonstrated both by the direct and the indirect method. Spasm recognized by the increased depth of the indentation made by the circular muscle fibres, which may entirely separate segments of bismuth. Atony is the opposite, viz: the obliteration of the characteristic colon in markings.

Diverticulitis is usually found in the sigmoid and descending colon, and usually residue shadows after the passage of the main bismuth mass is the sign sought. It is very difficult to distinguish from a new growth on account of the shadow of the inflammatory mass frequently around a diverticulum.

THE SACRO-ILIAC JOINTS.

J. C. Litzenberg, Minneapolis (*Journal A. M. A.*, Nov. 24, 1917), says that while there are those that dispute the true joint nature of the sacro-iliac synchondrosis, all agree that there is physiologic mobility during pregnancy, and this, some hold, may come on during other physiologic conditions. In such cases there are sometimes distressing symptoms, from simple backache to absolute inability to move without suffering. The writer declares that most women, except in the severe cases, believe backache to be a necessary part of their experience, to be endured with womanly fortitude, and he fears that too many physicians also have this view. He gives brief case reports illustrating certain phases of the subject, asserting that every pregnant woman is a potential sacro-iliac patient, while other gynecologic conditions frequently produce backache so that other causes of the pain may need to be treated. The point he wishes to emphasize is that backache may be an entity in itself and that it may by referred sensations even simulate pelvic disease. Much of the backache occurring during menstruation is in the sacro-iliac joints, being due possibly to relaxation or congestion at this period. It behooves the obstetrician and gynecologist to remember that not all lower backaches, even with pelvic symptoms, are due to pelvic disease. The general practitioner and the surgeon should also remember this possibility of backache independent of visceral or neurasthenic condition. The principles of treatment are simple, calling mainly for immobilization of the joints by adhesive straps, belts or other special devices described in orthopedic works. The more extreme cases often tax the skill of the best trained orthopedists, whose aid should always be sought in dealing with the more serious conditions.

SOME CAUSES OF DIFFICULT LABOR AND THEIR TREATMENT.*

By W. W. WELLS, M. D.

Instructor in Obstetrics, State University Medical School, Chief Obstetrician of Wesley Hospital and Holmes Home of Redeeming Love, Consultant to City Maternity Hospital, Oklahoma City, Okla.

The cause of most of the mortality and morbidity of child birth has been overcome by the intelligent application of asepsis and antisepsis. Now we rarely see a case of puerperal infection except in the case of the criminal or the grossly ignorant. This branch of medicine and surgery is being elevated to a place where, by greater accuracy in the diagnosis of position and greater skill in accomplishing delivery, the mortality and morbidity will be reduced to the minimum.

There are so many causes of difficult labor that I will not try to cover them all in this short paper, such as those caused by some change in the powers as inertia uteri, tetanus uteri, and precipitated labor. Then there are those caused by some abnormal condition of the passengers, as unusual presentation of the foetus, breech, footling, transverse, also the anomalies of the foetus as hydrocephalus, teratoid monsters, lastly and those to which we will confine our remarks almost wholly, are those due to some abnormal condition of the bony pelvis and the soft parts, such as generally enlarged (justo major), generally contracted (justo minor), flat pelvis, rhachitic flat pelvis, asymmetric pelvis from infantile paralysis and transversely contracted pelvis, or any combination of these.

A study of the general make up of the gravida will tell us a great deal. Full muscular women seldom have contracted pelves and if they do the type is usually masculine. Short, petite women may have generally contracted pelves. A woman that limps, or is a hunch-back or has crooked legs, may have a distorted pelvis.

Evidence of rickets should always be sought for in the rhachitic rosary, the square large head, enlargement of the epiphyses, bow legs, and curvature of the spine. A careful consideration of all information obtained enables the accoucheur to make a diagnosis of the case, to give a prognosis, and to recommend treatment.

First we will consider the equally enlarged pelvis, the justo major. This type of pelvis most often occurs in a masculine type of woman, the measurements are all enlarged. We use Leopold's method, all of the measurements are in centimeters,—the pelvis would be considered enlarged when they were 1 1-2 to 2 c.m. above normal, then any pelvis that measured 26½-29½-32½-22, this means that the interspinous is 26½ c. m., intercrestal 29½ c.m., intertrochanteric 32½ c.m., external conjugate 22 c.m. With this type of pelvis we may have a precipitate labor or mal-presentation of the foetus and this may mean for the patient, postpartum hemorrhage, inversion of the uterus, and laceration of the genital tract. For the foetus, death from prolapse of cord, rapid delivery, or striking against some solid object when delivered. The diagnosis is made early by external pelvimetry, seeing that the diameters obtained are equal to or greater than the measurements given.

I scarcely need say to such an audience as this, the treatment consists of instructions to the patient and nurse, that precipitate labor may occur and that as soon as pains begin the patient should be put to bed in the dorsal recumbent position with knees close together or better still turned on her side. This position would retard the labor and give the soft parts time to dilate. When the physician arrives he may give a light anesthesia and put moderate pressure on the presenting part, in this way retarding delivery. This is not a variety of pelvic abnormality that is likely to call for operative procedure unless we have a mal-presentation of the foetus.

The next we will consider is the justo minor, or first variety of contracted pelvis. A contracted pelvis, I need not say, is one in which any one of the im-

*Read at Lawton-Medicine Park, Okla., May 9, 1917.

portant diameters measures 1 1-2 to 2 c.m. or less than normal. In the justo minor pelvis, the measurements would be 23½-26½-29½-19 c.m. or less. Internal pelvimetry is necessary to confirm the diagnosis. An X-ray examination would show the pelvis equally contracted and it would also show any exostosis if present. We will consider the treatment of justo minor pelvis later, along with the treatment of other forms of contracted pelves.

The flat non-rhachitic pelvis is one of the most common forms in the United States occurring in about 43 per cent of contracted pelves. The transverse diameters (interspinous and intercrestal) remain the same while the conjugates are shortened. While in the rhachitic flat pelvis the interspinous is equal to or greater than the intercrestal. Thus these two measurements and the shortened conjugate with other signs of rickets would confirm the diagnosis of a rhachitic flat pelvis. This also holds good in the generally contracted flat rhachitic pelvis.

In these cases the external conjugate is shortened. As a clinical index to contracted pelvis, this diameter is unreliable. However, when the external conjugate is at or below 15.2 c.m., or even below 15.8 c.m., the pelvis is invariably contracted. If it measures 20.3 c.m. or more, there is ample room. In the treatment of contracted pelves we will consider them in regard to amount of contraction.

First, when the true conjugate is 7.5 to 9 c.m. or the external conjugate is 17.5 to 19 c.m., more than one-half of these cases will deliver spontaneously. Of course the history of previous pregnancies and the size of the foetal head will tell us what course we must pursue. In these cases if the head be firmly engaged after a fair test of labor, forceps should be applied. We never apply forceps to a floating head. Where the true conjugate is 7 to 7.5 c.m. or the external conjugate is 17 to 17.5 c.m.—this class of cases should be in the hospital, as they are very difficult cases and the mortality to the mother and child is great.

I scarcely need say to you after a fair test of labor without results, a Cesarean section would be indicated. When we come to the actual delivery, we find that it is not the measurements of the pelvis nor the size of the child that makes delivery difficult, but it is the narrowing of the pelvis, the position of the child and most of all, the ability of the part presenting to shape and conform itself to the pelvis. Still, in preparing ourselves for the delivery the only things we have to help us to determine the outcome are the past performance of the woman, her apparent strength and desire to do her part, the size of the child and the size of the pelvis.

In conclusion: The pelvimeter should be used as a routine in the examination of the pregnant woman. That high forceps are not indicated where the head will not engage from any cause, but rather Cesarean section, that even though we have a contracted pelvis with a favorable position of foetus which shows no overgrowth or deformity, the patient can well go on to labor. Of course the X-ray is a valuable asset in making the examination of the foetus and parturient. Notice also that unless there is a marked contraction of the pelvis the gravida should be given a fair test of labor, which consists of 4 to 6 hours of active labor.

But this should be in a hospital where Cesarean section could be performed if necessary. In a contracted pelvis Cesarean section is indicated where the foetal pulse is over 150 or below 110, or where there is a discharge of meconium in a head presentation.

Notice that the neglect of frequent observation of the foetal heart sound has cost the life of many a child. We should make the smallest number possible of vaginal examinations, one or two depending on external palpation for general information, and rectal for definite information. And that accurate pelvimetry is necessary in order to recognize the type of deformity. Notice also that pelvimetry without the estimation of the size of the foetus is of little value and that the most accurate foetometry is the test of labor. All border-line cases should be given the test of labor and the test should be in a hospital.

USE OF FORCEPS.*

By O. C. NEWMAN, M. D., Shattuck, Okla.

Gentlemen: Permit me to thank the committee for selecting me to write a paper on the use of forceps. Not that I feel equal to the occasion or capable of ably presenting the subject, but it has caused me to take the opportunity of reminding myself of things I have never known or have long forgotten. I may impart no knowledge but hope to stimulate enthusiasm, that this discussion may suggest points of usefulness by which we may be benefited indirectly by my efforts and may make it worthy of our time as well spent.

A few remarks may be interesting pertaining to the history of the forceps before discussing their use. It is not an ancient instrument and no record of many centuries past or crude appliances have been discovered from ancient relics that resemble forceps. We can readily conceive the idea why so little progress was made in obstetrics when we realize that the employing of midwives was general, and these for the most part were ignorant and filthy old women that had not had the advantages of the institutions for learning and no thought of assistance other than the process of nature and the routine procedure that had obtained from time immemorial. Educated accouchers were called only in extraordinary cases, but with progress the prejudice which excluded educated physicians from practice of midwifery, gradually gave way and there was opened for obstetrics a new era.

At an earlier period there were crude appliances devised apparently for the mutilation of the foetus, in delivering a woman and when instruments were necessary, always meant death to the child and more or less damage to the mother. Such as was the custom of a few generations past no doubt is the cause of the laity being prejudiced against the use of our modern appliances.

The first forceps were invented probably in 1580 by Chamberlain, and at that time no less than at present, we are impressed to believe that monopoly existed for personal profit or superiority in their sphere of usefulness and retained as a family secret and handed down from one generation to another. In 1723 at a meeting of the Paris Academy of Medicine, crude appliances for the delivery of women were presented and in discussing this question it was added that if by chance any one should happen to invent an instrument which could be so used and keep it secret for his own profit, he deserved to be exposed upon a barren rock and have his vitals plucked out by vultures, little knowing that at that time such an instrument had been in the possession of the Chamberlain family for nearly a hundred years. About 1753 Vischer and Von de Poll purchased the secret and made it public.

The obstetrical forceps rank among the most useful discoveries of modern surgery and while not in common use until a little over a century ago, it may be said that the invention has been the means of saving the lives of countless numbers of women and children. Of all obstetrical operations the most important is the application of the forceps. Nothing but practice can impart the operative dexterity which it should be the aim of every obstetrician to acquire. Yet when improperly used and on cases when not indicated it has made invalids of many women and caused the death of many a child. I have often stated, not in an egotistical way, that the physician not capable of introducing instruments without causing an extra pain to the mother without an anesthetic does not know how to introduce them.

The forceps are more commonly used as *tractors* and because the maternal forces are unable to expel the foetus on account of simple uterine or abdominal inertia.

There can be no set rule when, as to the time of use, as to stage of labor,

---

*Read before the Woodward County Medical Society, July 11th, 1917. Discussed by Doctors Wells of Oklahoma City and Tisdal of Elk City, by invitation.

though many advocate that after two hours of labor with no progress, the cervix dilated and proper presentation, the forceps should be used. They are used as *rotators*, but with great caution and then only from the natural axis, through traction as labor progresses. The forceps are used as *compressors*, though not so intended, yet with the head as a sphere and the blades of forceps only on two sides, and as traction is made sufficient to overcome resistance so required, we unavoidably have more or less compression. Some advocate applying the forceps through a partially obliterated cervix and assisting *dilitation* by traction upon the head, but better to stretch the cervix manually and not apply forceps until dilitation is complete.

In rare instances one blade of forceps may be employed as lever, but with great danger to injury to soft parts. We have learned incidentally in our younger days they have relieved us of many anxious moments by acting as irritators; when demonstrating our skill we have completely failed to introduce more than one blade which caused unusual expulsive pains and relieved us of our anxiety, to our great surprise, by causing birth of the child.

Forceps may be demanded either in the interest of the child or in that of the mother and in many instances these interests are combined under the head of maternal conditions, but secondarily the child also. A few of these may be mentioned, as eclampsia, heart disease, fever or infection during labor, pneumonia, typhoid, tuberculosis, edema of lungs, hernia, appendicitis and other intra-abdominal conditions, placenta previa. In the interest of child, prolapse of the cord, a foetal pulse 100 or exceeding 160 indicates the child is in danger and will perish if not promptly delivered.

In vertex presentations the amniotic fluid tinged with meconium interferes with placental circulation and imperfect oxygination, manifests itself by paralysis of the sphincter ani and sudden death of mother, etc. There are none of us who have not had prolonged and tedious cases who could not resist the temptation of using the forceps. At the same time it should be insisted upon that the operation should never be performed to save the physician time, but only when distinctly indicated by the condition of the mother and child.

The suggestions as enumerated for the use of forceps when indicated in distinctly selected cases, clearly suggest to our minds that the forceps have no competitor in the field of usefulness, shown by the vast number of mothers and children saved when skillfully handled and properly applied and manipulated.

Yet of recent years it has been suggested and advocated by many that in our armamentarium of therapeutics, we have been supplied by a product that has almost displaced the use of forceps, saved time to the busy accoucher and is a boon to the tired mother and her anxious attendants. This product is known as pituitrin. The experience I have had in my limited practice of obstetrics and the observations I have made from receiving stillbirth reports of Ellis County, confirmed me in the belief that the attempted use of forceps is safer in the hands of a physician without experience than a tube of pituitrin in the hands of a busy and skilled physician. After I had observed the effect of the product, even before I had at any time observed a remark of criticism in literature, regarding its use, I made the statement that it was not far distant when we would read in every medical journal that pituitrin had ruined the health of more women and caused more idiots in children in a shorter time of usefulness than all other drugs or appliances used in obstetrics.

This product is applied forceps by therapeutics, and properly comes under the use of forceps, as being demonstrated and advocated for its brilliant results and usefulness of today. No doubt I will be accused of giving too large doses, or not knowing how or when the product is indicated. This was true in the beginning, but fortunately I had no bad results, before I convinced myself that 1 c.c. was much too large and at present hesitate very much in believing that any amount that gives results is too large. I was unable to find my best articles on the contriindications and use of the preparation, but refer you to the Journal of A. M. A., June 2, 1917, paper written by Dr. J. J. Mundell.

Before closing I want to quote you an abstract in the Therapeutic Gazette, referring to a paper written by Dr. Allen G. Heard of Galveston, Texas, in the Texas Journal of Medicine, reporting three cases of his own and two cases of Bubis tending to prove: That the improper use of pituitary extract in labor is a cause of cerebral or meningeal hemorrhage in the new born; that hemorrhage in the nervous system of the infant resulting from the use of pituitrin in labor is productive of diffuse nervous lesions so extensive as to result in early death, or if the child survives, in terrible afflictions of paralysis, epilepsy and idiocy.

THE ROENTGENOLOGIC DIAGNOSIS OF TUBERCULOSIS.

By WALTER E. WRIGHT, M. D., Tulsa, Okla.

The roentgen examination of the chest for the diagnosis of pulmonary tuberculosis is not a new method in the history of roentgenology. Francis H. Williams of Boston, as early as 1896, reported cases of tuberculosis examined with the fluoroscope. Roentgen examination for pulmonary tuberculosis should assuredly be considered an important and necessary adjunct in modern medicine as a diagnostic factor. Valuable as it may be when used to confirm the positive clinical diagnosis, insofar as it points out indisputably the character, location and extent of the lesion, it has demonstrated its best power in those patients with suspicious clinical signs but negative sputum.

The intensity and penetration of the roentgen ray is in inverse proportion to the square of the distance and the ease of penetration lessens with increased atomic weight. As lung structure is so constituted that the air-containing tissue makes it possible to recognize by contrast slight changes in density even in small areas, it is readily understood why the changes which occur in pulmonary tuberculosis, in its earliest stages, are observable in the roentgenogram before it is possible to secure a physical diagnostic sign.

The bacillus tuberculosis produces specific lesions which take the form either of separate nodular masses or diffuse growths infiltrating the tissues; aggregations of these elementary tubercles give rise to large tubercular masses. Tubercles are small nodular bodies whose diameters range from .5 to 3 mm. and which undergo caseation and sclerosis. A roentgen observation of early pulmonary tuberculosis is the single calcified or caseated tubercle or groups of tubercles.

The examining methods used in the roentgen laboratory for the detection of tuberculosis are the fluoroscope and the stereoscopic roentgenogram. In fluoroscopy, it is possible to observe the moving parts, such as the excursions of the diaphragm, the pulsation of the heart and aorta, and the aeration of the lungs.

Stereoscopic roentgenograms are two plates exposed by such a method that when they are examined in a stereoscope they present a single image of the different densities of the chest in perspective. The anatomy demonstrated in stereoroentgenograms are the bones, ribs and spine, the diaphragm, the heart and aorta, the bronchial trunks, and the hilus shadow.

The earliest signs of pulmonary tuberculosis are noted in the hilus shadows, the bronchial trunks and linear markings extending to the periphery: these lines radiate from the trunks: the hilus shadow shows increased density with widened area, containing smaller shadows of marked density, while the increased fibrosis and lymphatic tissue is responsible for the increased hilus area. The bronchial trunks are heavier and broader than usual. The linear markings become less regular in outline, criss-crossing each other, coarsened and studded, sometimes forming a network of mesh: with increased consolidation within the lung, the whole area presents the appearance of a unified mass of increased density. There are three important manifestations of the disease recognized by the roentgenologist, the hilus lesions, peribronchial infiltration in the parenchyma further out around the bronchi, and their terminations.

In active cases, it is seen that the lungs have a thick, fuzzy, woolly appearance, or resembling clouds of tobacco smoke. Later as the condition advances there is a typical picture of calcified areas suggesting fibrosis, aerated spaces denoting the location of cavities resulting from the breaking down of consolidations, and distortion of the viscera.

The roentgen examination is the one means of bringing pathologic lung processes into view, and the interests of our patients are best served by the cooperation of the clinician and the roentgenologist.

BREATH SOUNDS IN EARLY TUBERCULOSIS.

A study of the breath sounds in incipient tuberculosis is reported by H. A. Bray, Ray Brook, N. Y. (*Journal A. M. A.*, Nov. 24, 1917). The object of the study was to ascertain the clinical importance of breath sounds in pulmonary tuberculosis with the hope of obtaining data for early diagnosis. A study was made of 124 cases of incipient disease confined to one or both apexes, and the comparative significance of the respiratory changes was considered both alone and in conjunction with other physical signs and diagnostic procedure. The writer desired the advantage of studying apical involvement alone instead of subjecting the patient to the greater physical strain of complete chest examination, because of the greater frequency of involvement of the apex. All conditions which might alter the character of the breath sounds at the apex were excluded. The findings are commented on at length, and the author reaches the following conclusions: "1. Abdominal breathing is an effective method for the differentiation of granular breathing, from those extrapulmonary sounds simulating this type of breathing. 2. The observation of the time interval and force of the respiratory act is essential in the differentiation of physiologic from pathologic alterations in the duration and intensity of the respiratory murmur. 3. The lung glides across the auscultated field during respiration. 4. Variations in the force of the respiratory act may profoundly alter the character of the respiratory murmur in the region of the apexes. 5. Expiratory alterations predominate at the right apex, inspiratory at the left apex. 6. Prolonged expiration, when more pronounced at the left than at the right apex, is a reliable sign of disease at the left apex. 7. Bronchovesicular breathing may be explained by contiguous areas of consolidated and aerated lung that alternately glide beneath the stethoscope during respiration. 8. The frequency with which alterations in the respiratory murmur occur over the healthy apex in unilateral disease deserves attention. 9. Physiologic respiratory modifications interpreted as pathologic represent the most frequent error in the physical examination in early tuberculosis. 10. A study of the breath sounds in early disease is often difficult and misleading, and for this reason should not be unduly emphasized in diagnosis."

EPIDEMIC MENINGITIS.

George Mathers, Chicago (*Journal A. M. A.*, Nov. 24, 1917), reports a case of mixed infection of epidemic meningitis in which the pneumococcus, as well as the meningococcus, was found in the spinal fluid. This case is similar to the cases reported by Metter and Salanier in a recent communication. The writer calls attention to the importance of such cases and their diagnosis. Of course they do not respond to the antimeningococcic serum injection but give the symptoms of the meningitis. Observations of this type emphasize the importance of frequent cultural examination of the spinal fluid in cases of epidemic meningitis. In the case reported, cultures showed a gram-negative organism with the characteristics of the meningococcus, together with the gram-positive typical pneumococcus.

OBSERVATIONS OF THE CARREL-DAKIN TREATMENT AT NEW YORK POLYCLINIC HOSPITAL.

By A. RAY WILEY, M. D.
House Surgeon, New York Polyclinic, New York City
Tulsa, Oklahoma

As with all new ideas in medicine, surgery or revival of an old idea, the literature is flooded with opinions pro and con and leaves the readers of less experience as much behooved as before. Such has been the case with articles on the Carrel-Dakin treatment, most of the authors condemning without trial or others carried away with enthusiasm and lauding it beyond reason.

The author's experience has been with all the cases at the Polyclinic Hospital since February, 1917, and observations at the Rockefeller Institute of Medical Research on frequent visits. This article is given as a summary and not a detail account of any series of cases.

The treatment is one of perfected detail technique, and unless the treatment is carried out in detail as explained by Dr. Carrel, only failure awaits your efforts. It is like mathematical precision, if one part is slighted or incorrect it just as well all be incorrect and one can only learn the technique by working with one with experience or in some institution devoted especially to this work, such as the War Demonstration Hospital at the Rockefeller Institute.

Too much is often expected of the treatment. Chronic osteomyelitis is not rendered sterile in 2 to 4 days and in some cases it takes that many months. The solution on the cutaneous surface is very irritating and unless the skin is properly cared for and strength of solution accurately gauged, causes the patient undue pain. The dressings, especially the daily changing of tubes, is painful and unless considerable care and diplomacy is exercised with your patient, you will lose their confidence completely.

The whole system of the treatment, including the bacterial counting, the making of the solution, the testing of the strength of the solution, the preparation of the apparatus and the dressings, cannot be carried out in a small hospital to the financial good of the hospital. It is only in a large hospital, a war hospital or large industrial hospital, and then with a corps of trained and experienced doctors and nurses that it can be carried out successfully.

The treatment is only adaptable to certain lesions and conditions and with its complicated technique, it really has a limited field. It should not be attempted by a small institution or individual as the number of cases would be too small to determine the virtues of the treatment and would incur considerable expense. What we should have is a large number of cases, say five thousand cases treated with Dakin's, then another series with as near similar injuries as possible and of near constitutional resistance treated with latest surgical technique in cooperation with a corps of notable surgeons as controls, or still another series treated with other antiseptics. Only after such series are carefully tabulated and compared for results, should we accept the treatment for what it is worth. Personally I believe the treatment would stand the test, which could be carried out in some of the base hospitals on the Western Front.

I am indebted to Major G. A. Stewart and Lieut. Sullivan of the War Demonstration Hospital of the Rockefeller Institute and Major Edward Wallace Lee of the Polyclinic Hospital for their personal interest in the cases I have treated and in observing the cases at the Rockefeller Institute. Drs. Stewart and Sullivan and others are cooperating very earnestly with Dr. Carrel at the War Demonstration Hospital in working out every detail of the treatment, but the number of cases are limited (less than a hundred) and no controls used of the ordinary surgical treatment. Various solutions and strengths are used to discover if there is any solution other than the original Dakin's that will better suit the demand. They are sincere workers and it is to be hoped that they are not pursuing a "will 'o the wisp," in the dark wilderness of medicine, but will point out a true light of real value.

PROCEEDINGS OF ST. ANTHONY'S HOSPITAL CLINICAL SOCIETY.

Oklahoma City, October 15, 1917.

DR. A. A. WILL, Pres.   DR. LEILA E. ANDREWS, Secy.

Dr. Edward F. Davis presented the following cases:

J. M., male, aged 34, farmer. While burning brush, got some foreign substance (probably ashes) in left eye which soon became congested and painful. In a few days a "scum" came on the cornea and vision was impaired. Had no special treatment for five weeks when examination showed a thin scar over lower part of cornea and an indolent ulcer above with considerable vascularization surrounding ulcer. There was little pain and only slight discharge. The ulcer resisted all ordinary treatment and was becoming larger gradually. The base was clean and slightly bulging and only the edge took fluorescin stain. One morning, he reported that he had had a sudden pain in the eye and a quantity of watery fluid escaped the preceding night. Inspection revealed an irregular line in the floor of the ulcer, indicating that it had ruptured. Following this, all symptoms abated, conjunctival congestion passed away and the corneal vessels disappeared in a few days. This case is shown on account of the fact that there was a spontaneous Saemisch operation. This incision was to have been made on this particular day but nature made it unnecessary.

Mrs. J., aged 72. Cataract extraction in right eye six months ago. Previous laboratory findings of blood, urine and conjunctival secretion was negative. Vision, at that time, merely perception of light. Recovery was rapid but vision was only about 10-200 and was not improved by glasses. The poor vision is due to a pre-existing choroiditis. The left eye was operated on ten weeks ago but recovery was complicated by a slow, painless plastic iridocyclitis with occlusion of the pupil and great thickening of the iris. An attempt was made to incise the pupillary membrane and to remove a part of the thickened iris but the new formation was so dense that this could not be done satisfactorily and no further efforts were made. In this case the patient is in no worse condition as a result of the operations on the second eye and the net result in the first eye is that she is able to get around which she could not do in safety before.

Report of case of Mrs. R., aged 51. Has been on Allen treatment for diabetes mellitus. She became sugar-free and at the same time developed a disturbance of vision so severe as to be unable to see an ordinary type written page. Examination showed a marked oedema of the optic nerve which gradually cleared up after she had been sugar-free some days and her sugar tolerance had been increased. This is a frequent finding in the cases reported by Joslin.

Dr. Smith reported cases of two men burned with steam following the bursting of a boiler. The men arrived at the hospital several hours after the accident occurred. Both had had their bodies and limbs bandaged and a hypodermic of morphine but on arrival complained very much of pain and were in a state of considerable shock. Very little time was spent in the removal of their clothing and superficial cleansing until they were put to bed, which was covered with a cradle and fitted with an electric light in such a way that none of the bed linen except that on which they lay came in contact with their bodies. They soon became warm and ceased to complain of such severe pain.

Both patients were badly burned. F. E. S., age 41, had burns of the first or second degree covering at least three fourths of the body surface. These burns were chiefly on the face, back, buttocks and limbs. The other patient, M. E. J., age 43, was burned over similar areas but the surface covered not being over two-thirds of the body surface.

Both patients were treated as follows: after they became warm they were bathed with a tepid dilute solution of sodium bicarbonate every two hours. Small quantities of a bicarbonate solution was given by mouth and large amounts of the solution was administered per rectum by the Murphy drip. F. E. S. on the third day developed a severe nephritic lesion as was shown by the urine analysis, however no acetone appeared. The heart muscle became weak, the pulse became rapid and the patient died on the fourth day followiug twenty-four hours of delirium.

The second patient, E. S. J., was nearly as badly burned as the first but his kidneys seemed to stand the severe toxemia better than those of the first. The urine analysis of this patient showed a slight nephritis. No acidosis developed but a slight glucosuria which cleared up in a few days. After four weeks stay at the hospital, with urine negative, a temperature practically normal, the patient feeling fine and in good condition except for some small areas over his legs and buttocks which required skin grafting, he was removed to the railroad hospital in St. Louis for further treatment.

We were greatly pleased with the open air method of treatment. We especially noted that the wounds became only very slightly infected, and the men complained very little of pain. The wounds of the man who recovered were deep and extensive and we feel quite sure that the constant use of sodium bicarbonate solution, both internally and externally, prevented a severe acidosis which superimposed on the kidney lesion which he developed would have caused the death of our patient. The open air method gives free drainage, preventing the necrotic material from being absorbed and is of vital importance just as it is in draining a pus cavity to prevent absorption of pus.

Drs. J. W. Riley, S. R. Cunningham and H. Reed in discussing the report recited similar cases in which most satisfactory results were obtained by the open air method.

Meeting of November 19, 1917.

Dr. G. A. LaMotte showed a very interesting case of tumor of the mouth, which seemed to have its origin in the hard palate. Had been growing for about 10 years, was softer than bone-tissue, was painless and was not causing much inconvenience. The case was not diagnosed.

Dr. O. J. Walker, Director of the Laboratory at St. Anthony's Hospital, then gave a splendid paper on "Acidosis and the Recent Methods, of Demonstrating It." This paper was accompanied by demonstrations by Dr. Walker and his laboratory assistants, and was most instructive. It marks the first of a series which he has promised us, showing to us and demonstrating for us the value of these laboratory aids—to our every-day work—no matter what the line of work may be. This paper will be printed in full in a subsequent issue.

DIET IN NEPHRITIS.

A. F. Chace and A. R. Rose, New York (*Journal A. M. A.*, Aug. 11, 1917), has studied the dietary requirements in patients suffering from interstitial nephritis by methods of blood analysis, and deduced dietaries which they published in tabulated form. They summarize their findings as follows: "A scheme of dietetic treatment for nephritis, based on the more recent advances in the field of nutrition, and tested in advanced cases of interstitial nephritis in this hospital, has had encouraging results thus far. The patients used in the test have been followed not only by the usual clinical observations at the bedside, but also by frequent chemical examination of the blood. The determination of creatinin and urea nitrogen affords an excellent and convenient means of gaging the kidney's capacity to eliminate nitrogenous waste products and noting the response of the nephritic to treatment. The plan provides a diet adequate in calories, protein, mineral elements and food accessories. To attain this, a variety in the menu has been insisted on. This insures a happier and more content attitude on the part of the patient, the inclusion of all the requisite vitamins and the complementing of biologically incomplete proteins. At least one hot dish is provided each day by giving a bowl of cream soup. Green vegetables are given to bring the iron intake in excess of 15 mg. per day. The sum total of the day's ash constituents should be decidedly alkaline in reaction and rich in calcium. * * *"

JOURNAL OF THE OKLAHOMA STATE MEDICAL ASSOCIATION

VOLUME XI   MUSKOGEE, OKLA., JANUARY, 1918   NUMBER 1

PUBLISHED MONTHLY AT MUSKOGEE, OKLA., UNDER DIRECTION OF THE COUNCIL

DR. CLAUDE A. THOMPSON, EDITOR-IN-CHIEF

ENTERED AT THE POST OFFICE AT MUSKOGEE, OKLAHOMA, AS SECOND CLASS MAIL MATTER, JULY 28, 1912

THIS IS THE OFFICIAL JOURNAL OF THE OKLAHOMA STATE MEDICAL ASSOCIATION. ALL COMMUNICATIONS SHOULD BE ADDRESSED TO THE JOURNAL OF THE OKLAHOMA STATE MEDICAL ASSOCIATION, 307-8 SURETY BUILDING, MUSKOGEE, OKLAHOMA.

The editorial department is not responsible for the opinions expressed in the original articles of contributors.

Reprints of original articles will be supplied at actual cost, provided request for them s attached to manuscript or made in sufficient time before publication.

Articles sent this Journal for publication and all those read at the annual meetings of the State Association are the sole property of this Journal. The Journal relies on each individual contributor's strict adherence to this well-known rule of medical journalism. In the event an article sent this Journal fo publication is published before appearance in the Journal, the manuscript will be returned to the writer.

Failure to receive the Journal should call for immediate notification of the editor, 307-8 Surety Building, Muskogee, Okla

Local news of possible interest to the medical profession, notes on removals, changes in address, deaths and weddings will be gratefully received.

Advertising of articles, drugs or compounds not approved by the Council on Pharmacy of the A. M. A. will not be accepted.

☞Advertising rates will be supplied on application. It is suggested that wherever possible members of the State Association should patronize our advertisers in preference to others as a matter of fair reciprocity.

EDITORIAL

THE RESPONSE OF THE AMERICAN DOCTOR.

A few months ago there was considerable perturbation in some minds over the possibility that the American Medical Profession might be found lacking in its response to the call of the Nation for aid in the War. A few, very few fleeting weeks have dispelled that idea in such an emphatic manner that "he who runs may read" and incidentally, interpret in the response, the very great ideals actuating the medical profession. Not weighing the matter as one of dollars and cents; not counting the losses, probably incalculable in a financial way, without regard to the inconveniences incident to wholly uprooting the daily habits of his life and taking up new burdens and labors, with which he was wholly unacquainted, the American Doctor, unaccompanied by the brass-band and the patriotic speeches, quietly boarded a train, at his own expense rode across the State, paid his own bills, underwent an examination, returned to his home to wait until ordered to go. It is said that now more than twenty thousand have been commissioned or are in process of receiving commissions. Under misinformation or misunderstanding hundreds of them gave up their offices in expectation of being called only to learn that months may elapse before they are called, if at all. It is said, too, that this number is more than adequate to care easily for an army far in excess of two million men. Add to this the known fact that thousands are ready to go at a later date when their services are apparently more pressingly required than now, and the scoffers who ignorantly talked of the possibility of drafting the doctor have their answer in eloquent and convincing action, action more convincing than any set of resolutions or talk.

To those who know him it is not necessary to introduce the American Doctor. His altruistic, self-sacrificing attitude on all State matters is only too well known to the observer. Mostly not in the draft age, deeply rooted by unusual ties to his surroundings, to him going to war means something indeed. We are proud to belong to that profession. Unboastingly, but with the greatest sincerity, we are able to say to the people, "we will do our share," more than that we will do all we can do, even exceeding the requirements wherever possible and prove the contention of our enthusiastic friends that we are the important part of American citizenship necessary to a successful conclusion of the War and the resumption and continuation of peaceful activities after the War.

THE MEDICAL ADVISORY BOARDS.

The principal new feature of the changed draft regulations provided for the creation of Medical Advisory Boards throughout each state. All registrants disqualified on physical grounds, those who think they should have been or should not have been so disqualified physically and certain others referred to the Board by the Adjutant General are to be reexamined, after the Local Board examiners have completed their examination. All registrants heretofore examined and disqualified and those disqualified at the cantonments from the first increment of the draft are also to be reexamined by the Advisory Boards. The only exceptions to this reexamination are in such cases where the registrant is obviously disqualified physically—in such cases as loss of an eye, limb, paralysis and other plainly discernable disqualifications. One change, seemingly one to be greatly desired, is the power of the Board to place the military physical fitness of the registrant either as wholly unfit, partially fit or entirely so. This last seems to be a very sensible arrangement, for many men who are unable to undergo the rigors of heavy outdoor labors in the field, etc., are able to render their country valuable service otherwise, thus releasing men who are tied up in performing inside, or less strenuous, work for the more necessary work of War.

BRUSHING UP OUR MEDICAL DEPARTMENT.

There is something commendable in the manner in which our Nation is entering the War. Aside from the usual vexations incident to the handling and classifying of thousands of physicians—placing them where they can do the most good in the niche into which they best fit, our directors of the medical activities are virtually postgraduating-hundreds of men in order to intimately acquaint them with the work they will be called to do. Our surgeons showing aptitude for such service are promptly sent to some center where skilled instruction in bone surgery and other needed branches is given by the best men. If he is an X-ray man he goes to a center where such is best taught, the laboratory man, the internist, in fact every branch is given all the help to perfect itself that may be had.

This augurs well for the final casting up of the services rendered by our profession and means that our men in the field will receive the best of treatment considering their surroundings and the opportunities present to relieve them from the injuries and illnesses.

PATRIOTIC LABORATORIES.

Drs. LeRoy Long, Dean of the Medical Department of the State University, and Walter E. Wright, head of the Walter E. Wright Laboratory, Tulsa, promptly placed their respective laboratories at the disposal of the newly created medical advisory boards of the State. They will perform or have performed all the necessary technical and complicated examinations they may decide is necessary to clear up any questionable point in the case of the registrant.

PERSONAL AND GENERAL NEWS

Dr. E. L. Underwood, Crescent, has moved to Oklahoma City.

Dr. W. B. Reeves, Wapanucka, is attending the Chicago clinics.

Dr. William H. Rogers, Tulsa, has been appointed City Physician.

Dr. J. R. Bryce, Snyder, was very ill in December with pneumonia.

Dr. M. K. Thompson and family, Muskogee, visited Galveston in November.

Dr. Amos Avery, Sapulpa, is nursing a broken arm due to automobile collision.

Dr. J. C. Taylor, Chelsea, visited the New Orleans hospitals and clinics in December.

Dr. J. C. Mahr, Oklahoma City, has been ordered to report to Ft. Oglethorpe for duty.

Dr. L. E. Inman, Oklahoma City, has been promoted to a Major in the Medical Reserve.

Dr. J. M. Bonham, Hobart, has been appointed a Captain in the Medical Reserve Corps.

Major R. M. Howard, M. R. C., paid his Oklahoma City friends a flying visit in December.

Dr. A. K. West, Oklahoma City, had his Ford Sedan appropriated by a thief while making a call.

Dr. W. B. Reeves, Wapanucka, is moving to Greenville, Texas, where he will make his future home.

Dr. J. C. Johnson, McAlester, is visiting the New York Clinics where he will remain for six weeks.

Dr. Raymond L. Fox, Altus, has been assigned from Ft. Sill to Chicago for special work in bone surgery.

Dr. C. H. Howell, Frederick, M. R. C., was ordered to report in San Antonio December 10th for assignment to duty.

Dr. M. F. Keller, Calera, is visiting the New Orleans clinics. He is nursing a broken arm received from an over active Ford.

Dr. J. A. Gregoire, a physician formerly residing in Cheyenne, it is said has been found guilty of first degree murder by a Kansas Court.

Dr. W. J. Whitaker, Pryor, has been invalided home for an indefinite period on account of illness. He will take up his old work in Pryor.

Dr. Z. G. Taylor, Mounds, is the latest sufferer from automobile theft. He recently lost his Ford and all attempts at recovery have failed.

Dr. T. L. Willis, Mangum, recently lost his car when the machine in some manner unknown caught fire while he was driving along the road.

Dr. W. B. Newton, Muskogee, is at home on indefinite leave from military service. An old ankle injury has been causing him much trouble.

Dr. A. D. Johannes, Oklahoma City, has changed his name to "A. D. Johns." The change was made to simplify spelling, according to the "News."

Dr. L. S. Willour, McAlester, Captain M. R. C., was detailed to study orthopedic surgery in the clinic of Dr. R. L. Hull, Oklahoma City, in December.

Dr. Robt. L. Hull, Oklahoma City, has been made a Major, M. R. C., and classes in orthopedic surgery are being assigned to him for instruction at Oklahoma City and Norman by the War Department.

Tulsa Chamber of Commerce heard from Drs. W. Forrest Dutton, A. W. Roth and J. N. Temples in an open meeting recently at which the "Necessity and Benefit of Medical Inspection of Schools" was discussed.

RESOLUTIONS PASSED BY THE OKLAHOMA COUNTY MEDICAL SOCIETY
ON THE DEATH OF DR. RUDOLPH F. SCHAEFER.

Whereas, Almighty God has called from suffering our beloved friend and professional brother, Dr. Rudolph F. Schaefer, we, the Oklahoma County Medical Society, desire to express our high appreciation of him as a man and physician. He was one whose efforts were for the good of the profession and of the community in which he lived.

We send our heartfelt sympathy to his family that they may know that we, his colleagues, mourn with them.

L. J. Moorman,
H. H. Cloudman,
Committee.

Craig County Medical Society banqueted Dr. W. R. Marks at the State Hospital, December 14, on the eve of his departure for war service. Dr. Marks has been in the Government Service previously in Alaska.

Drs. A. L. Blesh, M. E. Stout, J. Z. Mraz and D. D. Paulus are the four Oklahoma City physicians who have gone out of one office to War. They announce that the office will be closed for the duration of the War.

Dr. Claude Thompson, Muskogee, has been assigned to temporary duty as Aide to the Governor in establishing Medical Advisory Boards in Oklahoma. He was commissioned 1st Lieutenant M. R. C., for that purpose.

Dr. Ross Grosshart, Tulsa, suffered a great bereavement in the recent death of Mrs. Grosshart, who was suddenly stricken and died in a few hours. His many friends in the profession throughout the southwest will regret to hear of his loss.

Dr. G. P. Cherry, Mangum, has just cleaned up a law suit of many years standing, coming out the winner in a contest for post office rent that has been pending since 1912, the case going through all the perplexities of the law's notorious delays.

The Hygeia Hospital is now located in its new and larger quarters at 4733 Vincennes Ave., Chicago, Ill. Physicians who wish to refer cases of drug addiction and alcoholism to Dr. W. K. McLaughlin, Supt., for treatment, should make special note of the new location of the Hygeia Hospital, since the new quarters are located in a section of Chicago very far from the old address.

Miami has had to be reassured that its smallpox situation is well in hand and there is no immediate danger of a general quarantine on that account, by inspectors from the State Department of Health. May we soon have the day when smallpox will be treated either with wholesale vaccination or silent contempt. Public hysteria need never occur and does not among the intelligent vaccinated; it is questionable if the State should waste its money attempting to reassure the other kind.

Enid physicians have formed an arrangement to further specialize in the work of their respective fields. Occupying an entire floor of the Enid National Bank Building, they will attempt to refer their work in such a manner as to give the patient the benefit of individual study. The physicians composing the clinic are: Drs. W. L. Kendall, nervous diseases and orthopedics: E. N. McKee, X-ray and skin diseases; A. S. Piper, eye, ear, nose and throat; F. A. Hudson, general surgery; Julian Feild, diseases of children and obstetrics; Jas. H. Hayes, kidney, bladder and rectal diseases. This class of work will unquestionably produce good resilts.

CORRESPONDENCE

THE DERMATOLOGICAL RESEARCH LABORATORIES
Philadelphia Polyclinic and College for Graduates in Medicine
Jay Frank Schamberg, M. D., Director.

Philadelphia, November 24th, 1917.

Dr. C. A. Thompson,
  Muskogee, Okla.

Dear Dr. Thompson:

The United States Government is about to confer a license upon our laboratories to prepare and vend arsenobenzol. We are interested in the campaign for the suppression of syphilis and shall do all in our power to cooperate towards this end. The action of the Government enables us to again make our product directly available to the profession.

We are prepared to market arsenobenzol to physicians in 0.6 gram doses at $1.50 per ampoule, and in 0.4 gram doses at $1.25 per ampoule; 2 gram ampoules will shortly be supplied to hospitals (except private hospitals) at such a rate as to permit individual doses to be administered for less than $1.00.

Neosalvarsan is not being made by us at present.

Requests for arsenobenzol should be directed to the above address.

Very truly yours,
DERMATOLOGICAL RESEARCH LABORATORIES.

MISCELLANEOUS

MEDICAL RESERVE CORPS APPOINTMENTS, TO NOVEMBER 15th.

Waller Cornelius Threlkeld, Ada; Henry DeWitt Shankle, Afton; Charles Edward Thompson, Enid; Lyman L. Bunker, Ivanhoe; William McIllwain, Lone Wolf; Charles Ersey Smith, Muskogee; Claude A. Thompson, Muskogee; Gardner Henry Applewhite, Shawnee; Roy Keene Goddard, Supply; Grover Cleveland Moore, Wagoner; David Albert Beard, Westville.

ASSIGNMENT TO ACTIVE DUTY—MEDICAL RESERVE OFFICERS.

Much discontent is manifest throughout the country owing to uncertain conditions prevailing as to assignment to active service. To set the matter at rest and advise all concerned, the War Department has issued the following information with the request that all concerned give the matter the widest publicity.

1. Appeals for active duty accompanied by statements that officers have ceased all civil practice, have sold their homes and otherwise severed local connections, are continually reaching this office, leading us to the conclusion that some misunderstanding must exist as to the conditions under which appointments in the Medical Reserve Corps are accepted.

2. You are requested to give the widest publicity to the fact that the acceptance of a commission in the Reserve Corps does not necessarily imply immediate assignment to active duty; that the Reserve Corps has been organized to meet the conditions that will arise when our troops are more extensively engaged; and that until that time officers should continue their usual duties pending notice that orders are to be issued.

3. Up to within a short time ago it was possible to assign officers as rapidly as appointments were accepted, but for some time to come very few officers will be called out unless conditions materially change.

4. We have every reason to expect that the services of every available medical officer will be eventually required but it is manifestly impossible to utilize the entire Corps with the number of troops now serving.

5. All officers of the Reserve Corps on the inactive list will be given at least fifteen days' notice when first assigned to active duty. Until they receive such notice they should continue with their civil practice.

By direction of the Surgeon General.

R. B. Miller,
Lieut. Col. Medical Corps, U. S. A.

A LETTER TO ALL COUNTY COMMISSIONERS.
The University of Oklahoma, the School of Medicine, Oklahoma City, Oklahoma

Dear Sir:

I am writing you this letter to call your attention to our facilities for taking care of the poor people of your county at a very nominal expense to you.

We have on the faculty of the School of Medicine a great number of specialists in the different departments of medicine and surgery. Patients referred to us will receive the careful attention of the specialists into whose department they may go,—and in addition the advantages to consultation with any or all of the other departments. In case of poor people sent by you there is absolutely no charge for this service, the only charge being $10.00 per week to partly cover the actual expense of keeping patient in hospital. In cases in which X-ray examinations are necessary we charge $2.00 per plate, but X-ray examinations are not necessary in the majority of cases. Outside of this there is absolutely no charge whatever. The service of physician, surgeon, or specialists of whatever character, laboratory work, operating room, anesthetics, dressings, medicines, etc., are all rendered without extra charge.

There are many cases, partly those of a chronic surgical character that need not stay in the hospital longer than a couple of weeks when they are sent home cured and able to take their places as earning members of society. There are many cases of a medical character—many of them babies and small children—whose lives may be saved by proper attention to feeding and such medication as may be necessary. The expenditure of the nominal sum required to keep these people in the hospital in the hands of experts for several weeks is an economical procedure when it is considered that if they are not properly cared for they become burdens upon the people in the countries from which they come.

As the Medical Department of the State University we are anxious to render every possible service to the people in the different parts of the State. So far as the faculty of the School of Medicine is concerned we would be glad to have some arrangement through which we could take patients without charge even for hospital, but the State does not furnish us funds for that purpose for the reason that it seems to be fair to have each community pay the expense for service rendered. Patients sent us receive exactly the same professional care at the hands of the physician or surgeon given to private patients in any well ordered and well equipped hospital. Every effort is made to have the patients feel that the nurses and doctors have a personal interest in them and every effort is made to keep such patients from feeling that they are the recipients of charity.

We do not wish to interfere in the least with any hospital in your county. Some of the counties of the State have hospital facilities; many of the counties do not. We wish to offer you our service so that you may take advantage of the facilities in the care of your poor people if you are not able to secure the necessary facilities at home.

In sending patients all that is necessary for you to do is to send in an official order from your board to Mr. Paul H. Fesler, Chief Clerk, University Hospital, setting forth the fact that your board will be responsible for the expense incurred including the cost of transporting the patient home after leaving the hospital.

When patients are sent you may telephone the University Hospital, asking for some official, and if the patient needs an ambulance one will be sent to meet the train without extra charge.

In the case of patients coming without first advising hospital have them take a cab or street car and go to the Univeristy Hospital, 325 E. 4th St.

No one outside of those engaged in this work can realize how much good can be done for the people of our State in this field. I may say to you, too, that as we work at this problem of taking care of the helpless poor, the desire grows to be of more and more service. It is not a question of dollars and cents but it is the serious question of rehabilitating our citizenship and of bringing health and happiness to an unfortunate class of people.

I sincerely hope that we may count upon you to cooperate with us in carrying on this important work.   Yours truly,

(Signed) LeROY LONG, Dean.

To my son upon his departure for the war.

"DO THY BIT."

Go, my son, and do thy bit,
    The freedom of the world's at stake;
Autocracy has set claim to all,
    Destruction and slavery's in her wake.

Go, my son, and do thy bit,
    The world was not made for kings;
Help to set the universe free,
    And reap the reward it brings.

How oft have I huddled thee to my breast,
    And fondled thee on my knee;
How oft have I watched the hours go by
    When disease hovered o'er thee.

How anxiously have I watched the night,
    And cooled thy fevered brow;
And prayed the fates to save my boy,
    Just as I am praying now.

Through all thy years of childhood,
    I have kept vigil o'er thy life;
No father ever more fondly loved,
    Nor faltered less in strife.

But go, my son, and do thy bit,
    First born of my blood, depart;
God's richest blessings go with thee,
    Is the prayer of an aching heart.

I know you will come back to me
    From whatever foreign land,
With good report for absent years,
    And the ring upon your hand.

I know you will come back to me,
    Sometime, somehow, some way;
It may be in a rosewood box,
    Or in the judgment day.

But go, wherever duty calls,
    Be it in the trench or pit;
Give up all for freedom's sake,
    Go, my son, and do thy bit.
            —J. W. Echols, McAlester.

WOUND INFECTIONS.

M. D. Shie, Cleveland (*Journal A. M. A.*, Dec. 8, 1917), gives his observations made in an emergency hospital of a large manufacturing plant. All departments were represented by patients who came to the hospital. Out of fifty or sixty patients seen daily, from 8 to 10 per cent had furunculosis and 5 per cent had wound infections. It is observed, however, that all cases came from two machine shops and a further particular observed was that out of the 1,200 or more workmen only those who worked on lathes had multiple furunculosis and that 90 per cent of the infections occurred among the lathe workers. The number of infections varied with the number of lathes used. This led to the suspicion that some element in this particular kind of work must be the cause. There were two possibilities, the oil used and the cutting mixture. As regards the first, there was good reason for suspicion. The lubricating oils that were used automatically over and over again seem especially liable to produce "oil pimples" on parts of the body which come in contact with the oil. Cutting mixture is a compound of animal fats, petroleum oils, and, as a rule, acids used to facilitate the action of the cutting tool. It runs down over the work into drains beneath, which empty to a central reservoir from which it is pumped up to tanks near the roof, whence it flows down to be used over again. The men are accustomed to spit in the mixture below their machines and otherwise contaminate it, but it is used and re-used until it becomes so dirty it almost clogs the pipes. At least that was the condition before it was remedied. Each of these possible causes was investigated and the remedies sought for. Numerous disinfectants were tried, but only the coal tar products were found available, being not only cheaper but less liable to be toxic. Heat was also used for disinfection and found more or less effective. The cases of infection have been greatly reduced with the use of cresol and with education of the men and with the use of heat in combination with the disinfectant. The writer draws the following conclusions as to the cause of and remedy for furunculosis infection. 1. In a large manufacturing plant the vast majority of cases of wound infections and furunculosis were found to be localized among lathe workers in the machine shops. 2. The peculiar features of lathe work are the use of cutting mixture and oil, and the manner in which these circulate and are used repeatedly, thus making them extremely liable to contamination, which rendered them open to suspicion as factors in the causation of the wound infection and furunculosis. 3. These suspicions were borne out by bacteriologic investigation and animal inoculation, which showed the causative factor to be pyogenic organisms which were present in vast numbers in the cutting mixture and less numerous in the oil. Marked results were obtained. 4. Abundant portals of entry for these organisms were found on the arms of workingmen in innumerable small cuts and punctures made by flying chips of steel from the lathes. 5. The methods of prophylaxis possible are: (a) by heat; (b) by chemical disinfection, and (c) by a combination of the two. Various chemical disinfectants were tried, and the cresol group was found to be the most effective and the least expensive. 6. By use of chemical disinfection (cresols), wound infections have been reduced from 5 per cent to less than 0.5 per cent in the plant under consideration, and furunculosis has almost disappeared.

DIET OF PRISONERS OF WAR IN GERMANY.

American soldiers are in France and some of them have been and others inevitably will be taken prisoners, and a report of A. E. Taylor of Philadelphia (Journal A. M. A., Nov. 10, 1917), of his observations of prisoner of war camps in Germany will be of general interest. In the broad sense, says, one fundamental fact holds for the prison of war as well as other prisons. Prison life depends more on the character of the management than on the prison laws. But the prison of war problem is something more. The prisoner represents a reduction in the military forces of his country. He is industrially and politically a fact, and unfortunately can be made a weapon of defense in the hands of his captors, since he may be made the object of reprisal for the attainment of military ends. In a historical review, Taylor says, of the provisioning of the prisoner of war in Germany, three periods must be defined: the period of unorganization, the period of organization and the period of stringency. One must bear in mind also throughout the five accepted principles of the management of prisoners of war in Germany. (a) The possession of prisoners by Germany in greater numbers than those of her subjects in the hands of her enemies gave a situation of vantage. (b) The fact of a food blockade, as Germany could not secure manufactured commodities from the neutral world, gave her extraordinary rights over the labor of the prisoners of war. (c) The rules of discipline and control applying to her soldiers under her military law applied to prisoners of war under military rule. (d) Distinctions between prisoners of war of different nationalities were not recognized; the allies who fight together must as prisoners of war sleep together, eat together and work together. The Germans were taken by surprise, he says, by the number of prisoners taken in the fall of 1914, and in their confidence that their army would march directly to Paris, no special provision for the care of prisoners of war was contained in the campaign plans. Sometimes the quarters and food that were used were almost intolerable for several months, and the writer regrets to feel compelled from his personal observations to conclude that in some camps and under some commanders malice was a factor in the mistreatment. With the large number of prison camps the chances of getting a brute for an overseer were not few. His own personal experience only dates from March, 1916, and his information as to the earlier conditions was derived from testimony and records of the American Embassy and statements of German officials. The story of later conditions is more important. The fact that Germany has not declared war against the United States will not prevent the captured soldier from "getting his" if he should fall into the hands of a rancorous Prussian sergeant—a creature sui generis. The first subsistence arrangement for prisoners was by the contract system, which seemed the most feasible, and it was frankly admitted to Taylor by German authorities that in many instances the caterers grossly violated the trust imposed on them by the government, as was easy from the lack of inspection service, but openly the Germans usually denied more than nominal abuses. The first governmental regiment was issued in the spring of 1915, and was in a certain sense an admission of previous neglect. Under the commander of the camp operated a committee composed of subsistence officer, surgeon and paymaster. The service of the surgeon was limited to inspection of raw materials in stores and to a daily report on the taste of the midday soup. The details of the organization of the subsistence method are given, and as the expert of the prison nutrition office there was selected one of Germany's scientists who was better versed in the nutrition of animals than of his own species. In Taylor's first interview with Professor Packhaus, he learned that he was not conversant with a literature of human physiology, though well versed in animal nutrition from the old standpoint of energy equivalents. He was not conversant with modern investigations, and was practically unacquainted with the work that had been done on adaptation of the diet and had no conception of the psychology of rationing. He attempted to ration prisoners of war exactly as one would feed live stock. Taylor reached Germany in March, 1916, and left in October, and during this period Germany passed from closeness to stringency in food supplies, and so he had, therefore, plenty of chance to study the rationing of the prisoners of war during this period of transition. The two mistakes that were responsible for most of the difficulties were disregard for the psychology of the diet and the selection of potato instead of bread as the keystone for the dieting. In this way their own people suffered. Other evils were due to the mixing of nationalities among the prisoners. For what would do for a Russian, for example, would not do for English or French. The bread was according to our standards very poor, though it might not have been so easy for the Germans accustomed to rye bread to appreciate this, and the amount of food given to prisoners as officially stated to the writer was only that which was available for the poorest nonworking citizens of the empire. Much food, of course, was sent from home to the prisoners, and there was fear that any repression of the food parcels sent to Germany for the prisoners through Switzerland and otherwise would have a bad effect on the German prisoners in Russia, though there was a protest against what was sent to the prisoners from the German population. Ambassador Gerard was an important factor in preventing abuses, and this director of nutrition seems to have very narrow ideas. Tables are given showing the diets in the Prussian prison camps. It is apparent, Taylor says, from these figures, that the United States must undertake and organize the feeding of Americans that may be taken as prisoners of war and confined in Germany. This indeed has been already undertaken, but if food conditions become more stringent in Germany the military authorities there may decide to rob the prisoners, and the allies in that case could have no recourse except reprisal. Taylor advises against this, since the western allies could never in theory or practice follow the Germans in reprisals.

SHELL-SHOCK.

Henry Viets, Boston (*Journal A. M. A.*, Nov. 24, 1917), reviews the English medical literature of shell shock, making frequent quotations from the authorities to whom he refers. The first report of cases appeared in 1915 under the term of "shell-shock." The symptoms are varied, covering nearly all the functional and hysterical phenomena described by authors. The importance of the problem cannot be overemphasized and if it is possible, those subject to the disease should be eliminated from among the recruits before they are exposed to the perils of trench warfare. The neuropathology of the condition has been best studied by Mott. In the fatal cases, the symptoms of shell-shock resemble those of the gas poisoning, which most neurologists hold cannot alone produce shell-shock. The treatment is largely moral as well as physical and seems to have been well worked up in the British hospitals. The writer asks in conclusion: "What can the Medical Corps of the United States Army do toward the prevention of shell-shock? Obviously it must be checked at the recruiting station or in the cantonment camps before the men leave for France. There ought to be no question in the minds of the medical officers as to the advisability of checking this condition at the source, for no one who has seen the results of modern warfare on the unstable mind can do otherwise than urge such measures with utmost vigor. It becomes the duty of each medical examiner to weed out from the recruits such men as are liable to shell-shock. By so doing an enormously important advance will be made in our army, as judged by the experiences of the other armies of the Allies. We have been strongly advised by Osler to check the enlistment of the neurasthenic. It is obviously difficult to pick him from the crowd, as he may come up in good form, and be eager to go overseas. But it is not so difficult with the mentally deficient, the 'queer stick,' the 'boob,' and the butt of the practical jokers. He is soon observed by both officers and men, and if one singles him out and talks with him for five or ten minutes, one ought to have no difficulty in deciding his fitness for active trench warfare. One ought also to look with especial care into the past history of the depressed, the man who worries unnecessarily, the self-conscious, the shy, the high-strung, excitable man, the violent-tempered, the nervous, the timorous, the easily frightened, or the neurotic individual. Any or all of them may make poor first-line-trench soldiers. The task is difficult, but that in itself should not prevent us from trying. What an advantage it would be to our army officers, and what a saving of life it would mean to our men, if the shell-shock patients could be eliminated from our forces that will fight overseas! Such a utopia is probably impossible, but I feel confident that careful weeding out of the mentally unstable will certainly greatly reduce the numbers of shell-shock cases that are bound to appear in our casualty lists."

COUNCIL ON PHARMACY AND CHEMISTRY.

During November the following articles have been accepted by the Council on Pharmacy and Chemistry for inclusion with New and Non-official Remedies:

Farbwerke-Hoechst Co., New York, Salvarsan.

Borcherdt Malt Extract Co., Borcherdt's Malt Sugar.

NEW AND NON-OFFICIAL REMEDIES.

Para*D*n for Films (Surgical Para*D*n, Plastic Para*D*n).—Paraffin intended for application to burns, etc., should be more ductile and pliable than the official paraffin, and be liquid at or below 50 c. Thin films should be pliable at or below 28 c. and ductile at or below 31 c. and somewhat adherent to the skin. Paraffin for Films is used mainly in the treatment of burns. It is used also to prep re "paraffin covered bandages" and to seal gauze dressings. In the paraffin treatment of burns, the wound is cleaned and dried; a thin coating of liquid petrolatum or melted p raffin for films is applied, and is followed by a thin layer of cotton and another layer of cotton; another layer of melted paraffin is applied, and the whole then bandaged.

Stanolind Surgical Wax.—A brand of paraffin for films melting at 47 c., being pliable at or below 25 c. and ductile at or below 29 c. Standard Oil Company of Indiana, Chicago (*Journal A. M. A.*, Nov. 3, 1917, p. 1525).

Silver Protein-Squibb.—A compound of silver and gelatin, containing from 19 to 23 per cent of silver in organic combination. Like other silver protein compounds, it is used in from 1 to 25 per cent or stronger solutions for prophylaxis and treatment of the sensitive mucous membranes, particularly in gonorrhea, conjunctivitis and other infections of the urethra and of the eye, ear, nose and throat. E. R. Squibb and Sons, New York.

Arsenobenzol (Dermatological Research Laboratories).—A brand of arsenphenol-amine hydrochloride. Its actions, uses and dosage are the same as those of salvarsan. It is supplie in ampules containing 0.6 gm. The General Drug Co., New York City.

Acetylsalicylic Acid-Milliken.—A brand of acetylsalicylic acid complying with the standards of New and Non-official Remedies. It is sold only in the form of 5 grain capsules and 5 grain tablets. Jno. T. Milliken and Co., St. Louis, Mo.

Acetylsalicylic Acid (Aspirin), Monsanto.—A brand of acetylsalicylic acid complying with the standards of New and Non-official Remedies. Monsanto Chemical Works, St. Louis, Mo. (*Journal A. M. A.*, Nov. 17, 1917, p. 1695).

PROPAGANDA FOR REFORM.

"Patent Medicines" here and in Canada.—The federal law governing the interstate sale of "patent medicines" prohibits false and misleading statements in regard to composition and origin and false and fraudulent therapeutic claims. The Canadian law offers no protection against false, misleading or fraudulent statements that may be made for products of this class. As a result, many claims made for "patent medicines" when sold in Canada are not made when the same preparations are sold in the United States. An examination of Dodd's Kidney Pills, Doan's Kidney Pills, Williams' Pink Pills for Pale People, Paine's Celery Compound, Hall's Caturrh Medicine, Hoods Sarsaparilla, Dr. Chase's Nerve Pills, and Gino Pills as sold here and in Canada leads to the conclusion that the "patent medicine" industry as a whole is founded on falsehood, and that misleading and false claims will be made for such preparations, at least in the majority of cases, just so long as manufacturers are subject to no restraint except their own consciences (*Journal A. M. A.*, Nov. 10, 1917, p. 1636).

Shotgun Vaccines for Colds.—There is no reliable evidence for the value of mixed vaccines in the prevention or treatment of common "colds" and similar affections. The Council on Pharmacy and Chemistry accepted for New and Non-official Remedies mixed vaccines only on condition that their usefulness has been established by acceptable clinical evidence. So far it has not admitted any of the "influenza" or "catarrhal" mixed vaccines (*Journal A. M. A.*, Nov. 10, 1917, p. 1642).

Iodeol and Iodagol.—Iodeol and Iodagol (formerly called Iodargol) are the products of E. Viel and Company, Rennes, France. They have been widely and extravagantly advertised in the United States as preparations containing colloidal, elementary iodin, and with the claim, that because of the colloidal state of the iodin, they possessed the virtues but not the drawbacks of free iodin. As the result of chemical examination, pharmacologic, bacteriologic and clinical investigation and a study of the submitted evidence, the Council on Pharmacy and Chemistry declared the products inadmissible to New and Non-official Remedies because they did not contain the ammounts of iodin claied; because the iodin was not in the elementary or free condition but behaved like fatty iodin compounds, and because the therapeutic claims were exaggerated and unwarranted. The American agents, David B. Levy, Inc., announce that the sale of Iodeol and Iodagol has been discontinued (*Journal A. M. A.*, Nov. 17, 1917, p. 1725).

The Carrel-Dakin Wound Treatment.—Arthur Dean Bevan holds that the value of the Carrel-Dakin method of treating infected wounds has not been established. He has been forced to the conclusion that Carrel's work does not meet the requirements of scientific research. Bevan believes that the choice of antiseptics in the treatment of infected wounds is of little moment, and that the use of the Carrel-Dakin fluid, like Koch's lymph, Bier's hyperemia and the vaccine therapy of acute infections, will have a short period of popularity (*Journal A. M. A.*, Nov. 17, 1917, p. 1727).

Sphagnum Moss, A Surgical Dressing.—In England, sphagnum moss, or peat moss, is being used as a substitute for absorbent cotton. The dried moss is said to absorb twenty-two times its own weight of water, while absorbent cotton will not absorb more than six times its weight. For surgical use the dried moss is packed loosely in muslin bags which are then sterilized by heat or chemicals such as mercuric chloride (*Journal A. M. A.*, Nov. 24, 1917, p. 1790).

OFFICERS OF COUNTY SOCIETIES, 1918

County	President	Secretary
Adair		
Alfalfa		
Atoka		
Beaver		
Beckham		
Blaine		
Bryan	J. L. Reynolds, Durant	D. Armstrong, Durant
Caddo		
Canadian		
Choctaw		
Carter		
Cleveland		
Cherokee		
Custer	J. Matt Gordon, Weatherford	C. H. McBurney, Clinton
Comanche		
Coal		
Cotton		
Craig		
Creek		
Dewey		
Ellis		
Garfield		
Garvin		
Grady	D. S. Downey, Chickasha	Martha Bledsoe, Chickasha
Grant		
Greer	Nay Neel, Mangum	Thos. J. Horsley, Mangum
Harmon		
Haskell		
Hughes		
Jackson	T. H. Hardin, Oluster	W. H. Rutland, Altus
Jefferson		
Johnson		
Kay		
Kingfisher		
Kiowa		
Latimer		
Le Flore	E. E. Shippey, Wister	Harrell Hardy, Bokoshe
Lincoln		
Logan		
Love		
Mayes		
Major		
Marshall		
McClain		
McCurtain		
McIntosh	B. J. Vance, Cherotah	W. A. Tolleson, Eufaula
Murray		
Muskogee	J. G. Noble, Muskogee	A. L. Stocks, Muskogee
Noble		
Nowata		
Okfuskee		
Oklahoma		H. H. Cloudman, Oklahoma City
Okmulgee	W. C. Mitchner, Okmulgee	Harry E. Breese, Henryetta
Ottawa		
Osage		
Pawnee		
Payne		
Pittsburg		
Pottawatomie		
Pontotoc		
Pushmataha		
Rogers		
Roger Mills		
Seminole		
Sequoyah		
Stephens		
Texas		
Tulsa		
Tillman		
Wagoner		
Washita		
Washington		
Woodward	R. A. Workman, Woodward	C. W. Tedrowe, Woodward
Woods		

OFFICERS OF OKLAHOMA STATE MEDICAL ASSOCIATION.

Meeting Place—Tulsa, May, 1918.
President, 1917-18—Dr. W. Albert Cook, Tulsa.
President-elect, 1918-19—Dr. L. S. Willour, McAlester.
1st Vice-President—Dr. McLain Rogers, Clinton.
2nd Vice-President—Dr. G. F. Border, Mangum.
3rd Vice-President—Dr. Horace Reed, Oklahoma City.
Secretary-Treasurer-Editor—Dr. C. A. Thompson, Muskogee.
Delegate to the A. M. A., 1918-19—Dr. Chas. R. Hume, Anadarko.
Delegate to the A. M. A. 1917-18—Dr. M. A. Kelso, Enid.

COUNCILOR DISTRICTS.

1. Cimarron, Texas, Beaver, Harper, Ellis, Woods and Woodward; Councilor, Dr. J. M. Workman, Woodward. Term expires 1919.
2. Roger Mills, Beckham, Dewey, Custer, Washita and Blaine; Councilor, Dr. Ellis Lamb, Clinton. Term expires 1920.
3. Harmon, Greer, Jackson, Kiowa, Tillman, Comanche and Cotton; Councilor, Dr. G. P. Cherry, Mangum. Term expires 1918.
4. Major, Alfalfa, Grant, Garfield, Noble and Kay; Councilor, Dr. G. A. Boyle, Enid. Term expires 1919.
5. Kingfisher, Canadian, Oklahoma and Logan; Councilor, Dr. Fred Y. Cronk, Guthrie. Term expires 1918.
6. Caddo, Grady, McClain, Garvin, Stephens and Jefferson; Councilor, Dr. C. M. Maupin, Waurika. Term expires 1919.
7. Osage, Pawnee, Creek, Okfuskee, Okmulgee and Tulsa; Councilor, Dr. N. W. Mayginnes, Tulsa. Term expires 1920.
8. Payne, Lincoln, Cleveland, Pottawatomie and Seminole; Councilor, Dr. H. M. Williams, Wellston. Term expires 1920.
9. Pontotoc, Murray, Carter, Love, Marshall, Johnston and Coal; Councilor, Dr. J. T. Slover, Sulphur. Term expires 1918.
10. Washington, Nowata, Rogers, Craig, Ottawa, Mayes and Delaware; Councilor, Dr. R. L. Mitchell, Vinita. Term expires 1918.
11. Wagoner, Muskogee, McIntosh, Haskell, Cherokee and Adair; Councilor, Dr. J. Hutchings White, Muskogee. Term expires 1918.
12. Hughes, Pittsburg, Latimer, LeFlore and Sequoyah; Councilor, Dr. Ed. D. James, Haileyville. Term expires 1920.
13. Atoka, Pushmataha, Bryan, Choctaw and McCurtain; Councilor, Dr. J. L. Austin, Durant. Term expires 1920.

CHAIRMEN OF SCIENTIFIC SECTIONS.

Surgery and Gynecology—Dr. LeRoy Long, Oklahoma City.
Pediatrics and Obstetrics—Dr. T. C. Sanders, Shawnee.
Eye, Ear, Nose and Throat—Dr. L. A. Newton, Oklahoma City.
General Medicine, Nervous and Mental Diseases—Dr. A. B. Leeds, Chickasha.
Genitourinary, Skin and Radiology—Dr. W. J. Wallace, Oklahoma City.
Legislative Committee—Dr. Millington Smith, Oklahoma City; Dr. J. M. Byrum, Shawnee; Dr. W. T. Salmon, Oklahoma City.
For the Study and Control of Cancer—Drs. LeRoy Long, Oklahoma City; Gayfree Ellison, Norman; D. A. Myers, Lawton.
For the Study and Control of Pellagra—Drs. A. A. Thurlow, Norman; L. A. Mitchell, Frederick; J. C. Watkins, Checotah.
For the Study of Venereal Diseases—Drs. Wm. J. Wallace, Oklahoma City; Ross Grosshart, Tulsa; J. E. Bercaw, Okmulgee.
Necrology—Drs. Martha Bledsoe, Chickasha; J. W. Pollard, Bartlesville.
Tuberculosis—Drs. L. J. Moorman, Oklahoma City; C. W. Heitzman, Muskogee; Leila E. Andrews, Oklahoma City.
Conservation of Vision—Drs. L. A. Newton, Oklahoma City; L. Haynes Buxton, Oklahoma City; G. E. Hartshorne, Shawnee.
First Aid Committee—Drs. G. S. Baxter, Shawnee; Jas. C. Johnston, McAlester.
Committee on Medical Education—Drs. A. L. Blesh; A. K. West; A. W. White, Oklahoma City.
State Commissioner of Health—Dr. John W. Duke, Guthrie, Oklahoma.

STATE BOARD OF MEDICAL EXAMINERS.

Melvin Gray, M. D., Durant, President; B. L. Denison, M. D., Garvin, Vice-President; J. J. Williams, M. D., Weatherford, Secretary; O. R. Gregg, M. D., Waynoka, Treasurer; E. B. Dunlap, M. D., Lawton; Ralph V. Smith, M. D., Tulsa; W. LeRoy Bonnell, M. D., Chickasha; Wm. T. Ray, M. D., Gould; H. C. Montague, D. O., Muskogee.
Reciprocity with Georgia, Kentucky, Mississippi, Nevada, North Carolina, Wisconsin, Kansas, Arkansas, Virginia, West Virginia, Nebraska, New Mexico, Tennessee, Iowa, Ohio, California, Colorado, Indiana, Missouri, New Jersey, Vermont, Texas, Michigan.
Meetings held second Tuesday of January, April, July and October, Oklahoma City.
Address all communications to the Secretary, Dr. J. J. Williams, Weatherford.

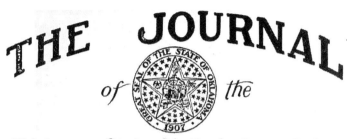

THE JOURNAL

of *the*

Oklahoma State Medical Association

VOLUME XI　　　　MUSKOGEE, OKLA., FEBRUARY, 1918　　　　NUMBER 2

ACIDOSIS AND RECENT METHODS OF DEMONSTRATING IT*

From the Wm. W. Bierce Clinical and Research Laboratory of St. Anthony Hospital,
Oklahoma City.

By O. J. WALKER, M. D., Oklahoma City, Oklahoma

The interest and study that has been centered upon acidosis during the past three years has been demonstrated, among other things, that it is an extremely common condition. Physiologically it follows violent exercise, or the sudden exposure to an atmosphere low in oxygen, as on a mountain top. Probably in most of our common diseases the severity, at least, is dependent more or less upon the degree of acidosis present.

Definition. Acidosis may be defined as a condition in which there is an increase above the normal of any of the acid elements of the blood, owing to an excessive production of acid products of metabolism; or, to a defective elimination of the same; or both.

In acidosis it is not meant that the reaction of the blood actually changes from the slightly alkaline, or neutral, reaction to acid reaction. Only in the very last stages of acidosis, just prior to death, does an acid condition of the blood occur and under no other circumstances. Any increase in the acid phosphate, or in the organic acids of the blood is, within certain limits, very promptly and completely compensated by a loss of CO_2 through the lungs. The term acidosis, then, implies only that the non-volatile acids (usually acid phosphates or organic acids) are increased, while the bicarbonate and carbonic acid are in compensation reduced.

D. D. Van Slyke[1] defines acidosis as "a condition in which the concentration of bicarbonate in the blood is reduced below the normal level." Naunyn (1906) first used the term "acidosis" to denote the abnormal metabolic condition in which hydroxy-butyric acid is formed. The departure from this use has been evolutionary. Apparently because the word acidosis is suggestive of acids in general rather than hydroxy-butyric in particular, when other types of acid intoxication were discovered they also were designated as acidosis. Henderson[2] and his associates have been mainly responsible for the broader conception of the term.

Physiology of Acid Regulation. In order that we may more fully understand the nature of acidosis, let us look for a moment into the physiology concerned. First the blood and in fact the whole body mass of tissue is maintained at a constant chemical reaction. Second, the respiration is a ready and prompt means of adjusting any changes in the constant chemical reaction of the body. Third, the kidneys are another means, though acting slower, in accomplishing this same

.*Read before St. Anthony Clinical Society, Nov. 19, 1917.

purpose. Thanks mainly to the works of L. J. Henderson[2] we now know the physical chemistry of the mechanism for the adjustment of the chemical reaction of the blood. The blood is conceived of as a delicately balanced complex of chemical radicals, all appropriately ionized. The alkaline radicals are mainly those of K., Na., Ca., Mg. and NH_4; and the acid radicals are the chlorides, sulphates, phosphates and some other mineral acids, carbonates, carbonic acid and various organic acids, such as lactic, B-hydroxy-butyric, diacetic, etc. Of these salts which affect the reaction of the blood, the phosphates (Na_3PO_4, HNa_2PO_4, H_2NaPO_4), carbonates (Na_2CO_3, $HNaCO_3$) and free carbonic acid are not only present in the greatest amounts but are so much the most important that no great error is involved in looking upon the blood as a solution of these salts alone. Due to the low degree of ionization of these radicals, a considerable number of acid free ions are capable of being bound without great change in the reaction being brought about. This, together with the proteins which also take up excess ions readily, endows the solution with the power, as it were, of soaking up the excess H-ions; it acts as a sponge, or as Henderson has so aptly termed it, as a "buffer."

The addition of acid to this complex results in a shifting of all the members present; some of the alkaline phosphate becomes acid-phosphate and at the same time carbonates become bi-carbonates; and some of the bi-carbonate loses its alkali and becomes carbonic acid. As a net result of this shifting all along the line there is, temporarily, more free CO_2 dissolved in the blood. This increased CO_2 stimulates the respiratory center with increased ventilation, and the extra CO_2 which has been formed is almost immediately washed out through the lungs and the reaction reduced to normal.

The mechanism may be illustrated roughly by a diagram[3] which, of course, must not be taken too literally as an exact representation of chemical facts.

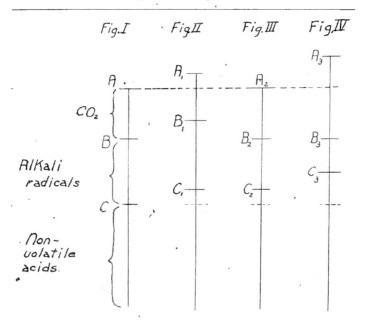

In Fig. I, let A-B represent the dissolved CO_2, or the divalent CO_3 ion. B-C represents the alkali radicals and the line below C the phosphates and all other acid radicals. Everything else being equal, these quantities will be proportional according to physico-chemical laws, which have been so admirably explained by Henderson. A change in one quantity will bring about a change in all. Thus, if there is added an acid, such as lactic, (Fig. II) the line C will rise to C1, and A will rise to A1, with a corresponding shortening of B1-C1. This increase in the amount of acids above the normal stimulates the respiratory center and the excess of CO_2 is quickly removed, bringing the line A1 back to its normal level A, or nearly so. As the excess of CO_2 is eliminated, there is a further interchange of H-ion from the phosphates toward the carbonates and the level of B1 will be correspondingly lowered. Any such condition as Fig. II is unstable and necessarily hardly occurs at all. since the increase of acid takes place gradually and the excretion of CO_2 so fully compensates it that the line A never rises appreciably above its normal level.

Fig. III represents the ordinary condition of acidosis. At this time the kidney begins to work overtime in its attempt to keep the non-volatile acids at the constant level C, so that within an hour or two enough acid phosphate, or other acid, will have been excreted in the urine to bring the line C2 back to the normal threshold of C (assuming of course that the addition of acid does not continue), and at the same time A2 and B2 will return to their normal level.

The importance of the singular power of the kidney of withdrawing the acid radicals from an alkaline medium and excreting them in acid urine, and the rapidity and delicacy of this function, has only lately been realized. The radicals withdrawn consist mainly of the acid phosphates, although if the acid production of the body is low, the alkaline phosphates and even bicarbonate will appear and the urine will become alkaline. Thus the kindey maintains a threshold value for acids above which acids ions will be excreted; and below which, in a similar manner, enough alkali will be excreted to keep constant the nornmal reaction of the blood. Although this level varies slightly between individuals, it remains remarkably constant in the same person. Also the total acid and therefore the amount of dissolved CO_2 remains constant in the same subject over many years.

The amount of alkali radicals which are available to neutralize acid (that is the tri- and di-sodium phosphates and the carbonates) is termed the "alkali reserve." The line BC in Fig. I represents this value.

Of course there is a limit to power of this respiratory and renal compensatory mechanism. Figures II-III represent a compensated acidosis. Fig. IV represents a condition which occurs only in the more extreme forms of acidosis (usually near death), where the level of C3 has become so high and B3-C3 (alkali reserve) so decreased that the most energetic breathing, or the most frantic efforts of the kidneys, cannot keep the total acid at normal level.

In the case of the blood it is mainly the salts of carbonic acid and partly the proteins rather than the salts of the phosphoric acid that furnishes the "buffer." Free carbonic acid is present in the body fluids in such concentration that it automatically converts into bicarbonate all bases not bound by other acids. The bicarbonate, therefore, represents the excess of base which is left after all the nonvolatile acids have been neutralized. In this sense it constitutes the "alkali reserve" of the body. Entrance of free acid into the blood reduces the bicarbonate to an extent proportional to the amount of the invading acid. The retained acid decomposes body bicarbonate, forming in its place the salts of the invading acid.

The normal concentration of the bicarbonate in the blood is so definite that it constitutes a physiological constant. The blood plasma of normal adults contains 55 to 77 per cent of its volume of CO_2 gas bound as bicarbonate. The limits of variation are similar in magnitude to those of the pulse rate. By utilizing as a standard the normal bicarbonate concentration, we can reduce the term "acidosis" to as definite a meaning as fever, or "tachycardia." In each case condition is indicated in which one of the physiological constants falls, or rises, to abnormal level. Like accelerated pulse rate, or increased temperature, it may occur temporarily even in health, e. g., as the result of exercise and consequent lactic acid formation.

It is not necessarily a pathological condition in itself, but is rather a symptom of disturbed function. Like fever or tachycardia, however, acidosis in itself becomes a danger when it has reached a sufficient degree of intensity.

Sources of Acid in the Blood. A word is not amiss here as to the origin of the various acids of the blood. Acid radicals come normally to some extent from bodily catabolism, but largely from the food. Meat is the great acid producer. Under normal conditions, however, there is often considerable acid production of bodily catabolism. Acid products always result from deficient oxidation. During vigorous exercise the muscles may not get sufficient oxygen and lactic acid is the resulting end-product, instead of CO_2, as normally. Again, lack of carbohydrate participation in the catabolism of fats results in a considerable quantity of diacetic and B-hydroxy-butyric acid.

It is evident from what has been said that acidosis may arise in one of two ways and the distinction is important: (1) By overproduction of acid, with which the kidney is unable to keep pace; (2) By failure of the kidney to excrete normal amount of acid even without overproduction.

Later Methods for Demonstrating Acidosis. Just as the thermometer and stethoscope are necessary apparatus in the diagnosis of fever and heart lesion, so do we need apparatus and simple methods for detecting acidosis. You are all familiar with the symptoms of acidosis starting with hyperpnea, ranging from a slight increase in lung ventilation to a marked air hunger; later there is headache, nausea and vomiting, coma, respiratory paralysis and death. It is extremely essential to be able to recognize the beginning of acidsosis before the stage of air hunger and coma.

The tests for early stages of acidosis fall naturally from what has been said into three classes, e. g., urinary and blood analysis and respiratory data. Practically all these tests, either directly or indirectly, constitute approximate determination of the bicarbonate of the blood.

Urinary Analysis. Here we have the methods for the determination of increased acid excretion and especially when the increase is due to any particular acid, as B-hydroxy-butyric, diacetic, etc. You are all familiar with the significance of these acid bodies in the urine. However, that we cannot absolutely depend on these tests is quite readily understood from what has been said of the kidney function in eliminating the non-volatile acids. Evidently quite a marked degree of reduction in the alkali reserve may have taken place before such acid bodies appear in the urine. Then again the kidney mechanism may be so injured that it is no longer capable of regulating the normal threshold of acid excretion.

Another fact has been brought out by Van Slyke[4] when he cites an instance in which he observed an excretion of 20 gms. of acetone bodies per liter of urine without an abnormally low plasma CO_2 capacity. The increased ammonia output is also of some value when present, but is one of the later manifestations and its absence by no means rules out an acidosis due to retention.

Respiratory Analysis. The alveolar air is in equilibrium with respect to its CO_2 content with arterial blood. Consequently, in accordance with the law of gas solubility, the concentration of CO_2 in alveolar air is directly proportionate to that of free carbonic acid in the blood. And the latter has been shown, with normal respiratory control, to be kept proportional to the bicarbonate concentration.

Of the methods for the determination of the alveolar CO_2 tension, that of Haldane and Priestly[5], that of Plesch[6] and that of Marriott[7] are the best. The latter method I wish to demonstrate before you this evening. In the words of Marriott, "The method depends on the fact that if a current of air containing CO_2 is passed through a solution of sodium carbonate, or bicarbonate, until the solution is saturated, the final solution will contain sodium bicarbonate and dissolved CO_2. The reaction of such a solution will depend on the relative amounts of alkaline bicarbonate and the acid carbon dioxide present. This is turn will depend on the tension of CO_2 in the air with which the mixture has been saturated and will be independent of the volume of air blown through, provided saturation has once been attained.

High tension of CO_2 changes the reaction of the solution toward the acid side. Low tensions have the reverse effect; hence the reaction of such a solution is a measure of the tension of CO_2 in the air with which it has been saturated.

The reaction of such a solution may be determined by adding to it an indicator such as phenolsulphonephthalein, which shows over a considerable range of reaction definite color changes. A certain color indicates a certain reaction.

Standard solutions of a definite reaction and indicating a definite CO_2 tension may be prepared by mixing acid and alkaline phosphates in definite proportions. Such solutions keep unaltered for long periods.

Collection of Alveolar Air. A rubber bag of approximately 1500 c.c. capacity is connected by means of a short rubber tube to a glass mouth piece. About 600 c.c. of air are blown into the bag with an atomizer bulb, and the rubber tube clamped off by a pinchcock. The subject should be at rest and breathing naturally. At the end of a normal expiration, the subject takes the tube in his mouth; the pinchcock is released and the subject's nose closed by the observer. The subject breathes back and forth from the bag four times in twenty seconds, emptying the bag at each inspiration. The observer should indicate when to breathe in and out. Breathing more frequently will not alter the results. At the end of twenty seconds, the tube is clamped off and the air analyzed. The analysis should be carried out within three minutes time, as carbon dioxid rapidly escapes through rubber.

The foregoing procedure applies to patients who are capable of cooperating to some extent. In the case of comatose patients, the initial amount of air in the rubber bag must be greater (1000 c.c. at least), and the period of rebreathing prolonged to thirty seconds. This is necessary, as it is not feasible that the bag be completely emptied of air at each inspiration; and therefore a longer time is required for the carbon dioxid tension in the bag and in the lungs to become equal. The initial amount of air in the bag should be such that it is at least one-half and preferably as much as two-thirds emptied at each inspiration. Since comatose patients cannot hold the mouthpiece, some form of mask is necessary. This may be a gas anesthetic mask, or one especially devised for this purpose by Marriott.

Technic of the Analysis. In analyzing a sample of air, about two or three c.c. of the standard bicarbonate solutions are poured into a clean test tube of the same diameter as the tubes containing standard phosphate solutions, but from 100 to 150 mm. long. Air from the bag is then blown through the solution by means of a glass tube drawn out to a fine capillary point, until the solution is saturated, as shown by the fact that no further color change occurs. The tube is stoppered and the color immmediately compared with that in the standard tubes. By interpolation, one can readily read the millimeters. Color changes are not so sharp above 35 mm. as at a lower end of the scale, but here changes are of less significance. In making the color comparisons, the solution being compared is placed between the two standards which it most nearly matches. When there is doubt as to whether the color of the solution is higher, or lower, than one of the standards, changing the order in which the tubes are placed in the comparison box will generally make the relationship clear.

The standard solutions are so prepared as to give correct results when the determination is carried out at a temperature of from 20 to 25 degrees C (from 68 to 77 degrees F.) When the room temperature is considerably higher, or lower, than these poitns it is advisable to immerse the tubes in water approximately 25 degrees C. during the blowing. They may be removed from the water for the color comparison, however, provided this is quickly made. The differences due to the ranges of temperature occurring under ordinary circumstances are practically negligible.

No correction for barometric pressure is required, as from the nature of the determination, barometric fluctuations are self-corrective. Variations in the temperature of the subject are never great enough to affect the value as much as 1 mm., and therefore may be neglected.

In normal adults at rest the CO_2 tension in the alveolar air, determined by this method, varies from 40 to 45 mm. Tension between 30 and 35 mm. are indications of a mild degree of acidosis. When the tension is as low as 20 mm., the individual may be considered in imminent danger. In coma, associated with acidosis, the tension may be as low as 8 or 10 mm. I have seen one case as low as 12 mm. and he died within an hour of making the determination. In infants the tension of CO_2 is from 3 to 5 mm. lower than adults.

The advantage of the method lies in its simplicity of operation and the fact that it is of small bulk and easily portable. It is rapid and sufficiently accurate for clinical purposes and therefore it is recommended as a part of the busy practitioner's outfit.

The disadvantages of this method are chiefly those of delicacy and accuracy. Any method that depends upon the comparison of colors is naturally open to a greater or lesser degree of error, depending upon the personal equation and kind of colorimeter. Simple comparison of comparts is the poorest of color methods. Then, too, other conditions besides acidosis may affect the CO_2 tension of the alveolar air. Thus stimulation of the respiratory mechanism by drugs (caffein) or intracranial lesions; or its depression by the same agents (morphine) may noticeably affect the tension of CO_2. Also any change in the lungs which affect their function will of neccesity affect the composition of the alveolar air and therefore the method is unsuitable in cases with pulmonary affections.

Blood Analysis. Of the methods of involving the blood, the determination the H-ion concentration has been used extensively. The gas-chain method has been the most used for this determination, but is long and difficult, requires delicate and expensive apparatus, and is therefore not applicable to clinical determinations.

Levy, Rountree and Marriott[8] have proposed a method which involves the well known principle that different indicators show their color changes at varying degrees of hydrogen-ion concentration. For example, methyl orange changes from pink to orange as the pH of its solution changes from from 3 to 5. At intermediate points, various colors may be obtained and certain color indicates a definite pH. Similarly phenolphthalein changes from a colorless to pink between pH6 and pH10 and can be used for measurement of the H-ion concentration between these two points. Standard solutions of known pH are prepared at H-ion concentrations approximating that of blood under normal and abnormal conditions. The known comparts are compared with the solution in question, i. e., blood.

In using the indicator method it is necessary to exclude the coloring matters of the hemoglobin and the proteins. This is done by dialyzing the blood through collodion sacs into a solution of normal NaCl.

Technique of Method. The work must be done in a room free from fumes of acids or ammonia. Blood is drawn with as little loss of CO_2 as possible. This is accomplished by drawing it under paraffin oil.

Approximately 1 c.c. of blood is pipetted into a dialyzing sac which has been washed inside and outside with normal salt solution and which has been tested for leaks by filling with salt solution. The sac is lowered into a glass tube, 100x10 mm. inside measurement, containing 3 c.c. salt solution and kept there until the fluid on the outside of the sac is as high as it is on the inside. From 5 to 10 minutes are allowed for dialysis. The collodion sac is then removed and .2 c.c. of .01 per cent phenolsulphonephthalein indicator solution added and thoroughly mixed with the dialysate. This unknown tube is then compared with a series of standard tubes until the corresponding color is found. Normal blood serum by this method gives a pH of 7.6 to 7.8. In acidosis the pH varies from 7.55 to 7.2.

The advantage of this method is that it is relatively simple and easy as compared with the gas-chain method.

The disadvantages of the method may be summed up as follows: (1) The dialysate does not necessarily have a reaction that is proportional to that of the original blood. (2) Such small quantities of acid and alkali are employed that it is very difficult to tell just when slight difference in tint has been produced. (3) The difference between the normal and acidosis figure (7.6 and 7.5 to 7.2) is so slight that very accurate readings of the color changes are necessary. With the prescribed method of using comparts and the personal equation involved, the required accuracy is seldom attained. (4) Even with the precautions prescribed above it is impossible to be sure that the amount of CO_2 in the different samples of blood is the same, which means, of course, a difference in pH value.

Determination of the CO_2 in the Blood. As was pointed out in discussing the physical chemistry of the blood, its bicarbonate concentration represents the alkaline reserve and is so constant normally that any variations from normal forms one of the most reliable and delicate means of determining the early evidences of acidosis.

D. D. Van Slyke[1] has devised a method of measuring the CO_2 capacity of the blood, which is so simple and easy of manipulation that it is eminently suited for clinical application, and at the same time is so delicate and accurate that it has already become a recognized method for accurate scientific work. The method depends upon the fact that CO_2 is liberated from a solution in a vacuum under the reduced pressure. The blood is acidified in order to liberate the CO_2 radical from its bicarbonate combination.

Complete extraction of the gas is not attempted, but the volume relations between the liquid and the free space of the apparatus being known, the residue remaining is calculated from the solubility coefficient of the gas.

The venous blood is saturated with CO_2, either from a tank at 5.5 per cent, or by air from the lungs of the operator, which is remarkably constant at 5.5 per cent. This gives us results which are approximately that of arterial blood and indicate the bicarbonate content of the latter.

Technique of the Method. The blood is drawn from the anti-cubital fossa with the patient at rest and without stasis of the blood by ligature. The blood is best drawn into a tube containing powdered oxalate and paraffin oil. The oxalate prevents coagulation and the paraffin prevents the escape of the CO_2.

Having centrifuged the fresh oxalated blood, pipette off the clear plasma and place it in a separatory funnel of about 300 c.c. capacity. Slight hemolysis does not affect the results appreciably, but hemolysis should be avoided as much as possible by immediate centrifugalization. In order to determine its alkaline reserve, the plasma is saturated with a carbon dioxid at alveolar tension. In other words, the operator blows vigorously through a bottle containing glass beads into the separatory funnel. If one blows directly into the separatory funnel, enough moisture condenses on the walls of the funnel to appreciably dilute the plasma. Close the funnel at stopcock S (Fig. V) and stopper T just before the stream of breath stops, and shake for one minute in such a manner that the plasma is distributed as completely as possible about the walls. After the shaking has lasted a minute, blow a fresh portion of the alveolar air through the beads into the funnel and shake for one minute.

The CO_2 apparatus (Fig. VI) is held in a strong clamp, e, which is lined with rubber, and the lower stopcock is supported by an iron rod, g, which is also covered with soft rubber tubing. The apparatus is completely filled with mercury. Care should be taken that capillaries a and b, which are above the upper stopcock, are also filled with mercury. There should be no air bubbles within the apparatus. Six dropping bottles, which contain the following solutions, should be at hand:

1. Distilled water. 2. Phenolphthalein (1 per cent in 95 per cent alchohol.) 3. Normal ammonium hydroxide. 4. Caprylic alchohol. 5. Normal sulphuric acid. 6. Mercury.

The mercury levelling bulb L should be hung by wire K on an extension about on the level with the lower cock f. The apparatus must be thoroughly

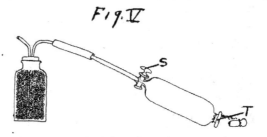

$Fig. \overline{V}$

cleaned before the determination is started. The apparatus can then be tested by allowing the mercury to run down and then forcing it up by raising and lowering the bulb L. The air is forced out and the mercury is caught in a bottle. (This is done until there is not a single air bubble in the apparatus). Add one drop of phenolphthalein to the upper cup a and a drop or two of the ammonium hydroxide. Now dilute this with about 1-2 c.c. of distilled water and draw off all except about two drops of the alkaline solution.

Now introduce 1 c.c. of the saturated plasma into the cup and allow it to flow under the alkaline solution, so that none of the carbon dioxide escapes. Turn the upper stopcock, c, so that a and d are connected and allow the plasma to run in until capillary is exactly filled. Add 0.5 c.c. of distilled water to cup a and then allow to run down to capillary. Repeat this, taking care that no air enters the apparatus with the liquid. Now admit into capillary, one drop of caprylic alchohol to prevent foaming, and pour about 1.5 c.c. of the sulphuric acid into the cup. Admit enough of the acid into the apparatus, carrying the caprylic alchohol along with it, so that the total volume in the apparatus is exactly to the 2.5 c.c. mark. Draw off the excess sulphuric acid. Now place a few drops of mercury in cup a and allow to flow down to capillary, in order to seal same and make it capable of holding an absolute vacuum. During the whole operation, the lower stopcock f should remain open, and when the apparatus is set up it should be in such adjustment that, if the wire K, which is connected to bulb L, is lowered to position 2, the mercury will run to the mark X on the figure, care being taken that the mercury will not run into fork j. Place wire K in Position 3, and allow the mercury to fall until the meniscus of the mercury has dropped to the 50 c.c. mark on the apparatus. This is controlled by stopcock f. The bubbles of CO_2 are now seen escaping.

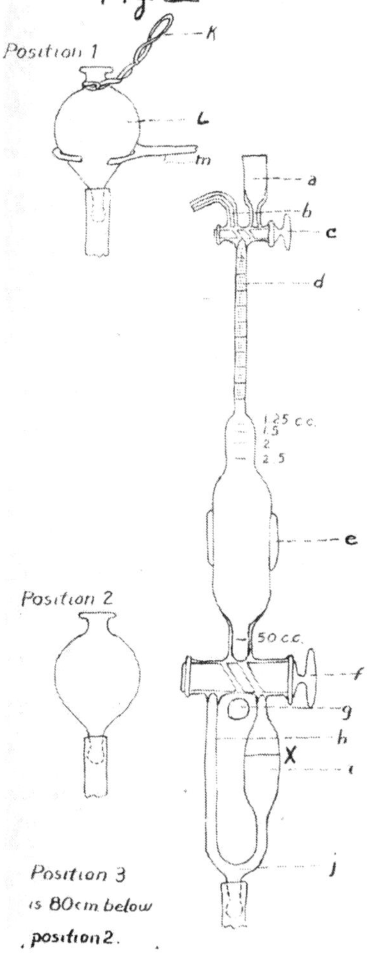

In order to completely extract the carbon dioxide, remove the apparatus from the clamp and shake by turning it upside down about a dozen times. (The thumb should be placed over cup a so as not to lose any of the mercury). Then replace the apparatus, the mercury leveling bulb L still being at the low level, and allow the solution to flow into the small bulb below the lower stopcock (right side). Drain the solution out of the portion of the apparatus above the stopcock f as completely as possible, but without removing any of the gas (the last drop being allowed to remain above). Now raise the mercury bulb L in the left hand, and with the right hand immediately turn the lower stopcock f so that the mercury is admitted to the upper part of the apparatus through the left hand entrance of the stopcock without readmitting the watery solution   Hold the leveling bulb L beside apparatus so that its mercury level corresponds to that in the apparatus, and the gas in the latter is under atmospheric pressure. A few hundredths of a cubic centimeter of water will float on the mercury of the apparatus but this may be disregarded in levelling. The calculation of the result into terms of volume percentage of carbon dioxide, bound as carbonate by the plasma, is quite complicated and is either accomplished by referring to a table devised by Van Slyke, or by using the direct reading from the apparatus, minus 0.12.

Plasma of normal adults yield 0.65 to 0.90 c.c. of gas which is the direct reading on the apparatus. If .12 were subtracted, the normal figures would be 53 to 78 in terms of volume per cent of carbon dioxid bound, chemically, by the plasma. Figures lower than 50 per cent in adults indicate acidosis. Figures aslow as 45 are normal for childrem. The exact calcula-

Fig. VI

Position 1

K

L

m

a

b

c

d

1 25 c.c.
1.5
2
2 5

e

Position 2

50 c.c.

f

g

h

X

i

j

Position 3
is 80cm below
position 2.

tion of the result into terms of carbon dioxide bound as carbonate by the plamsa is quite complicated and consequently the worker is advised to subtract 0.12 from his reading on the apparatus. The result thus obtained gives approximately (within 2 to 3 per cent) the volume per cent of carbon dioxide bound by the plasma.

The bicarbonate content of the blood is more desirable as a standard for measuring change in the acid-base balance than the H-ion concentration, for the reason that, while the bicarbonate decreases progressivley as soon as the normal excess of bases over acids begins to be depleted, rise in the blood pH is usually one of the latest changes to follow. The reason for this is that, until a large part of the blood bicarbonate has been exhausted the body can, by accelerated respiration, maintain the normal acid-base balance in the arterial blood. The H-ion concentration being directly proportional to this is therefore kept normal.

Clinical application of these methods for the early detection of acidosis may be made in a great variety of cases. They may be roughly classified as follows: (1) Overproduction of acid due to deficient oxygenation. Such cases include severe exercise, mountain sickness, acute anemias, gas poisoning and other forms of asphyxia, decompensated heart lesions, and poor circulation in general. (2) Primary lack of oxygen with compensatory raising of the threshold of acid secretion. Examples of this type are seen in acidosis of high altitudes and pregnancy. (3) Abnormal catabolism with production of large amounts of acids. These include diabetes, starvation, post-operative toxemias, and the diarrhoeas and cyclic vomiting of children, burns and septicemia. (4) Kidney insufficiency with retention of the normal acid output—i. e., severe nephritis, pus kidney, pneumonia, scarlet fever and other infections.

Treatment. There is still a great deal of uncertainty as to the treatment of acidosis. However, certain general principles are evident. The acidosis of high altitudes, anemia and pregnancy, call for no treatment as it here is a physiological compensatory mechanism. Alkalis are indicated in acidosis of the overproduction type, where the elimination is free. Allen and Joslin, however, warn against alkali therapy in diabetes. A free flow of urine is to be aimed at in all cases. Water is the best diuretic and glucose is probably next. Glucose is essential in diabetes, and probably many cases have been thrown into coma by the sudden withdrawal of sugar, which not only removes the very efficient diuretic but also leaves the fats to be improperly catabolized with the production of B-oxybutyric and diacetic acid.

When kidneys are damaged and unable to excrete acid, it is probably useless to add alkalis. Free purgation and elimination by skin is most effective here.

Meat is a great acid producer and should be avoided when there is danger of acidosis.

Fresh air blowing across the face probably attains its quieting effects in pneumonia by the relief of acidosis.

Finally, rest and the prevention of all activity which increases metabolism, is indicated.

1. D. D. Van Slyke and G. E. Cullen; Studies of Acidosis; Journal Biological Chemistry, XXX-291-1917.
2. Henderson, L. J.; The Theory of Neutrality Regulation in the Animal Organism; Amer. Jr. Physiology, XXI-427-1908: Ibid; Palmer and Henderson, Studies on Acid Base Equilibrum and the Nature of Acidosis; Arch. Int. Med., XII-153-1913.
3. James L. Whitney: Acidosis: A Summary of Recent Knowledge. Boston Med. and Surg. Jour., CLXXVI-245-1917.
4. Jour. Biol. Chemistry, XXX-296-1917.
5. Haldane and Priestly: Jour. Physiology, XXXII-225-1905.
6. Plesch, J; Z-Exp. path. u. Ther., 1907-VI-380.
7. Marriott, W. McKim, Jour. A. M. A., LXVI-1594.
8. Marriott, Levy and Rountree: Arch. Int. Med., XVI-388-1915.
9. Joslin, E. P.; Treatment of Diabetes Mellites, P. 394.

TONSILLECTOMY BY A MODIFICATION OF THE SLUDER TECHNIQUE*

By E. F. STROUD, M. D. Tulsa, Oklahoma.

For the past five years tonsillectomy has been universally adopted by all nose and throat men of note, in preference to tonsillotomy.

The question before the throat man of today is the most simple and quickest method of tonsillectomy. In my opinion, the best operation is the modification of the Sluder technique under general anesthesia, on account of: (1) The brief period of time required to perform the operation. (2) The small amount of hemorrhage during the operation. (3) Minimizing the chances of post-operative hemorrhage, and last, but not least, the preservation of both the anterior and posterior pillars of the tonsillar fossa.

The instruments used in this operation are a mouth gag, Freer's septum knife and a Sluder tonsillectome. The latter instrument is very similar to the old McKenzie tonsillotome, differing from it in the fact that it has a blunt blade and much heavier frame. The instrument is made in three sizes, viz: large, medium and small. I find that the medium sized instrument can be used in practically all cases over six years of age, while the small size should be used under that age.

The mouth gag should be either the Manhattan or Denhardt, as either of them give good leverage in forcing the mouth open, and is not in the operator's field. The Manhattan is the better for adults, as it has more leverage, and is the more powerful instrument of the two.

The technique of this operation in brief is as follows: The patient is placed in the dorsal position, and given a general anesthetic—after inserting the mouth gag, use the blade carrier of the tonsillectome as a tongue depressor, observe the tonsils thoroughly, then swing the instrument around so as to have the fenestrum posterior to the tonsil to be removed, having the handle of the instrument on the opposite side of the face—depress the handle of the instrument, by so doing the fenestrum of the tonsillectome is elevated and the tonsil is lifted out of the fossa, putting the anterior pillar on the stretch; in other words, the tonsil to be removed stands out above the fenestrum of the instrument. Then place the first finger of the free hand on the anterior pillar and force the tonsil through the fenestrum. Push the blade home behind the anterior pillar, being careful not to release hold on the tonsil, otherwise it will slip out of the fenestrum. After this, having engaged the tonsil, elevate the handle of the instrument and observe the uvula, in order to be sure that it is free. With a Freer's septum knife sweep the blade around the anterior groove of the fenestrum, at all times keeping it in contact with the blade of the Sluder. By doing this one cuts all fibres attached to the tonsil and frees it completely from its fossa with the result that no traction is made on the pillars.

The technique of the original Sluder operation is practically the same up to the point where the Freer's septum knife is used. After engaging the tonsil, the operator then makes traction on the tonsil and pulls it out in toto, breaking the fibres from the capsule. The objectionable points to this operation are: first, that it may distort both pillars on account of the great amount of force exerted in pulling the tonsil out of its fossa; second, that one may engage a small amount of anterior pillar in the instrument near the base of the tonsil, and when removing same may tear away quite a bit of mucous membrane, thus leaving a large amount of muscle tissue uncovered, which is slow to heal.

Some men advocate the use of an instrument with a sharp blade. My objection to this procedure is that once applied, and the blade pushed home, the instrument cannot be removed if the tonsil is not properly engaged, because the sharp blade cuts instead of crushes. Other men advocate the use of double bladed instrument, the sharp blade above the blunt. The technique of the operation

*Read at Medicine Park, Oklahoma, May 9, 1917.

by this instrument is the same as that of the Sluder up to the point where the tonsil capsule is freed from its fossa.   During my house service in the Post Graduate
Hospital in New York,· we tried this instrument thoroughly.   We found that
it left a nice tonsil fossa, but had a large number of post-operation hemorrhages
following.   The reason for this is the fact that the two blades of the instrument
are about 1-16 to 1-8 of an inch apart, and when the sharp blade is pushed home
it cuts throuh the network of veins surrounding the tonsil capsule.   Were the
sharp blade under the blunt one, the operator would leave the capsule in situ,
which at all times must be removed in tonsillectomy.

The Sluder method or any of its modifications can be used in 98 per cent
of tonsillectomies when in the hands of a man familiar with its technique.   I
have performed tonsillectomies on more than one hundred cases within the past
eighteen months, and have followed the technique I have described, in all except
two.   These two patients weighed over 180 pounds, had short thick necks and
gave histories of having had repeated tonsillar abscesses.

This operation is contra-indicated in malignancy of the tonsil on account
of the extensive dissection required in this condition.

In patients where ether, chloroform or local anesthesia are contra-indicated,
the operation I have described above may be done under gas oxygen anesthesia.

Discussion

Dr. H. C. Todd, Oklahoma City: After getting Dr. Stroud's paper, which
came just prior to my regular clinic at the University, I manned myself with the
proper instruments and went out there to try to execute this method and see how
it worked so I could discuss this paper a little more intelligently.   I think during
the whole period of my clinic I have had anywhere from two to a dozen for operation, but this last Wednesday when I went out there I found just one single, lone
medical student, and I didn't dare to use any new technique on him.

When the Sluder technique first came out, I became very much interested.
I had been taking out tonsils for many years, and I thought if there was a simpler
method and one better than I had employed, I wanted to know it; I wrote to Dr.
Sluder and asked him for all the material he had produced on the subject and he
sent me the reprints he had at that time.   I bought a Sluder outfit—what they
had at that time.   I got the original two sizes and I went out to my clinic and tried
it on 42 cases.   I realize that technique is not acquired in a day or in a week.
The percentage of failure was so great in my hands that I felt that either the operator or the technique was a dismal failure.   I tried to follow the technique prescribed—because Sluder says if you do not use that technique his instrument is
no good.   I wrote an article which some of you may have read, which appeared
in the *American Medical Journal*, and the thing that surprised me was the amount
of commendation I got from that little article, from men of some note over the country, showing that the Sluder method was not considered with a great deal of favor
at that time.

The reason I have not used the Sluder technique is the fact that in my opinion the most difficult tonsillectomies that we have cannot be performed by the
Sluder instrument.   Therefore I would rather keep the technique that I have
on the easy ones so that I will be prepared to operate on these difficult cases.

I do not believe, gentlemen, that there is any instrument devised that will
ever take the place of technique which puts the operator in positions that he will
know every minute of the time that he is operating, just exactly what he is doing
and just exactly what effect his instrumentation is having; and I do not believe
that this is possible with the Sluder instrument.   I am going to say this, after
five or six years of operating with the old McKenzie tonsillotome, which is similar
to the Sluder, that I did some mighty good work and I am going to admit that I
did some mighty poor work.   My great objection to the Sluder technique is that
you cannot engage a certain per cent of tonsils in the tonsillotome or is it possible

to get them out entirely without injuring adjacent structure, and a hemorrhage may result.

I am going to make this statement before I sit down, that I do not believe that the Sluder or any other instrument like it will ever come into universal use, and I believe that the Sluder instrument in a few years will be as *passe* as the McKenzie tonsillotome is today.

Dr. J. H. Barnes, Enid: I want to say that I have used the Sluder myself. What I like better than that is Beck's modification of the Sluder. I use that more than any other instrument. I use that in preference to the old Tidings method of snare. You will get less hemorrhage and less damage to the throat by using the Beck snare which he calls a modification of the Sluder. I would prefer that I use a clamp and knife rather than the manipulation that the doctor pleads for in his paper. The knife gets in behind, next to the posterior pillar, and you are not so apt to injure the pillar with a sharp knife. Those methods are good, I think, in the hands of those who have mastered the technique. I will say that 95 per cent of the tonsils can be taken out by the Beck system. You can take out the whole or pieces of the tonsils by the Beck.

Dr. L. A. Mitchell, Frederick: I wish to say that I have enjoyed the paper very much. I was glad to hear this discussion upon the Sluder instrument. Since I began using the Sluder instrument, my work has been much more satisfactory than ever before, and I have been able to develop so much better technique than I had ever had before that I would dislike to give up the use of the Sluder instrument.

In the past eighteen months, when doing some of my best work with the Sluder instrument, I have had the pleasure of working over some of my bum cases that I did prior to that time with the snare and other methods, getting out some of the remnants and pieces. I believe the doctor hit the keynote when he said that we ought first to get the technique. I had to get it before I was satisfied. I have never had an instrument that gave me as much satisfaction as the Sluder. The facts of the case are that before I got it I never went into a case as comfortable as I would like to be.

While it is true that, as has been said here, sometimes we do not get all of the tonsil—some little particle is left, but I have had the pleasure (as we all do) of seeing some of the other fellow's work, and I believe from what I have seen that those cases where the Sluder instrument has been used, show the cleanest work of all of them.

I want to say, too, that we must take into consideration that there is a lymphoid tissue in the throat that is external to the capsule of the tonsil and often it is thought that it is part of the tonsil left there when it is only a part of other lymphoid tissue—not tonsil tissue.

I believe that a man, in doing tonsil work, if he will, after getting his tonsil out, examine the tonsil, he can tell better what kind of a job he has done than by looking back into the throat. If you will examine your tonsil and find that you have your capsule complete you have done a complete job.

Unfortunately, when I first began the use of the Sluder instrument, I did something which should never be done; I used the instrument without seeing it demonstrated. I had never seen the instrument used and didn't use it right; I overlooked a careful reading of the technique. But that first time I did a dandy operation; it was one of those easy cases where, as we all know, it was ideal for the Sluder.

There is another thing: in the use of the snare I have always had trouble in dissecting the tonsil. As I have done it, and have seen it done, after you get your dissecting started, before you can tell much about it, your work is blinded by the blood. For that reason, I could not develop very much technique. In the Sluder operation we can get in and get out and have the tonsil cut before there is any blood there.

Dr. W. E. Dixon, Oklahoma City: I think in the tonsil work it is not advisable to ever give morphine before operation. I think what deaths have been caused have been due to giving the morphine. Prior to the operation, I use atropin.

Dr. Stroud, closing: In conclusion, I think that the work can be done where you have the patient completely relaxed and under the anesthetic. I have operated at least four or five patients within the past 18 months that have had a number of peritonsillar abscesses. One 30 years old and one 35, and both weighing over 180 pounds, had been heavy drinkers and smokers in their time. I was never able to relax them thoroughly and we had to dig out the tonsils as best we could. I think you can use the Sluder on any case you can use the snare.

ACUTE SUPPURATIVE OTITIS MEDIA*

By W. ALBERT COOK, M. D., Tulsa, Oklahoma.

During the changeable weather of the past. winter such diseases as influenza, scarlet fever, diphtheria, colds, and kindred troubles, have been so prevalent that. there has been an unusual amount of middle ear troubles and so it is worth our time to refresh our minds on this subject.

It is a lamentable fact that we can look around us and daily see the increasing number of deaf and partially deaf people—which might, to a certain degree, be remedied if the people generally understood the conditions better. There must be an education of the public to the fact that a trivial affair, allowed to run along, will eventually cause some damage which no treatment can remedy.

By suppurative otitis media we mean an inflammation of the tympanic cavity with suppuration; in some cases it is hard to distinguish between this and an acute catarrhal otitis, especially in the beginning.

The tympanic cavity is situated within the petrous portion of temporal bone about one-half inch long from the back, one-third inch high and about one-fifth inch from drum membrane to inner wall. This cavity is separated by thin bony plates from some very important structures. The brain above, the narrow floor separates it from the jugular fossa; the inner wall almost vertical, contains two openings, the round and oval windows which connect with the internal ear, the oval window being closed by the foot plate of the stapes; just above this window is the aqueductus Fallopii for the facial nerve, posteriorly above is the opening to the mastoid antrum; the aditus ad antrum; the outer wall of this cavity is composed of the thin elastic tympanic membrane and the. body ring, and just underneath the anterior wall lies the carotid canal.

Within the cavity is the chain of bones which are the connecting links between the sound receiving and perceiving apparatus. Anteriorly is the orifice of the eustachian tube, which not only is involved in these inflammatory conditions but is usually the canal through which the infection comes: so a few words regarding the tube, which is a direct connection between the ear and nose and throat. The tube in an adult is about 1 1-2 inches long. From the pharynx it passes outward, backward and upward; the outer third of the tube is a bony canal while the inner two-thirds is an elastic fibrous cartilaginous tube, lined throughout by ciliated mucous membrane, which is a continuation of the pharynx. The tube is narrowed at the bony and cartilaginous juncture. The cartilaginous portion is acted upon by two muscles, the levator palatii and the tenor palatii, whose actions under normal conditions are to dilate the tube and keep the air pressure in the middle ear equal to that in the pharynx, and because of the shortness of this tube and the comparatively large caliber in the child there is much more danger of infection being carried into the ear, thus the cavities of the temporal bone are looked upon by some as accessory cavities to the nose and throat, very liable to be involved or affected by inflammation of any kind involving the nose or pharynx.

*Read at Medicine Park, Oklahoma, May 9, 1917.

The cause of the inflammation may be traumatic, as from swimming, concussion of air, very loud noises and direct injury. Usually we see it coming from colds—especially in children, and usually these children are affected with some nasal obstruction and adenoids besides the congestion of the cold; also bad teeth are a source of infection, however, it occurs as a severe and frequently a destructive complication of many diseases, principally scarlet fever, diphtheria, smallpox, measles, typhoid fever, syphilis or tuberculous. The most frequent and destructive of these complications usually is scarlet fever; so rapid is it at times that only a few hours are necessary for almost complete destruction of the drum membrane and ossicles, and becoming chronic, is a source of constant annoyance and danger for years. Although it has been demonstrated that the micro-organisms are found in the normal ear which do no harm, yet suppuration usually exists before bacterial infection, and then we have first a single infection and later the infection becomes mixed with very many kinds of bacteria. In this pus we may find any of the following, and in many cases a large number of them: streptococcus pyogenes, pneumococcus, staphylococcus, typhoid, tubercular bacilli and influenza and many others. The streptococcus is most virulent and more frequently causes mastoid complications, in fact, when found, indicates a more or less serious condition, and by some is a diagnostic point in determining the necessity for a mastoid operation, even though the symptoms otherwise do not justify an operation.

An attack usually begins with pains in ear and head, chilly sensations, perhaps a chill and fever with temperature varying from 100 to 105. A child will roll its head about and toss and rub its hands over the ear and back of the ear, screaming and crying; sometimes the child may have convulsions, caused either from the high temperature or pressure. On inspection the drum membrane is seen to be more or less red and inflamed. The hearing is dulled and after a few hours or days there will be usually a bulging at some point of the drum membrane, at which point if allowed to run its course there may be a perforation; this may not be the point of election, but because it has been allowed to run on and perforate, the duration of the disease is perhaps lengthened and the final outcome is very much different from what it probably would have been if an incision had been made. The perforation being ragged in shape, heals more slowly than a clean cut wound.

After perforation or incision, the fever drops and the pain subsides and the patient is fairly comfortable and will usually remain so, except when the opening may become clogged; then there will be a repetition of former symptoms, pain and fever.

The majority of these cases are those which usually go on to the uneventful recovery after a few days or weeks, when the pus ceases and the opening closes slowly, taking weeks in some cases, and to this extent does the hearing remain deficient. Some of these openings remain open not only for a long time after suppuration ceases, but because of so great destruction of tissue never close, thus the prognosis depends upon the health of the individual, the severity of the attack, the kind of infection and the location. In the first stages of the disease the treatment would call for the relief of the intense pain and an attempt to abort the threatened attack.

For the pain, we try to give some relief by prescribing hot drops to be used frequently; these drops may contain carbolic acid, glycerine, atropin, cocaine, or some form of opium. Leeches are used by many. Externally, heat should be used in most convenient forms, with hot irrigations; after using heat, judgment and caution must be exercised or the trouble may be aggravated at that time or later. In spite of all this, it may be necessary to give something by mouth or hypodermic to relieve the excrutiating pain and nervous condition, though if possible this should be avoided, as the large per cent of these troubles comes from colds; this should be treated by the most approved methods, calomel and oil for children, and salines, restricted diet and, if necessary, sedatives and such other internal medications as the case demands.

In many cases, if there seems to be a fluid present after cleansing the nose, the eustachian tube may be opened and drainage established through the canal, and it may do wonders in removing the trouble. Some recommend very vigorous treatment of the postnares—when these attempts fail to bring about a cessation of the symptoms and the inspection shows that the case will go on to suppuration and the drum membrane is bulging, an incision of the drum membrane should be made; this should be made in bulging part or, better, in the posterior quadrant; some recommend a flap, but all advise a large opening. Menthol-phenol and cocain is recommended and used; it anesthetizes the inflamed membrane to the extent that there is not much pain during paracentesis. I have used and found as a very good substitute, cocain solution, 10 per cent first, and then campho-phenique acting equally as well, it is not usually necessary to give a general anesthetic except in children. In most cases at the time of incision, there will be seen only serum and blood, but in a short time there will be pus; usually there will have been hot irrigations and drops used which will have rendered the external ear clean, but if not, it should be cleaned as well as the inflamed condition will permit before the membrane is opened.

As soon as the immediate pain of opening the membrane ceases, there should be relief, but if later the symptoms recur, it may be necessary to enlarge the opening—however, if it is found that the infection has spread into the mastoid or the symptoms point to some other grave lesion, the patient must be put to bed and watched with proper treatment or operated upon for that particular involvement. After the drum membrane has been opened, a hot solution of boric acid or carbolic acid and glycerine, with or without an opiate, can be used; drainage being established, it is our aim to keep up a free and uninterrupted drainage which can only be maintained by keeping the canal clean and the surplus amount of pus kept out; this is best done by irrigation, which should be done with boiled water, with salt, boric acid or carbolic acid in it. The manner employed in doing this will depend upon the conditions to be met, age of patient and kind of pus. The pus can be wiped out very satisfactorily with cotton on an applicator, and I have found in small children that the little ones will remain much quieter from this method than from any other; also the wick is used satisfactorliy in some cases, but the one object is to drain freely. Some astringents may be used after cleansing. For many years there has been an epidemic of middle ear troubles during the winter months. The catarrhal bacilli is found in the early stages almost to the exclusion of any other micro-organism; these infections have shown some very painful and bad symptoms, but have usually cleared up without such serious troubles.

The mixed infection serums have taken a place in the treatment of these troubles and have found many advocates; but this method of treatment is not generally used, although in some cases the attack extent seems to have been shortened. For recurrent attacks of otitis, it is necessary to correct any nasal troubles which may exist, and also remove all adenoid tissue, especially around the mouth of the tubes whether there is any symptoms of adenoids other than the ear trouble. Enlarged or inflamed tonsils should be removed.

Discussion

Dr. L. A. Newton, Oklahoma City: I suppose I am doomed to always have something to do with suppurating ears, having read two papers before this association on this subject and now on the program to discuss this paper. I think it is a very excellent paper and, of course, it is one that is especially interesting this year because it seems to me there has been more complicated cases this year than I have ever seen, particularly those with mastoid symptoms.

The doctor speaks about doing a paracentesis. I have seen several cases this year that have not ruptured readily and these are the cases that give you mastoid symptoms. I believe the earlier we can get hold of these cases and do a paracentesis, the better. There are only a few cases having genuine mastoid disease. I had one case the past winter that was apparently a severe case of mastoiditis but it cleared up very nicely without operating. I have a case now, the patient had a very painful ear and every indication of mastoiditis. I used ice packs over the mastoid and it is clearing up nicely. The patient had sagging of the external canal and a very painful and tender mastoid with temperature. Recently I have been using hot, dry air in my suppurating ears. After I clean the ear thoroughly I use this superheated air, and I find that treatment splendid. They have all gotten well quickly. I don't know just where I got the idea, but I got it out of some of the current journals; but I am very enthusiastic about the hot, dry air. You can use it so hot that the patient will dodge and flinch from the heat.

Q. How long do you use it, doctor?

A. I usually heat the hot air plug or bulb five or six times and blow the air into the ear. I would like to have you try it. I believe the Victor people get out some instrument for that purpose. The fact is, I believe many of these cases would get well if you persisted in keeping the ear dry and clean, without doing a mastoid operation. I am relying more on alcohol than anything else as a medicine to be put in the ear. I usually make it about fifty per cent, depending on how well they can stand the pain, but I usually fill the ear full and then have them swallow several times in order to try and work it into the middle ear.

Dr. M. K. Thompson, Muskogee: I think after paracentesis has been performed the patient should be put to bed and the ear irrigated every three hours for the first twenty-four hours, and then if the discharge diminishes, reduce the irrigations to at least three times a day.

Dr. D. Worten, Pawhuska: I would like to ask what solution of alcohol do you use, glycerine or water?

Dr. Thompson: Water.

Dr. A. L. Guthrie, Oklahoma City: In regard to one part of the treatment, the doctor spoke of nasal or post-nasal troubles. Just what he means by active treatment, I don't know. Whether to use strong solutions during these attacks, I don't know, but I do believe in all these acute cases that the nasal cavity and the postnasal cavity should be thoroughly swabbed. The nasal cavity should be treated to prevent reinfections, or in other words, not strictly speaking, reinfections, but latent infections. I believe that hot irrigations or hot water should be used in the case of acute otitis media, through some small tube, so that it will get the effects of the heat more than the irrigation. I believe that boracic acid is best because pus is more soluble by boracic acid than anything else.

The treatment of mastoids is a very interesting subject to me and I differ considerably in the treatment of mastoiditis from some others. I believe in operating very soon. I have a case in mind now, say where it has gotten pretty far along. If that doesn't respond to ice packs in 24 to 36 hours, I am going to open that mastoid or somebody else is going to get the patient. I believe in early operations for the mastoid.

Dr. E. A. Abernathy, Altus: It is a very interesting paper and is a question with which we are confronted every day. My experience has been with them, the main thing to do is to have proper drainage. Another trouble we have is that the general practitioner sees them first and he uses laudanum and other things before we get them, and gets them in bad shape before the specialist sees them. If we get it early, and get the proper drainage, my experience has been we will not have any trouble at all. Dr. Guthrie spoke about the operation for mastoiditis and rather insists on that. I would not be quite so particular as he, because in a number of cases this season I have seen so many that looked like they ought to be operated on but were not and the result was a complete recovery with no bad results. Dr. Rutland was in a case with me a few weeks ago. It was my brother. I would have operated on him if he had not been a weak man. After a few weeks it cleared up entirely.

Dr. L. M. Westfall, Oklahoma City: There is no argument about opening a bulging drum. I have seen a number of cases in which the drum was decidedly inflamed and I could not see any bulging whatever, and the pain was intense. I have opened several drums, and after the immediate pain subsided they got relief. Perhaps because it let the air into the middle ear. I believe I have been fairly successful in the use of benzol. It burns terriffically for about thirty seconds, but it is splendid.

Dr. H. C. Todd, Oklahoma City: I want to express my appreciation for this paper. It is very timely, to say the least, since we have all been having a good deal of ear trouble to contend with in our practices. If you will pardon me, I want to say a few words regarding the discussion. The paper is so complete that I have nothing to offer specially regarding it.

The question of douching the ear is one that has given me a good deal of thought as to the advisability of trying to syringe the pus from the ear. I believe it was Stewart Lowe of London who made the remark in my presence that in his opinion we never gain anything by using the douche in the ear to remove pus. I am thoroughly convinced that Dr. Lowe is right. I think if those of you who douche the ear will just take notice, you will see how thoroughly you fail to clean out an ear after douching it. I think, moreover, that you take a chance on spreading the infection. I have made it a practice for ten years never to douche an ear for purulent otitis media. The pus is usually thick and difficult to remove and difficult to clean out, but it can be cleaned up very nicely. I think a great mistake is made in trying to wash the pus out of an infected ear.

Regarding the mastoid case especially reported by Dr. Newton. I should be very sorry to keep that patient without operation in view of the fact that a simple mastoid operation is not serious. What relief is to be given by sitting quietly by and waiting—in view of the fact that such grave complications may be present in many of these cases? I am speaking from a little bit of experience when I say this, because I recall that about four or five years ago (when I was perhaps a little more conservative along these lines), a young man of a good deal of promise came to my office with symptoms similar to those stated by Dr. Newton. I waited until he developed labyrinthine troubles which resulted in the death of that young man. What is the use in postponing the operation when serious symptoms present themselves? None whatsoever, so far as I can see.

It is a very interesting paper, and one which concerns all of us. I appreciate the fullness whith which Dr. Cook has presented the subject.

Dr. E. S. Ferguson, Oklahoma City: We all have our opinions about these cases and every man who treats them probably treats them in a different way. In the first place, it is always a question as to when you have a case confined to the middle ear and when it goes beyond the direct line and becomes a mastoid. I cannot agree that a tender mastoid ought to be opened. I cannot agree that mastoid operation is a simple procedure. I don't care how simple the operation is, I have never seen a case of acute mastoid trouble without tenderness of the mastoid, and I have never seen diseased middle ear without a tender mastoid. You go up from the periosteal region and I believe that an acute middle ear trouble will get well ninety-five cases out of a hundred with proper treatment.

There are always questions that come up with diagnosis, and particularly as to the typical mastoid. You might wait a long time in some cases. I am not going to say that it is not the case with those of us who wait. I have seen, I suppose, as many acute middle ear cases in the practice of otology as the average. I have operated on one mastoid this year. I have seen a dozen cases that I probably could have operated on and probably would be upheld by a number of men who would feel that it was perfectly justified. I have had one other case where I thought

I probably should have operated, and the day that I told the parents that it probably should be operated, the patient got well without any further trouble. I do believe that we ought to be careful and to let these cases extend beyond a certain limit. But the fact that the mastoid is tender is not sufficient reason for opening it.

The question of whether to use irrigation is one that has puzzled me a great deal. For a number of years I used irrigations and for a number of years I have not used them. I believe they get along better without irritation.

Dr. H. C. Todd: You will find it extremely difficult to wash that pus out of the auditory canal.

Dr. E. S. Ferguson: I have gotten apparently good results from irrigation, but I believe I get better results without irrigation. It has been my experience that my patients have done as well without irrigation.

Dr. W. E. Dixon, Oklahoma City: I operated on a case the other day. It is a mere matter of putting the hole in. It was full of pus and it was a mere matter of opening up the cortex. In that case it ran along and did not get well and the operation seemed the only thing. Dr. Ferguson expressed my opinion in operating on the mastoid. I have seen a number of these cases and have operated on some, but there are cases where you detect a tenderness in over the mastoid, not only right back of the auricle or center portion, but down the neck. In ninety-five per cent of these cases they will get well without operation.

Dr. A. W. Roth, Tulsa: I want to say a word on that Victor apparatus. It has a fibre tip and is constructed so that it keeps the air hot. You can heat it and then disconnect it, and still have the air as hot as you want it.

As regards otitis media, we have a good deal of it here in our country. I have had to operate three cases this year for mastoid so far, but I have had some very severe cases of acute otitis media where it seemed almost necessary to operate, and one young fellow whose condition continued for a number of days, and yet with the ice and with the irrigations in there and with the dry treatment, too, resulted favorably. The only thing is with the mastoid treatment you begin a long series of treatments and you are going to have your patient on your hands a long time, and if you can spare them the long treatment and also the perforation of the drum by allowing them to suffer just a little longer and using some ice and some local treament to the membrane, you are doing more service than to rush in and operate.

I believe that just as soon as you have had an opportunity to observe these cases there should be a paracentesis and a good one, but in most cases I believe in waiting some time before operating.

Dr. D. D. McHenry, Oklahoma City: I believe if it is a rule to discuss the discussion, I would like to say a word or two. I think the case outlined by Dr. Newton of the sagging of the mastoid, is certainly a case for operation, but there are two or three things which it seems to me we should take into consideration before operating.

First, is the type of infection such that we ought not to put off the operation? —and a great number of our emergency cases are of this sort.

Another excellent point is your white blood count, especially in the adult. If you have a white blood count, about 15,000, it is a pretty good thing to go into that mastoid. I had two severe otitis media cases: one had a white blood count of 22,000 and got well without the mastoid nicely; the other one 12,000, and when we got him on the table we questioned whether he would stand the operation, and found just pus in the mastoid, and very little granulation. The sagging antrum does not mean that we have pus back in the antrum. I have seen a few of those otitis media cases this year and have done three mastoid operations. I have had several others where there has been a tenderness and have had only a few where there is a sagging. I believe a good many of these can be gotten well without operation.

There is little danger to life, but the delay of a day or so makes the acute mastoid so very painful, at least all of my patients have complained of that, that I think we should avoid it if we can.

The other thing that I want to mention is suction. I find that a little suction increases the drainage. I believe that drainage is a thing we must have. It helps to keep the wound open. This question of irrigation has been a kind of joke because of the position taken by two or three of our men along this line. However, I see that one of them has changed his tactics. If you have once made it, and made it asceptically, I don't think it should be made as the average mother makes the irrigation when there are no postnares applications. I certainly endorse the strong postnares application. Personally, I haven't seen much results from the strong postnares application. I do not believe in the so-called radical treatments.

Dr. Cook, closing: This discussion has certainly been very interesting. The discussion of the paper has been rather limited but the discussions of the discussion have practically taken all the ginger out of the discussion that I wanted to discuss. One or two points were not made exactly clear. In the matter of suction—if the ear is wiped out thoroughly, I find you will get the drainage. I prefer the carbolic to the alcohol on account of the irritation and pain that the alcohol sets up.

The mastoid discussion I think we have had too much of already. I think it is a good idea not to bring up the tonsils and mastoid when we are considering acute otitis media.

MUSCLE GRAFTING

J. J. Nutt, New York, (*Journal A. M. A.*, Dec. 22, 1917), reports a study udertaken to determine whether function can be returned to a paralyzed muscle from poliomyelitis through the growth into it of the nerves from a neighboring sound muscle. He proposed to try splitting the sheaths of both the normal and the paralyzed muscles, scarifying the fibers so as to remove all obstruction offered by the sarcolemma to the growth and extension of nerves and then suturing the open surfaces of the two muscles. In one or two instances it has been his experience, and probably that of others as well, that after transplanting sound muscles to take on the function of the paralyzed muscles, notably after transplantation of the biceps to do the work of the paralyzed quadriceps, there has followed some return of power to the paralyzed muscle, possibly as a result of unintentional muscle grafting. The writer reports instances found in the literature. By experimenting on dogs he has sought to inform himself regarding the changes that occur after muscle grafting. He gives illustrations of the results obtained and reports his operations of this kind on patients in the State Hospital for the Care of Crippled and Deformed Children—sixteen in all. In conclusion, he says, "In four of them (the sixteen patients operated on), two paralyzed muscles each were operated on, making a total of twenty muscle graftings. Seven were complete failures, although one of these was opearted on as recently as July 27 and may yet prove to be of some value. Six patients show aslight return of power, which, however, is by no means sufficient to be of functional use. This slight power, as we know from similar results in muscle transplantation, may add to the strength of the joint and thus be of some benefit. Four cases have given fair results and three good results. The last seven cases give us the courage to report our work at this time, although we fully realize that much more will have to be done in both the laboratory and the clinic before the operation should be either unconditionally accepted or discarded."

IRIDOCYCLITIS DUE TO FOCAL INFECTION FROM A TOOTH*
Report of Case

By L. M. WESTFALL, M. D., Oklahoma City, Oklahoma.

To know a man thoroughly is to like him better, or to dislike him more. An extended acquaintance will bring forth qualities which we did not know he possessed. In the event that we find that his power is wielded for evil rather than good, we have him classified and are in a better position to cope with him. A superficial acquaintance with an individual does not bring out either his good or bad qualities.

So it is with infection. Not so long ago we were compelled in many cases to surmise the cause of conditions found. We were satisfied in a way, because we did not know of the possibilities that lay beneath the surface.

Focal infection, as related to the mouth and accessory structures, has only recently received the consideration that it deserves. During the tonsil and tooth crusade, no doubt some normal tonsils and teeth have been removed, nevertheless, the good that has been done by the removal of these diseased structures by far overshadows the injustice of the needless surgery.

Practically every movement during the course of its construction is likely to lose its equilibrium and is compelled to go through the "fad" or "hobby" stage. However, if the proposition has merit, it will eventually reach its proper level and serve its purpose.

This is true of medicine and surgery, as well as other lines. Hence when we are considering focal infections of the mouth, we may be inclined to believe that here lies the real cause of all the ills that the human may be heir to. This is not true, but the percentage of ills, directly traceable to primary infection of structures above the collar bone, is surprising to say the least.

The greater responsibility of detecting these points of infection lies with the oculist and aurist and dentist, the reason for which is self-evident. There are many diseases directly due to mouth infections which concern the general physician and surgeon, but it is not my purpose to discuss this phase of the subject. Reasonable care in the examination of these structures will bring its own reward. The X-ray is exceedingly useful in the obscure cases and without it, many focal infections would never be discovered.

In noting the various eye diseases which have been ascribed to mouth infections, the list includes practically every type of inflammatory and reflex condition with which we are familiar.

Eye diseases of secondary production to mouth infection occur in one of three ways: by bacteria or their toxines, reflex irritation, or a combination of both.

Many theories have been advanced to explain the mechanism of secondary involvement of the eye. Different observers have given as the course of the extension, venous, osseous, subperiosteal canals, perineural canals and the arterial system. Since the lymphatics of the mouth drain into the mandibular and cervical glands, this route may be eliminated. The most plausible course of extension would seem to be through the venous channels directly and the general arterial system indirectly.

Why organisms and their products, whose habitat is the mouth, should travel through the general blood stream and finally infect the eye, is questionable. If we accept the selective action theory, and this has been rather well proven by animal experimentation, that organisms of a given habitat, do have a special affinity for certain structures in other parts of the body, then the question is answered.

The following case, which is perhaps unusual in its severity and results obtained, illustrates very clearly what we may expect from infections of the mouth:

*Read before the Oklahoma Stare Medical Association, Lawton, Oklahmoa, May 9, 1917.

E. S. M. Age 33. Family history negative. Personal history: gonorrhea several times. No history of syphilis. Had rheumatism for the first time
about eight years ago and for five years the pain was constant. Three years ago
the patient took a vaccine treatment which relieved the pain but swelling
from the knees down remained.

About the middle of December, 1916, patient noticed that the left eye was
somewhat red and gave him some discomfort, but no actual pain. During the
next two weeks the eye became redder and developed moderate pain in the eyeball
and over the brow. Vision had steadily grown dimmer so that by the time two
weeks had elapsed, the eye was blind. Had bare light perception.

Examination showed the conjuctiva violently injected, with small vessels
encroaching on the cornea. Cornea somewhat clouded. Iris contracted and
muddy discoloration.

The light on attempted opthhalmoscopic examination produced profuse
lacrhymation. Media very cloudy and eye-ground could not be seen. Instillation of atropin produced an irregular pupil, but in time complete mydriasis
resulted. Pain during this time was intense, and light perception gone.

In the belief that this intense inflammatory condition was probably due
to the same infection that was responsible for the rheumatic condition, a search
was made for the focus. The nose, throat and teeth seemed to be negative. The
patient was sent to Dr. J. R. Caughron for an X-ray picture of the teeth. The
upper teeth all proved sound. The left lower third molar showed a decayed root.
The patient was advised to have this tooth extracted. In the meantime he was
seen by an oculist of unquestioned ability who advised the immediate enucleation of the affected eye, I am told.

The tooth was extracted, during which time the greatest pain was felt in the
eye. The patient stated that each time the root was touched, it produced extreme
pain in the eye. Two hours after this the pain had subsided sufficiently for the
patient to sleep without any opiate.

The results from this extraction were almost immediate. The inflammation
began to subside and three days later moving objects were perceptible. In a
week vision was 20-100. In two months vision was 20-20 and has remained so
since.

This man has had no return of his trouble except that recently rheumatic
pains in the feet have bothered some. Examination of the mouth at this time
shows a decayed tooth which may be responsible for this. Have examined the
fundus of this eye several times since the inflammatory trouble subsided and
found it normal.

Discussion

Dr. M. K. Thompson, Muskogee: This has been a very interesting paper
from the fact that we have all seen a good deal of this focal infection and have
had cases that would go on from month to month and go from oculist to oculist
and finally would have to be turned over to the dentist. I have in mind one case,
a doctor's wife, who had persistent headaches for years. She had muscular
imbalance, requiring a prismatic curve to give her any relief whatever, and
after an X-ray was made of the tooth showing a number of blind abscesses
which were drained, eventually she got relief entirely from that and could leave
off her glasses and had no headaches. We have seen numbers and numbers of
these cases, so we look for these conditions daily now. When we have cases
which show a condition that is hard to determine upon the face of super-
fical examinations, we go deeper and look for cases of focal infection. We find
them frequently in the tonsils and we look for that trouble quite often, but most
usually the trouble is outside of the eye trouble. So that it is necessary not only
for us to work along our chosen line of profession but also to call in these specialists in other lines.

We have all enjoyed this paper. It is only recently that these focal infections have been recognized so completely. There is not only just the one point of infection. You may have tonsillar conditions; may have the turbinates very much engorged, which makes it very hard sometimes to say just what is to be done. You follow along one line and find that you have to take up another. Just day before yesterday a patient from out of town came to my office with the history of having had trouble for years. She had been to Mayos', and they said it was sinus troubles, and coming off here I hardly had time to diagnose the case thorougly; but there is a little trouble in the sinus; however, it doesn't seem sufficent to produce the eye trouble she has. We are going to have an X-ray made of the tooth. There was some trouble with the tonsils. I am surprised that the Mayos didn't extract the tonsils. They said they would do that a little later on. If we do not find some abscesses on the tooth, I am going to insist on the tonsils coming out.

We find it is very difficult sometimes to look after these troubles alone and often have to call in help. I have two dentists next door with X-ray machines, and I think we are going to have to call in their help more and more.

Dr. W. H. Rutland, Altus: The case to which I refer is a school girl about 12 years old. She seemed to have had no trouble with her eyes until just recently and she came in on account of her failing sight; I looked her over and could not see anything unusual about the fundus or cornea, but her vision was about 20-70 in each eye; I examined her all over the best I could and did not find anything except a very much enlarged condition of the tonsils or the adenoids, and told the mother that I did not see anything else, but we would remove these with the hope that it would do the eyes good. She improved rapidly and in a month's time the vision had improved down to about 20-40 and now it is about 20-25.

Dr. W. Albert Cook, Tulsa: I do not know that I have anything to add to what has been said. I feel that it is coming into the limelight more and more all the time. These matters are very complicated. With so many local troubles we commence to look for the constitutional cause. By watching we can often find it. After everything else is eliminated, you decide that the trouble is possible rheumatism, and you take out the tonsils. If that does not prove to be the trouble, you then decide that the trouble is in a tooth; an infection will start there, and it takes some skilful work with the X-ray to locate these diseases, because I have had some cases that proved to be diseases where the X-ray did not demonstrate it. My imagination is not good enough to see all these cases that are pointed out by the X-ray. I believe we will find a great many more cases than we have heretofore found when we get more acquainted with the work.

Dr. J. H. Barnes, Enid: Mr. Chairman, this is a very interesting subject, "Focal Infection from the Teeth." I want to emphasize the kind of teeth in which we usually find these focal infections. In the first place, we should examine the teeth in all these cases where we have cyclitis. We will find that very often there we will have a history of syphilis. We will find this in a case of ureteritis. I have looked into this trouble with teeth with a dentist who has an apparatus and we have found where a nerve has been taken out and ground that that tooth is more apt to cause trouble. It is very seldom that a tooth with a live nerve will affect the situation. It seems that as long as the nerve is alive that the system —the local point—is able to take care of all the infection, but just as soon as that nerve is devitalized and removed, then is when we begin to have trouble. Another form that we have is pyorrhea. That is very common among our patients and we can get enough absorption in pyorrhea. If I should report one case, I could report several cases, of pyorrhea where the treatment was pushed to the limit because the patient refused to have the teeth cleaned up. These are the two main points, crowned teeth and pyorrhea, where we get the trouble.

One more thing with reference to taking X-rays of these. That is, they are very deceptive. Dentists have so many cases of that that they are skeptical and we should take them into our confidence and in having an X-ray made we should have someone who is not only expert in making the X-rays, taking and developing them, but we should have a man who is as interested in the work as we are and will study the case with us, and these men should have one position in which to take certain teeth, and that same tooth should be taken in that same position every time he takes an X-ray of it, and go through a regular routine in making an X-ray of a certain tooth—that they should be taken in the same position every time. Now we find that our men will not do that. The X-ray will take them first one way and then another. If we have a man who will take an interest in that work and take a picture the same way every time, we can read them much better and then the X-ray man will be able to help us out much better and we will be able to save some teeth that are causing the trouble.

Dr. W. E. Dixon, Oklahoma City: While attending the lecture of one of the good men of the East, the doctor made the statement that often it is necessary to pull good teeth with no pain at all—and that is fallacious. A lady had rheumatism and she had her tonsils removed. They perhaps had left a piece of that tonsil. The doctor sent her to my office. I tried each one of the teeth—no cavities, but I .insisted that she have an X-ray made. Four of those teeth were pulled and immediately she got relief.

Another case where following two weeks after some tonsil work a man, as he expressed it, had some nerves removed. He would go to one doctor and then to another. Each told him, "Yes, I can fix that." Finally he got on the train and was going to Mayos' and he was switched at Kansas City; there he went to a nose man, and then to a dentist, and finally came to my office for a nose operation. I insisted on his having an X-ray of his teeth, and I sent him to Dr. Caughron. We had the X-ray and pulled some teeth, and finally he came to my office with no results. I insisted that the place had not healed up, and he subsequently got relief when the operation was finally over and healed.

Focal infection is an interesting subject. Where it leads to we do not know. I think of an instance of skin trouble. I always call most skin troubles eczema. A skin man asked me to remove the tonsils of a child three years old. We did so and in ten days that child came to my office with the skin cleaned up.

During my absence last summer, Dr. McHenry had a case where a man had psoriasis of long standing. He removed the tonsils and afterwards the man told me that Dr. McHenry was a good skin specialist and that he had not had psoriasis for a long time.

Another case of skin trouble by removal of tonsils. A lady had been operated on and after she had dieted and her weight was gone, she had her tonsils removed and the focal infection removed. She got cleaned up. Ninety per cent of the people who die, do so from infection above the neck, and lots of it is focal infection. We do not know where the beginning is or the end is.

I enjoyed the paper, doctor, very much. I think it was a good one.

Dr. Westfall, closing: The subject of focal infection is such a broad one that when we start the subject we do not know where the end will be. Not all of the cases of focal infection are as simple as the one I reported. In fact, if we find one infection we may think the trouble is ended; but after that we find other causes which will cause reflex troubles. In many of these cases, perhaps, the failure to get results is due to the fact that we have not removed all the trouble.

IS THE MIDDLE TURBINATE BONE ESSENTIAL?

By L. C. KUYRKENDALL, M. D., McAlester, Oklahoma.

For the last three or four years my attention has been called to some phases of the treatment of the middle turbinate bone at the hands of rhinologists, as well as general practitioners. After what I have seen and comparing patients' experiences with my own, this thought came to my mind: Is the middle turbinate bone essential? I say it is, and the purpose of my paper is to try and prove to those who are of the opposite opinion that my theory is right.

When man was created, each bone, muscle, and organ placed in his body was without question placed there for a specific function or purpose, although in some instances this function has not been worked out; nevertheless, there is a function for that organ to perform, and when I say that the middle turbinate bone is essential, it is because it has a function to perform and it was not intended that it should be so wantonly sacrificed as I have observed from some operators.

In the submucous tissue of the membrane covering the inferior and middle turbinate bone, are venous plexuses which are known as the erectile tissue of the nose or "swell bodies." This erectile tissue is placed on the posterior ends of the middle and inferior turbinate bones and the inferior border of the inferior turbinate bone, and is placed there for the purpose of warming the inspired air, and regulating the amount of serous secretion. This is important because the lower respiratory tract does not secrete enough moisture for protective purposes, nor is it capable of warming the inspired air up to the body temperature without injuring its mucous membrane, therefore it stands to reason that the humidifying and heating portion of the nose must be in good physiological condition.

The sensory nerve supply of the turbinates are branches from the spheno-palatine ganglion. The hard and soft palates are supplied also from this ganglion.

The vessels of the mucous membrane and erectile tissue of the turbinate bone are supplied with vas-motor branches from the spheno-palatine ganglion. These are under the direct control of the vaso-motor centers of the medulla.

Asthma, when caused by reflex action coming from the nose, is caused by inflammation or other disease in the region of the distribution of the accessory nerves, especially the branches from the spheno-palatine ganglion. Asthma of nasal origin is caused also by the connection of association fibres (the connection between the vaso-motor branches of the spheno-palatine ganglion and the nuclei of the vagus), establishing between the upper and lower respiratory tract a physiological relationship. In this case it is well then to look for nasal polypus or ethmoidal sinusitis. The extreme sensitiveness of these areas' during an inflammation or where the turbinate is pressing against the septum is explained by this extensive distribution of the accessory nerve.

In rare cases the olfactory nerve extends down over the upper and median surfaces of the middle turbinate bone. The functions of the nose are olfactory, phonatory, respiratory, gustatory, and the ventilation of the nasal accessory sinuses.

If, as stated above, the olfactory nerve extends down over the median surface of the middle turbinate, it would be a very easy matter to lessen the acuity of olfaction through the removal of this bone. Don't understand me for one moment as being opposed to amputation of the middle turbinate bone, because I am not, but the plea I wish to make is more conservative surgery of this particular bone and your patients will not suffer the inconveniences I have witnessed, as well as experienced in my own case. Surgery as regards our particular line is assuming more and more the conservative and the day of radical has very nearly passed. I trust none of you are in the same class as a gentleman of this state who openly boasts of the number of turbinates he has removed. When such is the case,

*Read before the Oklahoma State Medical Association, Medicine Park, May 9, 1917.

I think of the man who boasts of the number of appendicitis operations he has had in the last year, and I am prone to think possibly some of it was unnecessary.

There are indications for the removal of the middle turbinate bone, and when they are present, remove it. But be careful to take off only enough to accomplish the desired results; the success of your operation will depend upon your knowing when to stop. On the other hand, do not subject your patient to unnecessary operations, as one physician I know has done, in that he would cut off a small portion of the mucuos membrane and wait a few days and repeat the process, until he had done this as many as ten or twelve times, each time charging for an operation, which made the bill much larger than it would have been had it all been done at once. That may be good business, but to my way of thinking it is not easy on the patient from a physical or financial standpoint, nor is it good medical practice.

In amputating or removing the turbinate bone, care should always be taken in order not to destroy or injure the swell bodies, because of the important function of these bodies. When there is indiscriminate removal of the turbinate, you destroy the warmth and moisture apparatus of the inspired air which has to do with the production of certain changes which allows for the normal transfusion of oxygen and carbon dioxide through the walls of the air vesicles. Also your have removed that portion of your air filter which catches and collects the finer particles of the air that have escaped the nasal hairs.

If the vaso-motor nerves which regulate the erectile tissue are disturbed in their function, the preparation of the inspired air for the lower air tract is imperfectly formed and the lower air tract is then exposed to the irritating influene of the inspired air and the irritation of the lining mucosa and the endothelial cells which line the air vessels of the lungs may result in bronchitis, while the transfusion of the gases, oxygen and carbon dioxide, may be disturbed in the air vesicles. Also the patient may experience a sense of stuffiness of the nose, or of a foreign body, or he may complain of an unduly open nose, and too much air in the nose does the sinuses no good whatever, but on the other hand may do a very great deal of harm.

While a student in medical school, I was operated on by one of the best rhinologists in St. Louis, and as a result of this operation (on both sides), I experienced all of the symptoms as given above, in addition to losing my sense of smell to a very great extent for four or five years, and it was very annoying, I can assure you. I have observed the same thing in my own early cases and in cases coming to me after having been operated on by other men. All of these things have caused me to know the middle turbinate bone is essential.

ARTHRITIS

The following is the summary of an article based on 1,100 consecutive necropsies by H. C. Clark, Ancon, Canal Zone, in negro laborers in the Panama Canal Zone (*Journal A. M. A.*, Dec. 22, 1917): 1. Gross lesions of arthritis were found in 15.6 per cent of 1,100 consecutive necropsies and less than one per cent. of those showing the lesions were considered "arthritic suspects." 2. All but two of the persons showing arthritis were hard-working adults, belonging chiefly to the negro race. A chronic degenerative type of arthritis included 129 of the cases. while 43 cases were well acute types of arthritis or some ill-defined acute and chronic types combined. 3. Chronic vascular diseases, such as syphilis and arteriosclerosis, and employment at hard labor are considered important etiologic factors in the production of chronic degenerative arthritis. 4. The focal degenerative arthritis found at necropsy in young adults offers the gross pathologist, in the writer's opinion, some additional presumptive evidence of syphilis, and the application of the laboratory tests for the disease is indicated.

MEDICAL NOMENCLATURE

By HOWELL B. GWIN, A. M., M. D., Tulsa, Oklahoma.

(Written for the Journal of the Oklahoma State Medical Association.)

Some years ago, while pursuing the study of anatomy at the University of Louisville, my attention was arrested by the unscientific, puerile and often absurd namings that exist in our medical vocabulary. There appeared to be about sixty or seventy-five parts of the human body having the names of men; besides these, there are many indefinite and nondescript names, such as acetabulum, for which I would suggest the name of *octoform*. Some of these names have been displaced and others are doomed.

Misnomers occur, also, as regards both diseases and their remedies. It is a mark almost of mental imbecility to continue such names as Addison's, Bright's, Potts', Graves' disease, etc. Some of the names of this class are properly supplanted, such as chorea for St. Vitus' dance, and erysipelas for St. Anthony's fire. Again, as regards remedies, surgical and medicinal, note Colles' fracture, Cesarean section or Sanger's operation, Loreta's operation, Waldrop's operation and Warburg's tincture, Blaud's pills, Buckley's uterine tonic, Dover's powder, Epsom salts, rochelle salt, etc. As an interesting study, track this false nomenclature through your medical dictionary. catalogues, and literature.

Few things are well defined, more are proximately described, but many are whimsically denominted, e. g., electricity from the Greek word elektron; amber, an agent from which it is supposed to have been derived; and in medicine, calomel, derived from the combined stems of two Greek words, meaning beautiful black. While such names are arbitrary, they are now fixed and have the force of proper names given to persons. I shun the role of a mere "purist," a stickler for an impossible accuracy, but as science advances, definitions and names will become clearer and more satisfactory.

It is proper to state that besides the sciences embraced in medicine, these *lacunae* of speech characterize all other sciences. Such imperfections inhere in every human mind, which, according to Emerson, has its limitations.

> Defects through Nature's productions run,
> We have spots, and spots are on the sun.

As examples, in geology many names are geographical; in botany many are personal or fanciful, such as Fuschia, named after a man, and Nasturtium, meaning a twisted nose. Finally, I make mention of a proposal of a fictitious name made by the friends of the sweet-singing poet of Georgia, who proposes his name, Lanier, for the Southern songster of the woods called the "mocking bird." Appreciation of Lanier is one thing and the destruction of the name of this charming bird is quite another—a name, as I discovered last summer, given 300 years ago by Captain John Smith, the early settler in Virginia, as the "mock bird."

Let us, as far as possible, repudiate the false, annul the whimsical, and exalt the true in all speech and literature.

MYOSITIS PURULENTA ACUTA

Masanaka Terada, Tokyo, Japan, (*Journal A. M. A.*, Dec. 22, 1917), reports a case of myositis purulenta acuta occurring in the course of typhoid fever and affecting the upper arm muscles. The clinical history is apparently not complete but the patient seems to have died. The necropsy report was given, as well as the bacteriologic and pathologic findings, which justify the diagnosis. The onset was marked by chills and high fever, but the temperature gradually fell to normal in about a week. Soon it rose again and was accompanied by the myositis as a partila symptom of ageneral bacteremia.

JOURNAL OF THE OKLAHOMA STATE MEDICAL ASSOCIATION

VOLUME XI   MUSKOGEE, OKLA., FEBRUARY, 1918   NUMBER 2

PUBLISHED MONTHLY AT MUSKOGEE. OKLA , UNDER DIRECTION OF THE COUNCIL

DR. CLAUDE A. THOMPSON, Editor-in-Chief

ENTERED AT THE POST OFFICE AT MUSKOGEE, OKLAHOMA, AS SECOND CLASS MAIL MATTER, JULY 28, 1912

THIS IS THE OFFICIAL JOURNAL OF THE OKLAHOMA STATE MEDICAL ASSOCIATION. ALL COMMUNICATIONS SHOULD BE ADDRESSED TO THE JOURNAL OF THE OKLAHOMA STATE MEDICAL ASSSOCIATION, 307-8 SURETY BUILDING, MUSKOGEE, OKLAHOMA.

The editorial department is not responsible for the opinions expressed in the original articles of contributors.

Reprints of original articles will be supplied at actual cost, provided request for them s attached to manuscr.pt or made in sufficient time before publication.

Articles sent this Journal for publication and all those read at the annual meetings of the State Association are the sole property of this Journal. The Journal relies on each individual contributor's strict adherence to this well-known rule of medical journalism. In the event an article sent th's Journal fo publication is published before appearance in the Journal, the manuscript will be returned to the writer.

Failure to receive the Journal should call for immediate notification of the editor, 307-8 Surety Building, Muskogee, Okla

Local news of possible interest to the medical profession, notes on removals, changes in address, deaths and weddings will be gratefully received.

Advertising of articles, drugs or compounds not approved by the Council on Pharmacy of the A. M. A. will not be accepted.

Advertising rates will be supplied on application. It is suggested that wherever possible members of the State Association should patronize our advertisers in preference to others as a matter of fair reciprocity.

EDITORIAL

DO NOT ROCK THE BOAT.

Of all the interviews and opinions given out with reference to the conduct of the War, the advice of Oklahoma's trenchant Governor, Williams, strikes us as worthy of close attention. In a few words he pointed out the monumenal task confronting the Nation, that we had done very well, should of course try to do better, but above all, this was not the time for captious criticism.

The War Department has been severely censured for the deaths occurring from pneumonia and other infections at the contonments, and this criticism falls ·directly on the medical profession having charge of the men. We do not believe for a moment that anyone with an atom of fairness will question the splendid ability of most of the men in the Medical Reserve and their superb qualifications for handling their problems, but it is hardly fair to criticise them for deaths following that great destroyer, measles-pneumonia, when the men are in incomplete camps or contonments, with many of the necessities not yet installed to give them proper care. When they come fresh from all quarters of the country, bringing with them infections ,thanks to our fixed principles of allowing the individual all the unsanitary and unquarantined license he wishes in order not to infringe on his "personal liberties", when an unprecedented number suddenly sicken and the hospitals are utterly unable to even house them, much less furnish adequate nursing service—we contend it is utterly unfair to hold anyone now in the army in any capacity responsible for the situation.

We do hold, with the ready-tongued wife of some Army officer, "The people listened to much to Bryan, now they are paying for it". Unpreparedness for anything was the fixed creed of thousands of our people. Senators and Congressmen from many states openly opposed, in compliance with the wishes of their Socialistic and ignorantly unpatriotic constituency, any preparation for Army or Navy improvement. Now we are in a fix. The blame—well, we need not try to place it, that is an utter impossibility. It is to be found in the right of every man to say what he pleases about anything or everything, regardless of his ability to handle the subject; in the low cunning of the cheap politician who wanted to "please the boys back in the Forks of the Creek" and appropriate money to build Bunkum Hollow a post office and make navigable Sawdust Creek instead of for the purpose of building guns to avenge the Lusitania or for properly outfitting our important National Guard; in the general tendency of the American people toward peaceful pursuits and their inability to see the potentialities of the struggle across the water, and of course in many other unusual conditions affecting our citizenship.

We cannot sit tamely by and allow aspersions to be cast on a noble profession on this account. We are better fitted to step into a uniform at once and take up multifarious military duties than probably any other profession, for the treatment of sick men is essentially the same under all conditions, but we insist we should at least have a place to put the sick man in and given an opportunity to render proper service before being unfairly censured.

A NOTE TO COUNTY SECRETARIES AND MEMBERS.

We feel it a duty to again call the attention of our county secretaries to the importance of collecting and remitting for all members during January. While every member has had his attention called to the necessity, if he would protect his interests, for paying dues during January, it is proverbial almost that our profession is careless bebyond belief in matters of business and in this particular it is not an exception.

The rule is that a man has the month of January to pay and if this little formality is neglected, even for a day, our Medical Defense committee has no discretionary powers to change the rule for the individual though the personal desire to do so is always very great, so it should be understood in advance that unless the dues of the member are in the hands of the State Secretary on the day the cause of the alleged malpractice occurs. no defense can or will be properly made.

. Our defense plan is so far working out excellently. Our members in trouble have already been largely assisted and are now being assisted by one of the ablest legal firms in the State and there seems to be no question that the number of these usually unfounded suits is decreasing. It is believed that as the individual physician realizes that he is a member of one of God's greatest professional brotherhoods, that hastily formed and expressed opinions, often not based on anything except wild hearsay, are usually the true cause of malpractice suits, they will almost totally cease to vex the tired and tried souls of the honest physician.

INDUSTRIAL COMMISSION DECISION REQUIRING SURGICAL OPERATION IN CERTAIN CASES

BEFORE THE STATE INDUSTRIAL COMMISSION OF THE STATE OF OKLAHOMA.

Pink Condren, Claimant,
vs.   Claim No. 4110.
Prairie Oil & Gas Company, Respondent.
(October 22nd, 1917.)

SYLLABUS.

I.

Under Workman's Compensation Law of this state an injured employee will be required to submit to a surgical operation when it appears from the facts that the operation involves no serious risk of life or health or extraordinary suffering, and if, according to the best medical or surgical opinion, the operation offers a reasonable prospect of restoration or relief from the incapacity from which the employee is suffering, then he either must submit to the operation or release his employers from further compensation,

II.

Refusal of claimant to submit to operation tendered by respondent under the facts was an unreasonable refusal; compensation will be denied from Nov. 1st, 1917, until he accepts an operation tendered by respondent.

III.

Claimant is entitled to an award of $7.21 per week from January 10th, 1917, until November 1st, 1917, and until further orders of the Commisssion.

Prentice & Mason, Tulsa, Okla., Attorneys for Claimant.
James A. Carroll, Independence, Kansas, Attorney for Respondent.

OPINION BY JACKSON, COMMISSIONER: The conceded facts in this case are, that claimant recevied an accidental injury on December 27th, 1916, while in the employment of the respondent and in the course of his employment; that his daily wage was $2.50; that he stuck a pick in his foot and is disabled from doing manual labor.

Respondent denies that his injury at this time is caused by the accident but that his continued incapacity for work is the result of his unreasonable refusal to submit to an operation.

Respondent tendered and offered claimant medical and hospital bill, and claim, if accepted, would relieve him of injury, and them from paying further compensation.

Claimant refused the operation on the grounds that he did not believe he would derive any benefit by having his foot operated upon. He admitted that since receiving the injury four pieces of bone had worked out of the wound. The respondent requested medical examination and by agreement claimant was to be examined by Dr. Fred Clinton of Tulsa, who was to examine claimant and report his findings to the commission. On October 1st, 1917, Dr. Clinton filed his report with the Commission, which reads as follows:

"The injury and deformity are both permanent until corrected. The permanent disability will depend of course upon the injury to soft parts already sustained and the thoroughness with which correction may be made of the displaced broken bone.

"Patient has sustained an open fracture of the metatarsal bone which has been followed by displacement of fragments, the upper of which is more marked. Fragments of bone are said to have worked out through this wound. Would suggest this wound be reopened and an effort made to bring the ends of the bones together and holding them there by such artificial aid as conditions would warrant after exposing them.

"In my opinion, after careful examination, Mr. Pink Condron should be operated upon with a view of correcting or minimizing his present disability, and it is my opinion further, that such an operation involves no serious risk to life or health, and offers a reasonable prospect of relief or recovery from the incapacity from which he is now suffering."

The question for consideration is, whether or not the action of claimant in refusing an operation is reasonable. Upon a careful examination of the authorities we find that the general rule of law, both in England and this country, under Workmen's Compensation Law is, that the question of an employee's refusal to follow competent medical advice, and the reasonableness of his acts is a question of fact to be determined in each case by a careful inquiry into the circumstances surrounding same. The main question for consideration is, whether compensation will continue when it appears from the facts that the employee's attitude towards medical and surgical treatment is the cause of his continued incapacity. We find the law to be where an employee unreasonably refuses to submit to medical and surgical treatment, where the operation will be attended with no danger of life or health or extraordinary suffering, and the best medical or surgical opinion is that the operation offers a reasonable prospect of restoration or relief from the incapacity from which employee is suffering, then he must submit to an operation or further compensation will be denied. In support of this proposition we offer the following authorities:

The general rule of law as laid down by the courts, both in England and state courts, under Workmen's Compensation Law is that compensation will not be awarded an employee for incapacity caused by his own misconduct. It is generally held that where his attitude towards surgical or medical treatment continues or increases incapacity from an injury, the courts will refuse compensation where it appears from the facts that the employee unreasonably refuses to submit to medical or surgival treatment, and if the facts show that the refusal caused the disability to be prolonged or aggravated, the employer will be exempted from paying compensation.

Warncken v. Moreland & Son, Ltd., 100 Law Time 12, 2 B. W. C. C. 350, 1 K. B. 184.
Paddington Borough Council v. Stock, 2 B. W. C. C. 404.
Dosker's Manual Compensation Law, 236-239.

A collier injured the middle finger of one of his hands. His employers paid him compensation for a time, and then discontinued it because he refused to undergo an operation for the removal of part of his finger. He had undergone one unsuccessful operation on the finger to effect a union of a tendon. The unanimous medical testimony was that the operation was advisable, would cause no serious suffering or risk, and would restore his original capacity for work; HELD: that the man's refusal to submit to the operation was unreasonable; that this continued incapacity for work resulted from his unreasonable refusal and not from the accident; and that he was not, therefore, entitled to further compensation.

An employe must use ordinary care in treating his ailments, and failing to do so, the employer cannot be held liable for increased disability because of such failure. In other words, increased disability occurring because the employee does not use ordinary care to cure and relieve his disability is not the proximate result of the accident, but is the result of an intervening agency, for which the employee, rather than the employer, must be held responsible.

Walsh v. Locke & Co., (Court of Appeal, England, January 22, 1914). (1914) W. C. & Ins-Rep. 98.

Negligence & Compensation Cases, 675. The court in handing down that opinion used the following language:

"SIR SAMUEL EVANS, P. If I had not the assistance of other decisions there might be some difficulty in this case, but the principle of the law on this point has been well established by the case of Warncken v. R. Moreland & Son, Ltd. (1909), 1 K. B. 184; 78 L. J. K. B. 332; 100 L. J. 12; 25 J. L. R. 129; 53 Sol. J. 134; 2 B. W. C. C. 350, which discussed the whole principle and was a direct approval of the decision of the majority of the judges in Donnelly v. W. Baird & Co. Ltd. (1908) S. C. 536; 45 Sc. L. R. 394; 1 B. W. C. C. 95. In Warncken v. R. Moreland & Son, Ltd., supra, Cozens-Hardy, M. R., said: 'I desire respectfully to adopt the views of the majority of the Scotch judges in Donnelly v. W. Baird & Co., Ltd., supra, and, particularly, if I may so, the judgment of Lord M'Laren'; and Lord Justice Farwell said: 'Lord M'Laren in Donnelly v. W. Baird & Co., Ltd., supra, has expressed my view exactly. He says: 'There is of course no question of compelling the party to submit to an operation. The question is whether a party who declines to undergo what would be described by experts as a reasonable and safe operation is to be considered as a sufferer from the effect of an injury received in the course of his employment or whether his suffering and consequent inability to work at his trade ought not to be attributed to his voluntary action in declining to avail himself of reasonable surgical treatment.' The law as laid down by Warncken v. R. Moreland & Son, Ltd., supra, was also followed in Marshall v. Orient Steam Navigation Co., Ltd. (1910) 1 K. B. 79; 79 L. J. K. B. 204; 101 L. J. 564; 26 J. L. R. 70; 54 Sol. J. 64; 3 B. W. C. C. 15; where Cozens-Hardy, M. R., said: 'The true test is, whether the continued disability is due to the accident or to the man's unreasonableness in refusing to submit to the operation.' The question of unreasonableness is one of fact or, of inference from fact.' "

A claimant, under Workmen's Compensation Act, providing the amounts payable for the loss of a member shall also be payable for its permanent disability, is under duty to submit to an operation, if it will not cause unusual risk, and it fairly and reasonably appears that its result should be real and substantial physical gain in capacity to use the injured member.

Floocher v. Fidelity & Deposit Co. of Maryland, Supreme Judicial Court of Massachusetts, 221 Mass. 54, 108 N. E. 1032.

Honald's Workmen's Compensation, 521. *Dosker's Manual Compensation Law*, 236.

"Where an injured employee refused to submit to an operation involving little danger or suffering, and which was not an experiment, the Industrial Accident Board erred in awarding compensation after the employer filed its petition to stop compensation until the claimant should submit to the operation, since, where a proposed operation is not dangerous and offers a reasonable prospect of restoration or relief from the incapacity from which a workman is suffering, he must either submit or release his employers from the obligation to maintain him."

Kricinovich v. American Car & Foundry Co. (Michigan), 159 N. W. 362.

The question of unreasonableness is one of fact. Refusal to undergo a simple operation unattended by dangerous consequences to remove the cause of disability, contrary to advice of competent surgeons, is unreasonable conduct and bars the applicant from further compensation.

Where at the time of making the award it seems probable that an operation will be necessary to remove the disability, compensation may be allowed conditioned upon submission to operation at the proper time.

Gordon v. Evans, 1 Cal. Acc. Com., Dec., 1914.
Haley v. Hardenberg Miss. Co., 1 Cal. Ind. Acc. Com., 127.

Under the facts in this case and the rule of law followed in the foregoing authorities, we are of the opinion that claimant's refusal to submit to an operation on his foot was an unreasonable refusal. Therefore, claimant will not be allowed compensation during his continuance of such refusal of an operation. There is no doubt about claimant's disability and that he is entitled to compensation to the time the surgeon filed his report and a reasonable time to submit to an operation; and if the operation should be unsuccessful, the same compensation for his disability he would be entitled had the operation not been performed.

An award will therefore be made in favor of claimant for the sum of $7.21 per week to November 1st, 1917, and claimant will be required to submit to an operation at the expense of the respondent. Upon his failure to take the operation, respondent will be relieved from paying further compensation, the Commssion reserving the right to review and modify the award when circumstances require it.

McDonald, Chairman, and Williams, Commissioner, concur.

PERSONAL AND GENERAL NEWS

Dr. D. Y. McCary has moved from Calvin to Holdenville.

Dr. and Mrs. O. R. Gregg, Waynoka, announce the birth of a son.

Dr. J. W. Adams, Chandler, is "short" one Ford stolen from his garage recently.

Dr. and Mrs. W. D. Phillips, Maud, visited Louisiana friends during the hollidays.

Lieut. J. Hoy Sanford, Muskogee, has been ordered to report for duty at Ft. Riley.

Dr. E. A. Leisure, Fairland, spent December at the Mayo clinics Rochester, Minnesota.

Dr. C. E. Clymer, Oklahoma City, was slightly injured in an automobile accident Christmas day.

Dr. N. R. Nowlin, Oklahoma City, motored to Dallas, Texas with a party of friends for the holidays.

Lieut. Floyd E. Warterfield, M. R. C., Muskogee, has been ordered to report at Ft. Oglethorpe, Ga., for duty.

Dr. J. M. Byrum, Shawnee, entertained visiting Medical Reservists and Shawnee physicians Christmas day.

Lieut. W. W. Rucks, M. R. C., formerly of Guthrie, is recovering from an operation performed at Ft. Sam Houston.

Dr. C. V. Rice, Muskogee, who has been doing special work in pediatrics in Chicago for six months, has returned.

Captain Rex G. Bolend, Oklahoma City, has been ordered to Camp Travis where he will be attached to the Laboratory.

Drs. J. W. Baker and A. L. McInnis, Enid, have been appointed County and Assistant County Physicians of Garfield county.

Dr. James C. Johnston, McAlester, and Miss Muriel K. Everett of Watertown, N. Y., were married in the latter city December 20th.

Dr. James C. Johnston, McAlester, has been appointed a member of the Local Board for Pittsburg County vice Dr. W. C. Graves, resigned.

Dr. H. H. Wynne, Oklahoma City, is trying the simple life and starts out by moving to a country home near Oklahoma City where he will in the future reside.

First Lieut. C. M. Ming, M. R. C., Okmulgee, for some time stationed at Ft. Sill, has been ordered to Cornell where he will take special work in X-ray diagnosis.

Dr. and Mrs. G. W. Hinchee, Oklahoma City, announce the marriage of their daughter Jessie to Mr. James II. Williams of Enid. The ceremony was solemnized December 30th.

Dr. C. S. Petty, Guthrie, narrowly escaped death when his car was struck by a freight engine. He sustained a fracture of the nose and three ribs and was otherwise painfully bruised.

Dr. Ira Robertson, Henryetta, is suffering from many bruises as the result of his machine turning over an embankment and pinning him underneath. The accident occurred when the doctor attempted to turn aside in order not to frighten a team.

Dr. Rex. G. Bolend, M. R. C., Oklahoma City, takes a fling at the Oklahoma nurses in the charge that none of then are responding from his city to the call for nurses for Army work. Miss Edna F. Holland, Superintendent of University Hospital and State Chairman on nurses service, thinks that about all is being done that may be considering the requirements laid down.

The State Hospital, which when completed, it is said will be the largest in State and one of the largest in the southwest, will soon enter the realm of realities. The State Board of Affairs, Architects Dean Long and others charged with its construction, have adopted the plans and selected a site about one mile southeast of the capitol and in the northeastern part of Oklahoma City.

Dr. James G. Rafter, Muskogee, takes a very proper shot at his political enemies who alleged as a result of their request that he resign as City Physician, that he was giving too much time to the Local Exemption Board of which he has been a member since its organization. The Doctor thinks his humble services to the city should not be placed above his duties as a patriotic citizen to his nation.

Ottawa County Medical Society is on a protracted spree of regeneration and progressiveness. They are now meeting once weekly, the members attending lunch together and having a scientific session afterwards. On invitation from local physicians they change their meeting place to other towns in the county, the last meeting being held at Picher where the members attended the dedication of Picher's splendid new hospital. The subject for discussion was "Miner's Tuberculosis".

Drs. H. T. Ballantine and H. L. Scott, Muskogee, have been appointed City Superintendent and City Physician respectively vice Dr. John Reynolds, removed, and Dr. J. G. Rafter, resigned. The appointments come as the culmination of a long recrimnatory and nauseating contest between the Mayor and Dr. Reynolds, each charging that the other played politics, mismanaged affairs, etc. An interesting sidelight is thrown on the political game as applied to public health matters in the admission of Dr. Reynolds under oath in a recent ouster suit seeking to remove the Mayor, that there was a definite trade between he and the Mayor before the election as to the office and the statement of the Mayor that he had to appoint the Doctor in order to hold a member of the city commission to his side.

CORRESPONDENCE

REPORTING OF ACCIDENTS FROM LOCAL ANESTHETICS.

To the Editor:—The committee on Therapuetic Research of the Council on Pharmacy and Chemistry of the American Medical Association has undertaken a study of the accidents following the clinical use of local anesthetics, especially those following ordinary therapeutic doses. It is hoped that this study may lead to a better understanding of the cause of such accidents, and consequently to methods of avoiding them, or, at least, of treating them successfully when they occur.

It is becoming apparent that several of the local anesthetics, if not all of those in general use, are prone to cause death or symptoms of severe poisoning in a small percentage of those cases in which the dose used has been hitherto considered quite safe.

The infrequent occurrence of these accidents and their production by relatively small doses point to a peculiar hypersensitiveness on the part of those in whom the accidents occur. The data necessary for a study of these accidents are at present wholly insufficient, especially since the symptoms described in most of the cases are quite different from those commonly observed in animals even after the administration of toxic, but not fatal, doses.

Such accidents are seldom reported in detail in the medical literature, partly because physicians and dentists fear that they may be held to blame should they report them, partly, perhaps, because they have failed to appreciate the importance of the matter from the standpiont of the protection of the public.

It is evident that a broader view should prevail, and that physicians should be informed regarding the conditions under which such accidents accur in order that they may be avoided. It is also evident that the best protection against such unjust accusations, and the best means of preventing such accidents consist in the publication of careful detailed records when they have occurred, with the attending circumstances. These should be reported in the medical or dental journals when possible; but when for any reason, this seems undesirable, a confidential report may be filed with Dr. R. A. Hatcher, 414 East Twenty-Sixth Street, New York City, who has been appointed by the committee to collect this information.

If desired, such reports will be considered strictly confidential so far as the name of the patient and that of the medical attendant are concerned and such information will be used solely as a means of studying the problem of toxicity of this class of agents, unless permission is given to use the name.

All available facts, both public and private, should be included in these reports, but the following data are especially to be desired in those cases in which more detailed reports cannot be made.

The age, sex, and general history of the patient should be given in as great detail as possible. The state of the nervous system appears to be of especial importance. The dosage employed should be stated as accurately as possible; also the concentration of the solution employed, the site of the injection (whether intramuscular, perineural or strictly subcutaneous), and whether applied to the mouth, nose, or other part of the body. The possibility of an injection having been made into a small vein during intramuscular injection or into the gums should be considered. In such cases the action begins almost at once, that is, within a few seconds.

The previous condition of the heart and respiration should be reported if possible; and, of course, the effects of the drug on the heart and respiration, as well as the duration of the symptoms, should be recorded. If antidotes are employed, their nature and dosage should be stated, together with the character and time of appearance of the effects induced by the antidotes. It is important to state whether antidotes were administered orally, or by subcutaneous, intramuscular or intravenous injection, and the concentration in which such antidotes were used.

While such detailed information, together with any other available data, are desirable, it is not to be understood that the inability to supply such details should prevent the publication of reports of poisoning, however meager the data, so long as accuracy is observed.

The committee urges on all anesthetists, surgeons, physicians and dentists the making of such reports as a public duty; it asks that they read this appeal with especial attention of the character of observations desired.

Torald Sollmann, Chairman
R. A. Hatcher, Special Referee
Therapuetic Research Committee of the Council on Prarmacy and Chemistry of the American Medical Association.

MISCELLANEOUS

NEODIARSENOL.

E. P. Zeisler, Chicago, (*Journal A. M, A.*, Dec. 29, 1917), discusses a recent series of twenty intravenous injections of neodiarsenol, a recent substitute for neosalvarsan marketed by a Canadian firm, which he gave patients in all stages of syphilis. He observed an unusually large percentage of severe reactions, such as fever, headache, veritgo, vomiting, nausea, faintness, thoracic, oppression sometimes extremely alarming, at least it was in one case. On account of his unpleasant experiences in the use of neodiarsenol, he has ceased to use it and has since employed the French preparation, novarsenobenzol (Billon), which has given satisfaction.

BEWARE OF SWINDLERS.

No doubt you may have seen the several notices, under "General News," in the *Journal A. M. A.* in several recent issues, entitled "Once More a Warning." These refer to swindlers operating in different sections of the country—various letters having been received from victims in Ohio, Colorado and other widely separated states. Now comes a letter from the well known publishing house of W. B. Saunders Co. of Philadelphia, saying a man under the name of E. T. Rogers, claiming to represent the University Progressive Club of Cincinnati, for medical and other journals, has been victimizing physicians in Illinois; and the same subscription swindler, or another under the name of Robert Wayne, has been relieving physicians of their well earned cash in the region of Gary, Ind. It is believed there is a concerted action, perhaps by an organized band, being taken at this time of the year, to victimize physicians on so-called "subscription" schemes. Every physician should decline to pay any money by check, or otherwise, to subscription agents not personally known to him, or for whom other physicians cannot vouch. Many of these so-called agents operate under the guise of students "working their way through college."

AMERICAN VERONAL.

In the Trading with the Eenmy Act recently passed by Congress, provision was made for the licensing of American manufacturers by the Federal Trade Commission to produce articles and substances patented in this country by enemy aliens. Already a number of chemical manufacturers have taken advantage of this provision, among them The Abbott Laboratories of Chicago, which has applied for and secured a license for the manufacture of Veronal, which, however, will be known hereafter by the name BARBITAL. This is the official name given by the Federal Trade Commission, and this name must be used as the principal title by every firm manufacturing it under license from our Government.

The Abbott Laboratories have already begun the manufacture of Barbital (formerly known as Veronal), and we understand that in short time it expects to have an abundant supply of this well known hypnotic, and that it will be made generally available through the trade. The quality of the product is guaranteed. Indeed, before a license is granted for the manufacture of any of these patented synthetics in the United States, the product must be submitted to rigid investigation at the hands of a chemist designated by the Federal Trade Commission. In this way Americans are assured of supplies of the American-made products at reasonable prices, and the manufacturer of fine American chemicals is given the stimulus which it requires.

Those interested are urged to communicate with the Abbott Laboratories, Chicago.

NEW METHOD AT BATTLE CREEK

The so-called fractional method of gastric analysis advocated by Rehfuss has been found to have such advantages that it has been introduced in the Battle Creek Sanitarium, where tests meets to the number of thousands are given each year. To the patients, the new plan is vastly preferable. Indeed, the swallowing of what was often called "the garden hose" was attended in most cases by actual suffering and in many by severe pain. Under the fractional method, a very small tube is used. An oval tip, made of metal and perforated, makes the swallowing easy. Of course, it is unconvenient to have to sit for an hour and a half or two hours without removing the tube, but there is no real distress. The usual test meal of two slices of toast and a glass of water is given, at intervals of half an hour, a small specimin of the gastric juice, 10 or 16 c. c. is taken, until the acidity curve begins definitely to come down.

Under the old method, the practice was to take out all the gastric juice at the end of an hour. At Battle Creek, the period had been lenghtened to an hour and a quarter because this was found to be the usual time of greatest acidity. A comparison of the two methods shows that the original plan was misleading in many instances. Under that procedure, cases would be set down as normal if the acidity was shown to be at the usual percentage one hour after the meal. However, as the fractional method proves, many patients who have the right acidity at that minute, many have too little or too much before and after the hour has passed. By studying the complete cycle of digestion, an accurate diagnosis may be made.

PNEUMOCOCCIC INFECTIONS.

C. C. Hartman and G. R. Lacy, Pittsburg (*Journal A. M. A.*, Dec. 29, 1917), publish a summary of their results in classifying pneumococci according to their biologic differences, using for the purpose the patients admitted from the Allegheny General Hospital and from Pittsburgh and its suburbs. Their technic was that used at the Rockefeller Institute and reported by Dochez and Gillespie, Cole, Avery, and others. The pneumococci were isolated from the sputum and blood cultures were taken when certain conditions, such as meningitis, lung abscess, etc., were present or developed. In several necropsies after pneumonia, cultures were taken from the lung and heart's blood and other accompanying lesions. The purpose of these various cultures was to determine whether pneumococci from various lesions in the body correspond with their biologic classification. Five of the patients of group I suffering from pneumonia were treated with a corresponding antiserum, two of them developing meningitis and receiving the antiserum, both intravenously and intrathecally. Blood cultures taken twenty-four hours later were positive three times in one case and twice in the other. Cultures of the spinal fluid after the serum was administered were also positive. Three of the patients treated recovered under the treatment. A table setting forth the incidence and mortality or pneumococci in 112 patients, including thirteen unclassified, suffering from strepococcic and other infections, gives a mortality of 23 per cent. for the unclassified group. If the unclassified cases are excluded and only those of the four groups of pneumococcus infection are included, the mortality is 35:3 per cent. The incidence of the various groups of pneumococci seem to agree closely with that observed by Cole. Details are given as to the culture findings of the various groups and localities. A recurrence and second infection occurred in two patients both in group I. The report shows that the incidence of the various groups of pneumococci occurs in a ratio similar to that of pneumonias generally. Those cases with positive blood cultures are more serious than the others. It would seem that most cases of meningitis are due to organisms of group I. Cultures taken from several sources in the patient invariably belong to one single group.

OSTEOPATHY IN THE ARMY.

There were 235 deaths in our training camps during the week of January 11. More than half of those—to be exact, 149—were due to pneumonia. As is well known, only practitioners of the old school of medicine are admitted to the army medical corps. The osteopaths, for example, are excluded. A bill is now before congress to admit osteopaths to examination for commissions in the army. And since osteopathy claims to treat pneumonia successfully, and can cite a fairly good record to substantiate that claim, it does seem as if this bill should be passed. For it is clear, from the figures given above, that the present treatment for pneumonia in our training camps is not successful.

No layman will presume to say that osteopathy could have prevented any one of those 149 deaths from pneumonia. That is not the point. The point is that osteopathy is recognized by public opinion and practice as a legitimate school of healing. The scope of its efficacy is steadily broadening. For example, it now maintains a sanitarium for the treatment of insanity where it is said to have had excellent results. It can lay an arresting hand on a vegrant vertebra and—presto! One's hay fever is only a sniffling memory. We haven't the slightest idea how osteopathy does those things, but it does them.

Now, if osteopathy can cope with pneumonia, the boys in our training camps are entitled to the benefit of that treatment. We all know how the so-called conventional school of medicine looks down upon every other branch or system of therapeutics. It might view with disfavor the advent of this newer school. There might be friction between the M. D. and the D. O. The public cares nothing about that. It has no concern at all with professional jealousies. It is vitally concerned with giving those boys in the training camps the best possible defence against all adversaries, whether germs or Germans. If osteopathy can help meet camp or trench requirements the army doors should be opened to it.—The Oklahoman.

We respectfully suggest that the writer of the above call on the Chiropractic, Christian Science, Naturopathic, Divine Healers and a few other of the especially well fitted schools of medicine to help us out of our grave National dilemma. Any one of the above claim, and, as logically too, to do all the osteopath does and more, so let's be fair and give them all an opportunity to save the day.—Ed.

IN FAVOR OF MEDICAL SUPERVISION.

Of course the Tulsa County Medical Society is in favor of medical supervision of the public schools. Did anybody ever know of a medical society that was not in favor of any supervision that could be attained, provided the money was forthcoming to pay for it? It was a foregone conclusion that the members of the society would be in favor of supervision of the schools and right away somebody estimated that it could be done at the trifling expense of $25,000 a year.

Medical inspection in the schools in most places simply provides a salary for a physician, who also adds to his income by his private practice. Then the position can be handed around among the physicians and it usually proves to be a good thing. The physician inspecting the schools makes the.

rounds once a month. He looks over the children in a herd and to prove that he is working at the job requires a few of them to put out their tongues. He inspects them by merely looking at their bright faces. Mostly medical inspection in the schools is a farce, pure and simple. The little children themselves know it.

In addition there are persons in every city—parents, rather—who have advanced beyond the stage of taking medicine or having it given to their children. The regularly ordainded and ethical physicians may contend that these parents have retrograded instead of having advanced, or that they are off on the wrong track, but the law recognizes practitioners of other cults to scme extent. If they do not want medicine poured into their children by the medical inspector of the schools, they have the right to enter an objection.—Tulsa Democrat.

This classical piece of libel emanates as indicated from the Tulsa Democrat, a sheet odorously known by newspaper men generally, by quite a distinctive and humilating title not necessary here to mention. We do call attention to the fact that the article was written by one who is either grossly ignorant of what school inspection is or one who desires to purposely misstate the function of inspection. Inspection and taking or giving medicine have nothing in common, as every intelligent person knows. An ordinarily informed farmer knows today the value of inspection, not only of his children but of his cattle and nursery stock, his seeds, in fact of every form of life going to make for his prosperity and security. Inspection has for its sole object the discovery of incipient diseases in such time as will prevent the infection of other children. It is based on the common sense principle of law that no one must unnecessarilly expose another to his infections, as would be, and is the case in communities where inspection is not had in order to weed out the dangers.—Ed.

COUNCIL ON PHARMACY AND CHEMISTRY—REPORT IN PART.

NEW AND NONOFFICIAL REMEDIES.

Borcherdt's Malt Sugar.—A mixture containing approximately maltose, 87.40 per cent.; dextrin, 4.40 per cent.; protein, 4.35 per cent.; ash, 1.90 per cent., and moistere, 1.95 per cent. It may be used when maltose is indicated in the feeding of infants, particularly in the treatment of constipation. The Borcherdt Malt Extract Co., Chicago. (*Journal A. M. A.*, December 1, 1917, p. 1875).

Tyramine Roche.—A brand of tyramine hydrochloride complying with the standards of New New and Nonofficial Remedies. The Hoffmann-LaRoche Chemical Works, New York, (*Journal A. M. A.*, December 1, 1917, p. 1875).

Atophan.—A proprietary brand of phenylcinchoninic acid complying with the standards of the U. S. P., but melting between 208 and 212 C. For a description of the actions, uses and dosage, see New and Nonofficial Remedies under Phenylcinchoninic Acid and Phenylcinchoninic Acid Derivatives. Atophan is sold in the form of pure atophan and atophan tablets 0.5 gm. Schering and Glatz, New York, (*Journal A. M. A.*, December 8, 1917, p. 1971).

Arsphenamine.—The Federal Trade Commission having adopted the name "arsphenamine" as the term to apply to 3-diamino-4-dihydroxy-1-arsenobenzene, first introduced as salvarsan, the Council on Pharmacy and Chemistry voted to adopt this abbreviated name in place of arsenphenolamine hydrochloride now in New and Nonofficial Remedies.

Arsenobenzol (Dermatological Research Laboratories).—A brand of arsphenamine. It has essentially the same actions, uses and dosage as Salvarsan. It is supplied in ampules containing, respectively, 0.4 gm. and 0.6 gm. Manufactured and sold by the Dermatological Research Laboratories, Philadelphia Polyclinic, Philadelphia, Pa.

Salvarsan.—A brand of arsphenamine. Supplied in 0.6 gm. ampules. Manufactured and sold by Farbwerke-Hoecsht Co., New York.

Chloramine-T.—Sodium paratoluenesulphochloramide. It has the actions, uses, dosage and physical and chemical propperties given in New and Nonofficial Remedies, 1917, for chlorazene.

Chloramine-T (Calco).—A brand of chloramine-T. Manufactured by the Calco Chemical Co., Bound Brook, N. J.

Novocaine.—The monohydrochloride of paraminobenzoyldiethylamino-ethanol. Actions, uses, and dosage, see New and Nonofficial Remedies, 1917, p. 31. Manufactured by Farbwerke-Hoechst Co,, New York (*Journal A. M. A.*, December 22, 1917, p. 2115).

PROPAGANDA FOR REFORM.

Some Misbranded Mineral Waters.—Shipments of the following bottled mineral waters were seized by the Federal authorities, and on prosecution declared misbranded under the provisions of the U. S. Food and Drugs Act: (1) Baldwin Cayuga Mineral Water; (2) Bowden Lithia Water; (3) Carbonated Colfax Mineral Water; (4) Chippewa Natural Spring Water; (5) Crazy Mineral Water; (6) Crystal Lithium Springs Water; (7) Gray Mineral Water; (8) Henk Waukesha Mineral Spring Water; (9) Seawright Magnesian Lithia Water; (10) White Stone Lithia Water, and (11) Witter Springs Water. The "lithia" waters (Nos. 2, 6, and 10) were in each case declared misbranded in that they did not contain sufficient lithium to warrant the term "lithia" in the name. A number (Nos. 1, 3, 5, 6 and

11) were declared adulterated in that they contained filthy or decomposed animal or vegetable substances of an excessive number of bacteria. Most of the waters (Nos. 1, 3, 4, 6, 7, 8, 9, and 10) were declared misbranded because the curative claims made for them were found unwarranred, false or fraudulent (*Journal A. M. A.*, December 1, 1917, p. 1901).

Salvarsan Manufacture Authorized in U. S. The Federal Trade Commission has granted orders for licenses to three firms to manufacture and sell arsphenamine, the product heretofore known under the-trade name of salvarsan, patent rights to which have been held by German subjects. Provided conditions of the license are accepted by the firms, the following will be authorized to make and sell arsphenamine: Dermatological Research Laboratories of Philadelphia; Takamine Laboratory, Inc., of New York, and Herman A. Metz Laboratory of New York. The license stipulates that the name arsphenamine be used in connection with the trade name, that the product must be submitted to the U. S. Public Health Service for examination before sale, and reserves the right to fix the price. (*Jour. A. M.A.*, Dec. 8, 1917, p. 1989.)

Anasarcin and Anademin. These are the twin nostrums of cardiac pseudotherapy. Cardiac disease with its resultant renal involvement is frequently encountered; and running, as it does, a chronic course, it offers an almost ideal field of exploitation for the typical nostrum vendor, who is more familiar with human credulity than with his preparation. Anademin is said to consist of apocynum, strophanthus and squill with elder—an irrational mixture of three heart drugs with inert elder. Anasarcin has been stated to contain sourwood, elder and squill. Anasarcin is a dangerous remedy in the hands of the average clinician, and its use is at all times to be condemned. In view of the dangers attending the incautious use of any member of the digitalis group of drugs, it is impossible to condemn sufficiently the recommendation that the use of Anasarcin should be continued without cessation until all symptoms of dropsy have disappeared. In the present state of our knowledge of cardiac drugs it is indisputable that digitalis and tincture of digitalis are best suited for the treatment of cardiac diseases except in those few cases in which intramuscular or intravenous administration must be employed temporarily for immediate effect (*Journal A. M. A.*, Dec. 8, 1917, p. 1992.)

The Carrel-Dakin Wound Treatment. From observations of the results of the treatment of wounds by the Carrel method, Wm. H. Welch is convinced that Carrel deserves credit for calling the attention of surgeons to the possibility of the sterilization of infected wounds by chemical means. The Carrel method actually accomplishes sterilization sufficiently for surgical purposes. The destruction of surface bacteria without injury to the body tissues is of primary importance (*Journal A. M. A.*, Dec. 8, 1917, p. 1994.(

Strandgard's T. B. Medicine. The resident physician of a Canadian sanatorium states that Dr. Strandgard's Medicine Company of Toronto, Canada, is attempting to sell its "consumption cure," called Strandgard's T. B. Medicine, to Canadian soldiers who are being treated at the sanatorium (*Journal A. M. A.*, Dec. 15, 1917, p. 2060.)

Pepto-Mangan. Physicians having served the purpose of popularizing it, Pepto-Mangan (Gude) is now advertised in newspapers. In consideration of the established facts in regard to the absorption of iron and its utilization, all posslble excuse for the therapuetic employment of Pepto-Mangan, in place of iron, has vanished. False claims regarding the efficiency of the preparation have been circulated by its promoters, and about two years ago the Council on Pharmacy and Chemistry reported that while the statements were no longer made, they had never been definitely admitted to be erroneous by the Breitenbach Company, and that Pepto-Mangan was then being exploited to the public indirectly. From the reading of the present advertisement in a medical journal, one can only suppose that this was intended to mislead physicians. The physician who prescribes Pepto-Mangan as a hematinic shows ignorance of the most rudimentary facts of iron therapy, and the intelligent patient soon perceives his limitations. "Useful Drugs" contains a list of iron preparations that are suitable for all conditions that call for iron. William Hunter discusses the subject of anemia and its treament at considerable length in "Index of Treatment," Edition 6, p. 17-37, and gives many prescriptions containing ron for use under different conditions (*Journal A. M. A.*, Dec. 29, 1917, p. 2202).

NEW BOOKS

PRACTICAL MEDICINE SERIES—VOL. VII.

Obstetrics. Edited by Joseph B. Delee, A. M., M. D., Professor of Obstetrics, Northwestern University Medical School, with the Collaboration of Eugene Cary, B. S., M. D., Assistant Gynecologist, St. Lukes' Hospital; Instructor in Gynecology, Northwestern University Medical School. Series of 1917. Illustrated. 224 pages. Price $1.35. The year Book Publishers, 608 South Dearborn, Chicago.

PRACTICAL MEDICINE SERIES—VOL. VIII.

Pharmacology and Therapeutics. Edited by Bernard Fantus, M. S., M. D., Associate Professor of Medicine, Subdepartment of Therapeutics, Rush Medical College, Chiacgo, Ill.

Preventive Medicine. Edited by Wm. A. Evans, M. S., M. D., L. L. D., P. H. D., Professor of Preventive Medicine, Northwestern University Medical School. Series 1917. Illustrated. 384 pages. Price $1.50. The Year Book Publishers, 608 South Dearborn, Chicago.

TECHNIC OF THE CARREL METHOD.

Technic of the Irrigation Treatment of Wounds by the Carrel Method. By J. Dumas and Aune Carrel. Authorized Translation by Adrian V. S. Lambert, M. D., Acting Professor of Surgery in the College of Physicians and Surgeons (Columbia University), New York, with an introduction by W. W. Keen, M. D., L. L. D., F. A. C. S. Illustrated. 90 pages. Price $1.25. Paul B. Hoeber, 67-69 East 59th St., New York.

So much has recently been written descriptive of the Carrel method of wound treatment by the application of sodium hypochlorite solution, that it seems unnecessary to issue a monograph on the subject, but inasmuch as constant reiteration of what most of us understand to be the rule is necessary to get the best results from the greatest number of users, this issue is justifiable. The tenchic of application, with the necessary apparatus, the examination bacteriologically of secretions and other phases is discussed.

DISEASES OF THE HEART.

A Clinical Treatise for the General Practitioner. By Edward E. Cornwall, Ph. B., M. D., Attending Physician Willisamsburgh and Norwegian Hospitals; Consulting Physician, Bethany Deaconess Hospital; Formerly Professor of Medicine, Brooklyn Post-Graduate Medical School; Fellow of the American College of Physicians, The American Congress on Internal Medicine, etc. Linen cover. Illustrated. 127 pages. Price $1.50. 1917. The Rebman Company, New York.

This book contains much indicative of the individuality of the author, is very readable and entertaining. The style is quite different from works usually issued and attracts the attention of the reader without effort. Considerable attention is devoted to the dietary, to heart stimulants, especially digitalis, strophanthin, strychnine, morphine, caffeine, etc. Attention is also directed to the general application of exercise, baths, bleeding, prophylaxis. The consideration of acute inflammatory heart conditions (infections secondary to other involvements) is very judicially administered and in such a manner as to be helpful to the general practitioner in the trying situations accompanying such complications. The uses of the strophanthus group is so nicely discussed we shall forgive the author for the statement that it is "more readily execrated" and assume he referred to the excretion of the drug.

TALKS ON OBSTETRICS.

By Rae Thornton La Vake, M. D., Instructor in Obstetrics, University of Minnesota, Obstetrician in charge of the Out-Patient Obstetric Department of the University of Minnesota, etc. Cloth. 157 pages. Price $1.00. 1917. C. V. Mosby Company, St. Louis.

The author frankly states this to be neither text book or compend but hopes it to stand as a frontispiece in the study of obstetrics. It is a discussion of the commoner phases of obstetrical practice and the complications met in such, interspersed with many suggestions from experience at the bedside. Sepsis, the toxemias of pregnancy and hemorrhage in obstetrics are given the leading place. Other Complications—heart lesions and tuberculosis, use of forceps, version ceserean section, etc., with many minor affairs are treated of.

GENITO–URINARY SURGERY AND VENEREAL DISEASES.

By Edward Martin, A. M., M. D., F. A. C. S.; John Rhea Barton, Professor of Surgery, University of Pennsylvania; Benjamin A. Thomas, A. M., M. D., F. A. C. S., Professor of Genito-Urinary Surgery in the Polyclinic Hospital and College for Graduates in Medicine, Instructor in Surgery, University of Pennsylvania, and Stirling W. Moorhead, M. D., F. A. C. S., Assistant Surgeon to the Howard Hospital, Philadelphia, Pa. Illustrated with 422 engravings and 21 colored plates. 10th editoin. Cloth. 929 pages. Price $7.00. 1917. Philadelphia and London, J. B. Lippincott Company.

This formidable work is to be properly termed a library on genito-urinary surgery and venereal diseases. The very profuse and applicable illustrations of operative procedure and technic render it an immensely valuable contribution to the literature and will doubly arm the physician interested in the subjects. The authors in searching for material descriptive of the rarer conditions have had access and used it freely, to that great storehouse of medical and surgical lore, the Philadelphia College of Physicians. Every condition incident to sexual life, its diseases and abnormalities is copiously noted, while the very important needs met in a wide range of work such as surgery of the prostate, bladder, kidney, testicles, cord, vesicles, urethra, both male and female, the ureters, nephrolithiasis, infections, tuberculosis and tumors is considered.

The portions devoted to syphilis contain more than 200 pages and consider all phases including the tried remedies, such as mercurials and arsenicals.

OFFICERS OF COUNTY SOCIETIES, 1918

County	President	Secretary
Adair	A. J. Sands, Watts	A. J. Patton, Stilwell
Alfalfa	H. A. Lile, Aline	W. H. Dersch, Carmen
Atoka		
Beaver		
Beckham		
Blaine	J. B. Leisure, Watonga	J. A. Norris, Okeene
Bryan	J. L. Reynolds, Durant	D. Armstrong, Durant
Caddo	A. H. Taylor, Anadarko	Chas. B. Hume, Anadarko
Canadian	P. F. Herod, El Reno	W. J. Muzzy, El Reno
Choctaw	V. L. McPherson, Boswell	E. R. Askew, Hugo
Carter	F. W. Boadway, Ardmore	Robt. H. Henry, Ardmore
Cleveland	J. J. Gable, Norman	Gayfree Ellison, Norman
Cherokee		
Custer	J. Matt Gordon, Weatherford	C. H. McBurney, Clinton
Comanche	E. R. Dunlap, Lawton	General Pinnell, Lawton
Coal		
Cotton		
Craig		
Creek		
Dewey		
Ellis		
Garfield	H. B. McKenzie, Enid	A. Boutrous, Enid
Garvin		
Grady	D. S. Downey, Chickasha	Martha Bledsoe, Chickasha
Grant		
Greer	Nay Neel, Mangum	Thos. J. Horsley, Mangum
Harmon	W. T. Ray, Gould	R. L. Pendergraft, Hollis
Haskell		
Hughes		
Jackson	T. H. Hardin, Olustee	W. H. Rutland, Altus
Jefferson		
Johnson		
Kay		
Kingfisher		
Kiowa		
Latimer	E. B. Hamilton, Wilburton	E. L. Evins, Wilburton
Le Flore	E. E. Shippey, Wister	Harrell Hardy, Bokoshe
Lincoln		
Logan		
Love		
Mayes	J. L. Adams, Pryor	L. C. White, Adair
Major		
Marshall		
McClain	J. W. West, Purcell	O. O. Dawson, Wayne
McCurtain		
McIntosh	B. J. Vance, Checotah	W. A. Tolleson, Eufaula
Murray		
Muskogee	J. G. Noble, Muskogee	A. L. Stocks, Muskogee
Noble		
Nowata		
Okfuskee	J. S. Rollins, Paden	A. O. Meredith, Bearden
Oklahoma	John A. Reck, Oklahoma City	H. H. Cloudman, Oklahoma City
Okmulgee	W. C. Mitchner, Okmulgee	Harry E. Breese, Henryetta
Ottawa	A. M. Cooter, Miami	Blair Points, Miami
Osage	G. W. Goss, Pawhuska	Benj. Skinner, Pawhuska
Pawnee		E. T. Robinson, Cleveland
Payne	E. M. Harris, Cushing	J. R. Murphy, Stillwater
Pittsburg	T. H. McCarley, McAlester	J. A. Smith, McAlester
Pottawatomie	R. M. Anderson, Shawnee	G. S. Baxter, Shawnee
Pontotoc		
Pushmataha		
Rogers		
Roger Mills		
Seminole		
Sequoyah		
Stephens		
Texas	W. H. Langston, Guymon	R. B. Hays, Guymon
Tulsa	H. D. Murdock, Tulsa	W. J. Trainor, Tulsa
Tillman		
Wagoner	C. E. Hayward, Wagoner	S. R. Bates, Wagoner
Washita	D. W. Bennett, Sentinel	A. S. Neal, Cordell
Washington	G. F. Woodring, Bartlesville	J. G. Smith, Bartlesville
Woodward	R. A. Workman, Woodward	C. W. Tedrowe, Woodward
Woods	G. M. Bilby, Alva	D. B. Ensor, Hopeton

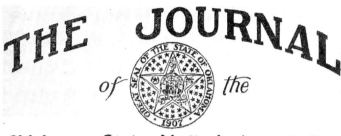

Oklahoma State Medical Association

VOLUME XI   MUSKOGEE, OKLA., MARCH, 1918   NUMBER 3

GASTRIC ULCER.*

By J. A. WESTFALL, M. D., Supply, Oklahoma

A gastric ulcer is more or less a destructive process, beginning in the mucosa, and extending to and even through the stomach wall. It occurs only where the gastric juices are found, that is in the extreme end of the oesophagus, the stomach proper and that portion of the duodenum above the common bile-duct and in rare occasions in the jejunum, after gastro-jenjunostomy. It may be acute or chronic. The acute ulcer is well defined and has-clear cut edges, the chronic ulcer is more or less irregular. Most ulcers, however, have become chronic before they produce any appreciable symptoms.

History of cases suggesting peptic ulcer are found as far back as the tenth century. Mathew Baillie in 1795 was the first to write a clinical description of this disease, but it was Cruveilhier some forty years later who first pointed out that it was a distinct pathological entity.

The subject of gastric and duodenal ulcers has received a very prominent place in medical literature within the last ten years, but statistics vary considerable as to age, sex and location. Gastric ulcer is more frequent in females and duodenal more frequent in males. The ratio of gastric ulcer to duodenal is one to three, according to the latest Mayo records. The average age is about 40 years, although some authors put it from 20 to 39 years. Some ideas of the frequency of gastric and duodenal ulcers may be obtained by the fact that about five per cent. of autopsies in England show healed or unhealed ulcers and about four per cent in this country.

·The cause of gastric ulcer is not known, but many interesting theories have been advanced and much work is being done at the present time. Martin in a study of the subject in Osler's System of Medicine, where he reviewed the work of sixty-three authors, found that only nine agreed. Most of the work is on the retention and infection theories. It has been a question for some time, whether the retention of food and increase of Hcl. were the result or were concerned with the cause of the ulcer. Chronic appendicitis-and other chronic foci of infection is considered a prominent factor by Billings and Mayo Robson, by carrying infection by metastasis; and in many cases a history of co-existing appendiceal trouble can be found. Excessive carbohydrate diet is offered as a theory by some, while the Mayos believe that the custom of drinking very hot and cold liquids play an important role in the etiology, as they pass directly into the stomach before they have time to cool or warm in the mouth.

*Read before the Woodward County Medical Society, June 6, 1917.

W. W. Hamburger, of Chicago, summarizing the causes of gastric ulcer, arrives at this conclusion: "Frequently small acute lesions or abrasions occur in the stomach from food traumatism, emboli, or bacteria, and under usual conditions they promptly heal with little or no evidence of ever having occurred; but under unusual conditions as hypersecretion and hyperacidity, from neurotic causes, from motor insufficiency, from recurring pylorospasm, from diseases of appendix, gall-bladder, and from decayed motility, from atonic stomach, enlarged liver, distented gall-blader, pancreas or colon; that under these unusual conditions acute ulcers are prevented from healing and become chronic."

In considering the etiology of ulcers, some mention must be made of its relation to cancer. Mayo says that gastric ulcers frequently undergo malignancy, but duodenal ulcers seldom do. McCarter, in the pathological study of 280 cases of chronic gastric ulcer in which there were no symptoms or physical signs of malignancy, found in 63 per cent. atypical cells, but as the author points out this does not prove that these were ever anything but cancer from the beginning. We do not know that cancer is very apt to develop in any tissue that is subject to constant or repeated irritation, especially where there is a predisposition to cancer. Any case that does not respond to ulcer treatment and management in four or five weeks, malignancy must be considered. According to White, cancer is not yet diagnosed early enough to determine a preceding ulcer.

The symptoms of ulcer usually present a rather definite picture. Discomfort or pain after eating, nausea, belching, hyperacidity, bloating and vomiting, all with definite food relations. The pain may be gnawing, boring, sense of heaviness, and sometimes even sharp in character, and comes on from one-half to two hours after meals. Time of pain may be varied according to nature of the meal; proteins with a longer interval than the carbohydrates. It is usually located just left of the median line, in the epigastrium. One characteristic of the ulcer pain is that it is relieved with small quantities of food. Hemorrhages occur in many cases and occult blood can be found in about 25 per cent. Benign ulcers bleed intermittently. In pyloric and duodenal ulcers, in which complications are not very far advanced, periodic remission will always occur; nervous and physical fatigue, exposure, indiscretions in diet, and acute infection bring them on. Symptoms of ulcer of the stomach proper may not be so clear cut, but duodenal and pyloric ulcers have definite symptoms. The longer the period between pains and the intake of food the lower the ulcer, vomiting usually affords relief.

Severe pains in the abdomen, profuse sweating, evidence of shock, tenderness in epigastrium, abdominal rigidity, together with the history of ulcers, indicate perforation.

While the symptoms of most cases are typical, yet an accurate diagnosis of gastric ulcer is by no means a simple matter, and has only been made within the last six or seven years. Diagnosis is based on the following: History and clinical symptoms, X-ray, physical examination and the laboratory. Wm. Mayo considers their importance in the order named. The characteristic burning, gnawing, or boring pain with a constant relation to intake of food, together with the history of chronicity and remissions are the cardinal symptoms of a diagnosis. Attacks are more liable to come in spring and fall.

In all gastric disturbances except cancer, where there is a decrease in Hcl. there is a hypermobility of the stomach. As retention occurs in from 70 to 90 per cent. of both ulcer and cancer, if we neutralize the stomach contents, in the ulcer the retention of food will disappear; in cancer it will not be affected. Primary cancer usually begins in from the fourth to the sixth decade and a previous history is practically absent, while ulcer gives history of chronic gastric disturbances. In cancer there is usually decrease or absence of Hcl., and ulcer shows an increase, although many ulcers, 18 per cent in some statistics, show normal acidity. In considering hyperacidity as a point in diagnosis, we must remember that a functional increase of Hcl. may be due to nervous strain or to some disturbances of gall-bladder, appendix, and in some cases of gastritis. Organic conditions as cholecystitis and cholelithiasis and appendicitis, which frequently obscure diagnosis, there is no regularity of symptoms, especially to food. In doudenal ulcers pain does not occur so soon, but usually two or three hours later and is more often a typical hunger pain. However, the smyptoms of gastric and duodenal ulcer are so closely associated that a differentiation is very difficult.

About 50 per cent. of the diagnosis can be made by X-ray in the hands of an expert, using the bismuth meal to study retention and outline of the ulcer. The laboratory is an important help in diagnosis in determining occult blood, the per cent. of Hcl., pus cells, streptococci, and staphylococci in the stomach contents.

Einhorn lays considerable stress on the thread test. A button is attached to the end of a silk thread and patient swallows thread to a point measured so button will pass through stomach. In about twelve hours thread is removed, and if dark red stain shows on thread, it indicates an ulcerated process. Positive test is of considerable importance, but a negative test indicates nothing, as the thread may not come in contact with the ulcer.

All cases of gastric and duodenal ulcers should undergo a rigid and routine medical treatment as soon as the diagnosis can be made.

The principles of treatment are: Rest of stomach until acute symptoms disappear, arrest secretions as much as possible and neutralize the present secretions. Simple ulcers without stenosis should be put in bed for three or four weeks with four more weeks of added rest from all work. All foci of infection should be carefully looked for and removed if possible. First day patient should receive little or no food, second day he should take three ounces of milk and cream every hour, in three or four days he should receive three soft eggs daily, one at a time, and nine ounces of some cereal well cooked. Cream soups and other soft foods should then be added to diet rather rapidly as anemia tends to cause ulcers to become chronic, but at no time should over six ounces be given at one feeding. Diet should be sugar free as possible. Most cases with no stagnation of food are usually controlled by feeding every hour and ten grains of magnesia and sodium bicarbonate, alternating with bismuth and cerium oxalate. Large doses of bismuth are required. In many clinics Einhorn's duodenal tube is used for the first two weeks, giving the stomach complete rest. Raw eggs, milk and lactose are given every two hours in those cases that do not yield to older methods. Thompson advises not to pay attention to constipation for the first week in order to suppress peristaltic movements of stomach. Ice cap on abdomen will relieve considerable pain.

Recent work of Hamburger has shown that pain is caused more by increased distention and peristalsis than by direct action of Hcl. on ulcer surface. For this he gives small doses of atropin or belladonna to control peristalsis. Silver nitrate in one-fourth to one-half grain pills three times daily is recommended by some authors.

It might be well to mention the treatment of Dr. Hart, of London, who, working on immunization theory, introduces 10 c.c. of normal horse-serum by mouth. He reports three complete recoveries after several years.

Most of the results of medical treatment can be obtained in four or five weeks and if at the end of that time an apparent cure at least cannot be affected surgery must be resorted to. I will not take up the surgery of gastric ulcer but will merely outline indications for surgical intervention as laid down by Einhorn.

1. Perforation demands immediate operation.
2. Recurrent profuse hemorrhage.
3. Frequent small.hemorrhages, not influenced by treatment.
4. Constant continuous hypersecretion not yielding to treatment.

5. Severe pains not influenced considerably by repeated and prolonged treatment.

6. Stricture of pylorus.

7. Ulcers accompanied by tumor formation and suspected malignancy.

Gastric and duodenal ulcer is a disease with grave pathology and the prognosis is always uncertain. Cases yielding but indifferently to treatment are in constant danger of perforation, pyloric stenosis, hour glass stomach, and fatal anemia. Relapses occur in about two-fifths of all chronic cases which have been supposed to be cured.

In conclusion I wish to recall a few important points. The cause of gastric ulcer is not known, but infection and retention theories are coming into prominence. These ulcers have more or less typical symptoms and great care should be taken to determine a constant relation to pain and intake of food. The concensus of opinion among recent authors shows that there is a close relation between gastric ulcer and cancer. Absolute rest in bed for three to four weeks is necessary in all medical treatment. And, as Leube has shown, one-half to three-fourths of all cases will be cured in four to five weeks by medical treatment, but if not cured then they they will not be without surgical aid. ·

INSTRUMENTS OF PRECISION IN DIAGNOSIS.

The Thermometer.

By GEO. F. GARRISON, M. D., Oklahoma City

In the fifth century, Cardinal Cusanus, a Roman Catholic churchman, made some timely suggestions as to the possible clinical value of weighing the blood and the urine, and of comparing the frequency of the pulse and respiration in disease with that in a normal control, as estimated by the water clock. These, however, were not put into effect or carried into practice, and remained unnoticed by succeeding generations. Between 1593 and 1597, Galileo had invented a rude thermometer, and as early as 1600 Kepler had used pulse-counting to time his astronomic observations. Later Galileo conceived the idea of using his own pulse to test the synchronous character of a pendulum's vibrations, which led him to the converse proposition of measuring the ratio and variation of the pulse by a pendulum. These ideas were appropriated and utilized by Sanctorius, who describes a clinical thermometer and pulse clock of his own devising about 1625, inventions which soon passed into the limbo of forgotten things for nearly a hundred years.

During the eighteenth century there were some noteworthy attempts to employ instruments of precision in diagnosis. In 1707, Sir John Floyer published his "Physicians' Pulse Watch," which records the first effort in a century to revive the forgotten lore of Galileo, Kepler, and Sanctorius.

Floyer broke the ice in that he tried to get the pulse-rate by timing its beat with a watch, which run for exactly one minute. He tabulated his results, but his work was neglected or its intention vitiated by a revival of the old Galenic doctrine of specific pulses, a special pulse for every disease. It was not until a later day, and under the influence of the great Dublin School, that the familiar figure of the doctor, watch in hand, came to be commonplace.

The clinical thermometry dreamed of by Sanctorius, and coquetted with by Boerhaave, Halter, and deHaen was revived in "Essays and Observations" (1740) of George Martine, of Scotland, which is the only scientific treatment of the subject before the time of Wunderlich.

Martine's ideas were carried into practice in the "Medical Reports" (1798) of James Currier. Long before Brand, Currie used cold baths in typhoid fever and checked up his results with the clinical thermometer.

It was not, however, until 1849 that William Thompson had worked out the mathematical relations of the laws governing heat transformations, and had established his "absolute scale of temperature," without which no thermometers could be reliable.

Upon this hint, Wunderlich made many careful observations of temperature in diseases, tabulating his results. He published his treatise on the relations of animal heat in disease in 1868. By utilizing the advanced thermodynamic knowledge of his time, Wunderlich made his book a permanent scientific classic, and thermometry became a recognized feature in clinical diagnosis.

But the thermometer did not come into general use until long after that. Neither Keen nor Tyson saw a thermometer or a hypodermic syringe during 1862-1865. Billings, however, in taking care of the wounded from seven days battle before Richmond (1862), had provided himself with both. We are told that the clinical thermometer was regarded as a novelty at Guy's Hospital as late as 1870.

FOREIGN BODIES IN THE AIR PASSAGES.*

By E. S. FERGUSON, M. D., F. A. C. S., Oklahoma City

In 1897 Killian gave the profession the first demonstration that a foreign body could be successfully and safely recovered from the bronchi through a tube passed along the natural air passages. At first this procedure was rarely done and for several years only a few cases were reported. At the present time the technic has been very thoroughly worked out by Chevalier Jackson, Killian, Bruening, Johnson, and others, and in almost every state some one or more men have equipped themselves for the work, and still only comparatively a few of the American laryngologists will attempt it.

The men doing the most practice in this line more fully than any others, agree, with Dr. Killian, that this procedure is not everybody's business. Accidents frequently occur and can only be minimized by each individual using the utmost care, and keeping in mind at all times that he is working in the extremely delicate tissues of the lungs and bronchi. Also if the foreign body has been in the air passage for a considerable time, the tissues become more easily injured and perforated because of the accompanying inflammation.

The mortality from foreign bodies in the lungs previous to the bronchoscopic period was very high, by some statisticians given as high as 52 per cent. and even, in those cases, not fatal impaired health was invariably the rule. There are a number of cases relieved by coughing out the invading substance but unless the object is small no such good luck can be expected. Generally, if expelled by coughing at all, it is very early after the accident, when the spasmodic coughing is the most severe. And again in some few cases where there is breaking down of the encysted mass, by abscess formation, and expelled during evacuation of the necrotic tissue.

Since endoscopy has been more or less perfected, the mortality has been reduced to such an extent that we must look upon the procedure as one of the great achievements in medicine.

Kahler reported 290 cases with 27 deaths, 9.6 per cent, and of these a number were due to accidents not directly attributable to the manipulation of instruments in the lungs. Others who have gathered statistics show mortality ranging from this up to 20 per cent.

The author has had fifteen or sixteen cases in the last six years and has had the privilege of assisting Dr. McHenry with a couple of his patients. I am also indebted to Dr. McHenry for his assistance in a few of my cases. It has been my misfortune to lose two of these cases, one I believe from too long an operative

*Read at Medicine Park, Okla., May 9, 1917.

manipulation and the other from pneumonia, the foreign body having been in the lung for about a week before attempt at removal. I also had a death in a young infant seven months old, following the removal of a whole peanut from the larynx. No effort was made to pass the bronchoscope as the child was almost strangled to death when brought to the hospital. A rapid tracheotomy was performed and the nut recovered, giving instant relief to breathing. The child was allowed to remain quiet for a little time and when apparently fully recovered from its hard struggle for air was picked up by the nurse to be placed in bed, when with a gasp respiration stopped and all efforts at resuscitation failed. We were unable to assign a definite cause for death unless it was sudden dilation of the heart brought about by the desperate effort at breathing for three hours before relief was given. A great many accidents have occurred while working in this new field of surgery, but we may look for better results as the tenchic is improved and the instruments for manipulation perfected.

Henry Hall Forbes of New York, in an excellent article in the December number of *Annals of Otology, Rhinology and Laryngology*, recounts the various accidents occurring during bronchoscopic work. He divides the accidents into three divisions in the analysis of his cases as follows:

First: Those occurring during the anesthetic stage,

Second: Accidents during the instrumentation, either for operation or examination, and

Third: Accidents occurring in the post-operative stage.

In the first stage the accidents happen from the effect of the anesthetic, sudden dyspnea due to a change in the position of the foreign body or a dislodgment of the foreign body, it taking a different position entirely.

During the second stage, accidents occur from collapses, sudden cessation of respiration, perforations of the oesophagus, asphyxiation, hemorrhages, opening of abscesses in the lungs, emphysema of skin, shock, breaking of instrument. This accident occurring in one of my own cases. After grasping a small nail in the right bronchus with forceps the small forceps tip broke, leaving not only the foreign body in the lung but the broken part of the instrument as well. I was able to remove both successfully in a few minutes after the accident happened. This gives the operator rather an uncomfortable feeling when the realization comes upon him that he has to deal not only with the original foreign body but in addition the broken instrument. In a child where every minute counts for so much it is a serious matter and instruments should be carefully inspected before beginning this operation.

Many of the fatalities during instrumentation occur from too long a manipulation, particularly in young children.

Jackson, in an article published in the *Annals of Otology, Rhinology and Laryngology*, states that bronchoscopy ordinarily should not be continued longer than 20 minutes in a child five years of age; nor longer than 30 minutes in one under twelve. Unless found necessary, the operation should not be repeated sooner than five days in children five years of age. In young infants 15 minutes is as long as manipulation can be safely prolonged. It is much safer to take three or four sittings at intervals of three or four days than to prolong the operation for an hour at a time.

The post-operative dangers are numerous and apparently successful operations are followed by serious complications. Oedema of the larynx is the most frequent accident, particularly in the young cases. In adults you need not fear this complication unless a great deal of trauma has been produced.

Jackson calls attention to the fact that some of the cases of supposed oedema are simply the accumulation of bronchial secretions flooding the air passages. He suggests that the tube be passed and these secretions sucked out before doing a tracheotomy unless true oedema exists. Many of the cases of oedema are no doubt due to forcibly passing a tube too large for the larnyx in these very young children and great force should never be used in the passing of tubes. If your light is good, it is about as easy to locate your foreign body through a small tube as it is through a large one and the danger from an accompanying swelling greatly minimized.

While it is unfortunate to have to do a tracheotomy, if the patient is dyspneic, it should be done at once and not put off until the patient becomes exhausted from an effort at breathing. Some operators favor operating through a tracheal opening rather than run the danger of a sub-glottic oedema. In my work, I have found that I could do the work much quicker through a tracheal opening in very young children and thereby lessen the dangers coming from prolonged operative procedure.

Again, if the symptoms of dyspnea are marked, a tracheotomy may be performed and still pass the bronchoscope perorally. There is less danger of infection than in working through the trachael opening and you have more freedom in the use of your instrument.

Pneumonia, while not as frequent a post-operative complication, is more fatal and is always a possibility. By raising the foot of the bed, the bronchi will drain much better in children, and in adults, particularly in those cases where morphine has never been given and coughing somewhat arrested, this position is of benefit.

Shock is not an infrequent accident and is probably in many cases due to prolonged instrumentation in the hands of inexperienced operators. Still we find frequently that shock occurs without our being able to account for it in any way other than to the lack of resisting power in these patients.

There are no contra-indications to the use of the bronchoscope, if a foreign body is present in the lungs, but great care must be used if there is an enlarged thymus or aneurysm present and you would hardly be justified in its use, if these conditions are present, for diagnostic purposes, in disease.

The majority of cases occur in children and if given a correct history of the accident, it will be found that the patient has had the object in the mouth and by a sudden inspiration, very likely in laughing, is drawn into the larnyx or down along the trachea and bronchi. The symptoms are those of obstruction to breathing, or bronchial irritation. The most constant symptoms is violent coughing, paroxysmal at first in an effort to expel the object from the air passages, and later, will continue from the irritation or inflammation set up by the foreign body. Dyspnea is usually present and, if the foreign substance is large, may be very alarming or even fatal. After a time swelling is apt to add to this difficulty. As time goes on the throat becomes more tolerant but there will remain a constant cough accompanied by a considerable amount of secretion, leading frequently to a diagnosis of tuberculosis. If the foreign body lodges in the larynx the voice will be greatly impaired, but if it goes on down into trachea and bronchi this symptom will likely be absent. If the diagnosis has not been made early the history of spasmodic coughing, with dyspnea, continued for sometime and then followed by a persistent cough, a little fever and loss of flesh suspicion should be aroused. Chills may be present and quite frequently there is pain. Should there be any history leading to the possibility of a foreign body, an X-ray picture is advisable. If the picture is well taken, there are very few articles that will not give the shadow.

Occasionally where vegetable substances are inhaled, the value may be questionable, but in most cases it will show a suspicious spot. Of course, should dyspnea be marked and delay dangerous, the tube should be introduced at once without waiting for the picture.

Surgical cleanliness is extremely necessary and should be carried out as carefully in this as in any surgical procedure as far as is possible in working about the mouth.

This operation is done under either local or general anesthetic in most cases. Young children do not stand cocaine well and some operators remove the foreign bodies in infants without any anesthetic at all. Where possible, though, ether should be used in children and either ether or cocaine in adults. The practice of giving a large dose of morphine just before the operation will help during the manipulation but in children at least, narcosis enough to prohibit coughing for some time may be dangerous, owing to accumulation of mucous in the lungs which can only be thrown off in that way.

Upper bronchoscopy, or the introduction of the tube through the mouth, can be done in most cases, but in case of a young child where haste is necessary, or the object low down, working through a tracheal opening may be advisable.

The cases coming under my observation are as follows:

In the right bronchus, shirt button, upholstering tack with large head, finishing nail about one inch in length, pumpkin seed. In the left bronchus, at second bifurcation, persimmon seed (Dr. McHenry's case), small tack loose in trachea or at bifurcation, sand burr, cockle burr, small fence staple, tin box corner binding, grain of corn, and one supposed corn, not found. In larynx, or just below cords, two sand burrs, one ordinary straight pin, backbone of fish 3-4 of an inch in length, peanut, and an open safety pin with point up.

In this list I have not mentioned several foreign bodies recovered from the oesophagus, the most interesting of which was a silver dollar which had proceeded on its way as far as the opening of the diaphragm fourteen inches from the lips. In conclusion, I will give a short history of the last case, operated on about a month ago which emphasizes many points brought out in the paper. Master E., age 8 years, referred by Dr. Lea Riely; family history negative, always had good health; during Christmas week, while playing, with a safety pin in his mouth, in some manner sucked it into larynx, very likely by laughing. Was not followed by paroxysm of coughing but voice immediately became husky. He went to school until about middle of March. About two weeks after the accident passed blood from bowels. Of late he developed a slight cough and loss of weight. Began to run temperature. It was suggested that he was developing tuberculosis owing to these symptoms, together with the hoarseness. When Dr. Riely saw him he had temperature 104, pulse 110, respiration 20 with diffuse ralls over both lungs, tongue coated. W. B. C. 23,000, differential 79.

Dr. Riely had X-ray taken which showed pin open in lower part of larynx; point sticking into post wall. Under ether, pin was removed through bronchoscope with considerable difficulty, owing to the fact that the pin was open and point upward.

Gentleness must always be practiced and be sure that force is never used, after grasping any object which may produce trauma of the mucous membrane.

Discussion.

Dr. D. D. McHenry, Oklahoma City: There is one thing that a great many of the general practitioners have an idea about and in which I myself do not quite agree and that is the examination of the bronchus for foreign body is very simple, and not a dangerous, procedure. In the hands of such men as Jackson, Castleberry, or two or three others I might mention, this is probably true, and there is very little danger probably, but in the hands of us who see only two or three cases in a year, I think there is a good deal of danger.

Just a few weeks ago I was called up to the hospital. A child living right there close had swallowed a safety pin, or it went down some place and they called and asked me to bring my bronchoscope and get it out. We made two or three X-rays and could not find a sign of the safety pin and were quite certain that the child was mistaken about it. The X-ray saved that child an operation. An X-ray should always be taken and I think our X-ray machines will show a shadow with most anything unless it is a glass object. I have gotten several pieces out of the oesophagus but these pieces can be easily gone past with the bronchoscope. These cases are very interesting but there is hardly enough to keep us in practice. It is dangerous work to search very long for these foreign bodies.

Dr. W. E. Dixon, Oklahoma City: Having heard the paper before, I had occasion to look up a little of the statistics and I find that Dr. Jackson reports 170 cases of different kinds through the country with a mortality of 5.3 per cent. and with 156 successes in removal of foreign bodies. Dr. Jackson reports 182 cases with 3 deaths, or 1.7 per cent, or rather four deaths; the fourth being an advanced case of kidney trouble. Three of them had been operated before and had tracheo-bronchitis, and in Dr. Jackson's work of 706 cases, he never did a tracheotomy. He tried the bronchoscpoe but advised against it for the reason that anatomically it would be much easier to find the foreign body through the tracheotomy opening, and he says you have just as good movement through the mouth as you do through the tracheal opening. He does not use it any longer. He reports 36 cases of infants under one year of age where he successfully removed foreign bodies and in these cases he has had no accidents. In 26 cases of infants one year of age, where they were normal, the temperature did not rise to 100. He advises working only fifteen minutes under six months of age. I think the danger is more in the instruments than in the length of time. Jackson never uses anything over a four millimeter tube for a child one year of age, and never over five to six years of age. With a small tube the bodies can be seen well and we are not likely to do the damage that we are with larger instruments.

The father of this work, Killian, has devised some instruments of 4, 4 1-2, 5, 6, and 7 millimeters in the last few years and he uses the Curston headlight. Browning came along and devised a method using an instrument with a light on the proximal end. Of course the smaller tube is harder to illuminate. Of course in my limited experience, having learned to work with the Bruening collar, I discarded this and sent in my instruments, and now I am using the Jackson.

It is wonderful to open up the trachea so you can see and get your mouth, trachea and larynx right in the direct light. After using the smaller tubes I discovered the other way seemed to me a very complicated proposition. I had a case where I used a bronchoscope every other day for two or three months in treating tracheal bronchitis, and the patient was never inconvenienced except being hoarse for a little while. I think when we get our technique down we can pass these tubes without any anesthetic. I enjoyed the paper very much.

Dr. W. A. Cook, Tulsa: I have never had any experience with the bronchoscope. I have never had the price to buy the instrument. I do not think anyone should undertake it unless he has sufficient practice so that he can develop the technique because the mortality is so high that it is very dangerous.

I had an interesting experience with a foreign body in trachea. The child was brought to me after having fallen down stairs and swallowing a ring. The ring had been made out of glass beads like the Indians use strung on a wire. This ring dropped down into the throat and the child cried from fright and said he could not breathe well. The mother tried to get it out, and failed. We had it X-rayed and got an outline of the wire. It showed to be in the trachea. The child was given a general anesthetic and by holding the vocal chords separated we were able to get down between the chords and get the ring out. There was very little inflammation with a complete restoration of the voice in about thirty days.

Dr. E. A. Abernathy, Altus: I had a case brought to me sometime ago of a little girl eight years old who had a pin in her mouth and in some way she claimed she sucked this down into her windpipe. The father and mother consulted the family physician and he referred them to me. This little girl had had trouble, so they said, with her breathing. The first thing I had done was an X-ray, which disclosed no foreign substances, and I was thoroughly convinced that there was no foreign body there and also convinced the child there was no foreign body there, and she went on home and never had any trouble whatever. The

family physician and father and mother had questioned the little girl so often
about her breathing that this child from the standpoint of nerves had worked
herself up until she had 99 1-2 temperature and could imagine most anything was
the trouble.

Dr. L. A. Newton, Oklahoma City: I think that the X-ray should be used
a great deal, even more than it is used, and that a man should have experience
along this line if any.

Dr. T. J. Horsley, Mangum: I want to speak of the importance of making X-
rays. I recall a case about two years ago, in my practice, that impressed that upon
my mind. I was called to the country to see a two year old boy. The doctor told
me I would have to go probably to do a tracheotomy for diphtheria. He said
he had given about 10,000 units of antitoxin. The child was breathing well
when I got there so I advised his diagnosis was probably correct. The child was
running a temperature of 99 1-2 or 100, so I didn't do anything. I told him I
thought he had done all that was necessary, collected my outfit, and went home.
Two days later he phoned he was bringing the child in, to be ready to operate at once.
He brought the child in to the hospital, but again the child was breathing well by
the time he reached the hospital. He had been given antitoxin, about 20,000
units in three days. I examined the child and didn't find anything wrong with it
especially. So I left it in the hospital. A couple of days later they moved it out
in the city. It had no trouble at all with low temperature, and one night late in
in the night it developed a little difficulty breathing and again they called me a
second time to see it; gave it more antitoxin and the next morning I called in
counsel. That physician found her breathing pretty badly and said to give the
child more antitoxin. The third one we called in said to keep giving antitoxin.
The child finally developed bronchial pneumonia and became very much emac-
iated. Finally it got better and they took the child home; in about three weeks
from the time they took the child home during a paroxysm it coughed up a half
peanut,—and got all right. So if we had had an X-ray made in that case it
would have saved a lot of trouble. A peanut will show in the X-ray possibly because of the oil in the nut.

Dr. A. W. Roth, Tulsa: I saw Dr. Ballinger one day take a peanut out of a
child. The X-ray was such that you could not locate the peanut after it came
out, not much larger than the head of a pin. You could see it very nicely in the
X-ray plate.

Dr. E. S. Ferguson, Oklahoma City: My experience has been with older
children except one, which was six or seven months old. The others have been
about four years of age, and I have been rather successful in getting the objects.
The seeing of the foreign body is not always the difficulty. You might remember
that. After you have seen your object, then your trouble begins.

You have to pass your forceps through that tube and getting the foreign body
after you locate it is much more trouble than locating it. If you have some of
these many things with a sharp point, you are up against a pretty hard proposition. It is not easy to get it out. You can get out a fence staple as easily as you
can a safety pin, with the delicate instruments you operate with.

My experience has been that it is hard to get along without an anesthetic to
avoid the coughing and struggling. You don't know when you are going to get one
of the coughing cases. I have had one or two adult cases done under cocain, but
the children are frightened to death and you have to deal with them forcibly, so
that I think it is much better to give a general anesthetic. These men like Jackson get to be experts so that they do not take long enough to require such preparation, but when we only have a case occasionally I think it is best to have the anesthetic. In the larynx you can just take it out with the laryngoscope.

THE DIAGNOSTIC VALUE OF NYSTAGMUS.*

By AUSTIN L. GUTHRIE, A. B., M. D., Oklahoma City

In the following short paper we do not attempt a complete discussion of the subject of nystagmus but shall confine ourselves to that which may be of diag- nostic value.

Definition: In order that nystagmus may be of value from a diagnostic standpoint we must limit our definition of the subject to those ocular movements characterized by regular, quick, short movements of two components, a quick and a slow, oscillating about a central point with the eyes directed in a natural forward or primary position.

These oscillations may be rotary, horizontal, vertical, or oblique, or any combination of the same, and they·vary in width from the slightest perception to five or six m. m., and in frequency, from one to five a second. As a rule they are very symmetrical and bilateral.· Their frequency, width, direction, and· relative time of each component is the same in each eye. Exceptions to this rule, however, have been reported, ·but personally I have never seen any.

· It is seldom that we see a case of nystagmus where the above characters are constant. They are usually intermittent and show in the same individual a tendency to vary, e. g., excitement or depression, mental concentration— especially during an examination of the eyes—and ocular fixation, physical exertion, alcoholic stimulation or any other condition predisposing to sudden change in blood pressure or cranial hyperemia, or the abatement of the original cause or its inhibitory action may cause a decided change in the character of nystagmus.

Types: We have two types: a physiologic and a pathologic. Physiologic nystagmus is never spontaneous, being manifest only after some artificial irritation of the vestibular apparatus. Due to the fact that both labyrinths send out equal impulses, the normal individual has no nystagmus unless these impulses are relatively disturbed by some external agent such as the application of heat or cold, or electricity, or a physiologic irritation induced by turning movements to the right or left.

Heat has a stimulating effect upon the endings of the vestibular nerve, producing an inequality of impulses, the stronger being from the side stimulated, causing a nystagmus towards that side. Cold has an opposite effect to heat, producing nystagmus to the opposite side. The cathode pole of a galvanic current has a stimulating or irritative effect while the anode has an inhibitory effect. Therefore, if the cathode is applied to the right ear we will get a nystagmus to the right; if the anode is applied to the right ear we will get a nystagmus to the left. A current of six milliamperes is used for this test.

Rotation Tests: There will be a primary nystagmus to the right while the patient is being turned to the right; the after nystamgus will be to the left, and vice versa. When the head is maintained in the upright position the nystagmus will be horizontal, due to a stimulation of the horizontal canals. If the head is inclined 90 degrees to the shoulder, the posterior vertical pair will be stimulated with a vertical nystagmus resulting. If the head is inclined forward or backward, the anterior vertical canals will be stimulated, causing·a rotary nystagmus. For accurate testing of the character of the nystagmus, the patient should wear frosted glasses so there will be no fixation of vision.· E. P. Fowler claims that nystagmus will last twice as long if the eyes remain closed.

The average time of the after nystagmus following ten turns will be 24 seconds, possibly lasting from one to three seconds longer when turned to the right than when turned to the left. The turns should be made at the rate of one or two seconds. The rapidity of the turns will have but little, if any, effect upon

---

*Read at Medicine Park, Okla., May 9, 1917.

the duration of the after-nystagmus, but the intensity of the nystagmus may be increased by rapid turning. Some writers have claimed that the duration will be longer after twenty turns, but this statement has been much disputed. In dancers who habitually turn to the right, the after nystagmus is much less in duration than when they turn to the left.

All tests in order to be accurate should be made with the eyes directed forward behind opaque glasses and the direction, duration, and plane of rotation closely observed.

In contra-distinction to the previously mentioned symptom known as nystagmus, we have certain ocular movements known as pseudo-nystagmus that vary from the true form in that they are not regular but very jerky; they rarely occur when the eyes are in the primary position but are manifest when the eyes are turned away from the primary position, especially when nearing the limit of rotation. The movements are from this point and return to it but never pass it; in other words, there is no central point of oscillation. This form, although usually bilateral, is more frequently unilateral than the true nystagmus. The pseudo-nystagmus is found in several nervous disorders, the most common of which is multiple sclerosis and Freidreich's ataxia.

Etiology: The true nystagmus may be hereditary, congenital or acquired. The hereditary and congenital forms are rare and are only mentioned in order that we may not forget them as etiological factors. The acquired forms are various and complex and require considerable study if this one symptom is to be of any value to us in making a diagnosis. Any condition producing bilateral amblyopia—unilateral amblyopia rarely—in early infancy may cause nystagmus in a patient whose history may indicate that the lesion is congenital, this being due to a lack of proper observation of the infant during the first few weeks of life. The most frequent of these causes are corneal opacities following ophthalmia neonatorum. Other conditions occurring later in life, such as the various forms of squint, possibly high degrees of astigmatism, and certain occupations that cause excessive eye strain due to improper illumination and abnormal position of the eyes, may be causative factors. The classical instance is the coalminer.

Nystagmus is of frequent occurrence in multiple sclerosis, being one of a triad of symptoms which definitely identifies this disease. It is also found in syringomyelia in sufficient number of cases to be considered a symptom of that disease. Several writers have found nystagmus associated with various other nervous lesions, but much doubt has arisen as to its differentiation from the pseduo-nystagmus, or an accurate elimination of ocular abnormalities, congenital defects or vestibular lesions.

Nystagmus may be caused by a toxic dose of the following poisons: Arsenic, lead, quinine, cocaine, ergot, etc. It is frequently seen during ether anesthesia.

Probably the most frequent cause for nystagmus is to be found in pathologic conditions of the labyrinth and the vestibular nerve together with its brain connections. It is here that the different types of nystagmus and the various tests are of special value in making a differential diagnosis.

First let us consider a case of circumscribed labyrinthitis. There may or may not be spontaneous nystagmus. If present, it will usually be rotary in character and may be to either side, due to the fact that both labyrinths are still functionating. The rotary, caloric, and galvanic tests will be normal.

Should the inflammation become diffuse the nystagmus will become more constant. If serous in character, it will be rotary and to either side—more likely to the sound side. If to the diseased side, it shows that the lesion is only irritative and not destructive. When to the diseased side, the cold caloric test applied to the diseased side will diminish the nystagmus. If applied to the sound side, it will be increased. If the nystagmus is to the sound side and the cold applied to the diseased side, the reaction will be negative; if applied to the sound side, the nystagmus will be diminished. The hot caloric test has an opposite reaction to the cold. The galvanic reactions will be quite similar to the caloric reactions.

In the serous form the pointing errors and falling tendencies are usually quite negligible, but if present, they will be away from the side of the quick component. If the nystagmus is to the sound side, the cold caloric to the sound ear will diminish the tendency to fall and correct the pointing error. If used on the diseased side, the reaction will be negative. If the nystagmus is to the diseased side, the reactions will be the same as in the circumscribed irritative form. If the nystagmus is very marked, there will be a tendency for the patient to lie upon the side of the quick component. In most cases where the exudate is serous, the symptoms will be less intense and our tests less decisive than in the purulent form.

In the acute suppurative labyrinthitis, the functionating labyrinth is suddenly destroyed, leaving no part to react to the physiologic tests. The nystagmus will be stronger and our tests positive and more reliable. The nystagmus will be rotary—possibly rotary and horizontal—and always to the sound side. Caloric to the diseased side will be negative; to the sound side it will diminish the nystagmus and correct the falling tendencies and pointing errors which usually are pronounced and to the diseased side. The position in bed will be on the sound side. When the destruction has been complete, the nystagmus will disappear within a period of from three to fourteen days. The rotary test with the head upright will cause vertigo unlike that experienced by the patient, but with the head flexed at 90 degrees, a similar vertigo will be experienced.

In the subacute and chronic forms the nystagmus may be to either or both sides. It will be weak and not always spontaneous or constant. The caloric tests on the diseased side will be reduced or negative, depending upon the direction of the nystagmus. The falling tendencies and pointing errors are seldom present; if present, very inconstant. The nystagmus gradually diminishes in strength and constancy but does not entirely disappear as soon as in the acute suppurative form.

Should intracranial complications occur, the nystagmus may shift from the sound to the diseased side until the pathological process passes from the irritative stage to that of destruction of the vestibular nerve, when the nystagmus will return to the sound side. I have observed this change in a case of acute purulent otitis media involving the labyrinth and later the meninges.

In meningitis the nystagmus is horizontal and strong and may be to either side as stated above. The caloric tests are positive on both sides—unless there is an associated labyrinthine lesion— and have no influence upon the pointing errors or falling tendencies which are always toward the diseased side regardless of the direction of the nystagmus. The position in bed will be on the side of the quick component. The rotary test with the head upright will produce vertigo similar to that experienced by the patient. The nystagmus increases with the progress of the disease.

Tumors: In tumors of the cerebello-pontine angle, spontaneous nystagmus is likely to be late in developing but increasingly pronounced with the development of the tumor. There will be a loss of vestibular irritability on the affected side due to an interruption of the nerve impulse along its way to the brain centers. In cerebellar tumors involving the cortex, nystagmus may be an early symptom, but in the deeper seated growths is usually absent. In other words the intra-cerebellar tumors rarely produce nystagmus; the extra-cerebellar tumors usually produce nystagmus. In tumors involving the vestibular nerve or its intracranial connections, causing partial deafness, the cold caloric to the sound side will greatly reduce the nystagmus. If deafness is complete and associated with symptoms of intracranial pressure, such as chocked disc, you may not be able to induce nystagmus by syringing the unaffected ear with cold water. This diminished vestibular irritability was originally stated by W. P. Eagleton as a sign of increased intracranial pressure. Spontaneous nystagmus has been reported in cases of tumors of the cerebrum where there was no auditory disturbance whatever. These cases are exceedingly rare and may have been associated with some undiscovered lesion posterior to the cerebrum.

In certain circumnuclear lesions—multiple sclerosis and syringomyelia—the nystagmus may be very marked and never disappears. In other lesions, such as neuritis and cerebellar abscesses, the reactions will be the same as in meningitis. In fibromas, the nystagmus lasts months and also in gliomas, but since the glioma is a pedunculated tumor the symptoms may change with a change of position of the head, i. e., the change of position of the tumor may relieve the pressure on the vestibular nerve.

Nystagmus will be coarser and more marked in subtentorial lesions than in labyrinthine disease and their differential diagnosis will become comparatively easy if we are fully acquainted with the labyrinthine tests and reactions.

After repeated experiments, I. Leon Meyers and J. Muskens claim that nystagmus is essentially of vestibular origin, being due to a pathologic condition of the vestibular complex or its oculo-motor tracts. Whether this theory covers the entire etiology or not, we feel assured that a great percentage of cases may be traced to this origin. If the symptoms of nystagmus are to be of any value to us in making a diagnosis, we must thoroughly understand the physiologic labyrinthine tests and make accurate observations of the character, direction, and duration of the nystagmus. First, determine whether it is physiologic or pathologic in type; second, localize the lesion to one or the other side; third, separate the labyrinthine from the intracranial lesions; fourth, ascertain if possible the character of the causative agent.

Discussion.

Dr. E. S. Ferguson, Oklahoma City: Dr. Guthrie's paper is an extremely interesting one, on a subject too few of us put to practical use. It is only by frequent application of the tests that they are of any real value, because you fail to recognize the significance of the signs of nystagmus in the diagnosis of the intracranial lesions unless thoroughly understood. I have found that it is necessary to refer to my notes when applying the tests, because I do not have occasion to examine cases frequently enough to carry the table of signs in my head.

While in Vienna I had the pleasure of taking a course under Drs. Ruttin and Barany and was struck with the ease with which they could defferentiate different lesions in the brain, by the scientific examination of the nystagmus. Let us all study the cases of head lesions more carefully and use the knowledge placed at our command for making a diagnosis early, when medical or surgical interference may be applied with some hopes of success. Dr. Guthrie has outlined clearly the method of applying these tests and given us a definite meaning of the nystagmus signs, and I thank him for presenting this subject and calling our attention to the value of a close study of the signs in making a diagnosis in diseased condition about the head.

Dr. Guthrie: If irritative, you will keep in mind that lesions of the labyrinth are no different from the lesions of the nervous system. These tests will be very simple; that heat has a stimulating action, that cold has an inhibitory effect; the hot caloric test has an opposite reaction to the cold.

Dr. Barnes asked the question, "What would be the effect if the labyrinth is destroyed?" You would get no effect at all; except with a strong galvanic current. Heat or cold at the proper temperature, say cold at 70 degrees and heat at 110, will not give any reaction.

The point that I wish to emphasize chiefly in this paper is that in a case of nystagmus (practically all of us as oculists have a patient of this sort) we should first differentiate between the true and false nystagmus—the tests are simple. Of course the differential points between multiple sclerosis and syringomyelia are more difficult to remember.   You can make out a small outline which will differentiate them very easily.

PURPURA HEMORRHAGICA.*

Report of Case.

By WILLIAM W. TAYLOR, M. D., Oklahoma City

Hemorrhagic diseases of the newborn, infantlie scurvy, and hemophilia are fairly definite and distinct disease entities.   Purpura is not a disease.   The term purpura only designates a symptom-complex in which there is a tendency to spontaneous hemorrhage under the skin from the mucous membranes and a low platelet blood-count.

For convenience purpura may be clinically divided into symptomatic and primary.

Symptomatic purpura is seen in such diseased conditions as are associated with infections, toxemias, diseases of the blood itself and some nutritional disturbances.   The toxins may or may not be of bacterial origin.   It is claimed by some that they are by-products of intermediary metabolism.   Both are probably true at times.

In primary purpura, as Dunn says, the primary is equivalent to "of unknown origin"; and inasmuch as we cannot assign a cause for them, as we can for the symtomatic purpura, as well as for other reasons, we may class them among the disturbances of nutrition and metabolism which, at the present time, are not very thoroughly understood.

The hemorrhage itself results from some abnormality of the blood   which lessens its coagulability; also from some abnormal condition of the blood vessels themselves produced by a degenerative change affecting the intima of the smaller ones.

According to the view of the majority of observers, this condition is due to toxic substances which get into the circulation.   These toxins are due to metabolic changes and to bacterial infections, many of them of obscure origin.   These poisons produce degenerative changes in the blood vessel walls, making them permeable.   Also they interfere with the coagulability of the blood itself by changes in the elements of the same.

All these types are characterized by cutaneous hemorrhages and in the so-called hemorrhagic purpura we have in addition, hemorrhages from any of the mucous membranes of the body—that of the nose, mouth, throat, stomach, intestines or of the genito-urinary tract.

Report of Case.

Chas. B., 5 years old, was child of healthy parents.   There were three other children, all healthy.   Mother had lost no children and had had no miscarriages. He had never been a robust child.   Had whooping cough six months previously but made a good recovery.

For the past two weeks his mother noticed that he had not been quite as well

Read at Medicine Park, Okla., May 9, 1917.

as usual. Did not care to play and at times would lie down during the day, which was unusual. For several days complained of his legs paining. The mother thought there was no temperature, no evidence of gastro-intestinal disturbances except that he did not care for his food. Drank buttermilk in small amounts to the exclusion of other things. At about this time the mother noticed purple spots over his body about the size of a pea; first appearing on his legs and then over abdomen and chest. This condition had persisted for one week before he was brought into the University Hospital.

His tempreature was 100 F., pulse 130. The urine showed nothing abnormal. He was not constipated—his mother said his stools had been thin and black—several daily.

Physical examination showed a child rather thin, somewhat underdeveloped and pale, tongue was coated, teeth were perfect. The gums were reddened, somewhat swollen, from which oozed blood. The mucous membrane of the throat was injected. Heart, though rapid, was normal as were the lungs. Abdomen was flat, showing no distention; was not sensitive to palpation. No muscular spasm. Extremities were normal. No Kernig's sign. No enlargement of peripheral lymph nodes. Rectal examination showed nothing. There were numerous cutaneous hemorrhages over both legs and abdomen. In some areas almost as thick as a measles eruption. Hemorrhages from mucous membrane of nose, mouth, throat, stomach and intestines. He at times complained of intense abdominal pains. Vomited four times during the first day in the hospital. The vomitus consisted of mucuos and dark blood. The bowel movements, five in number, contained dark and bright blood mixed with mucous. The abdominal pains, spasmodic in nature, were so severe that they required paregoric to relieve them.

The symptoms improved to some extent for three days, then he began to appear more ill in every respect. The hemorrhages increased; he became more or less stupid the greater part of the time; developed a septic appearance; the pulse became more rapid and weak; the temperature going to 103 F. The hemorrhages from the mucous membrane increased alarmingly on the third night, the child dying the next morning just as we were preparing to give a transfusion. The attacks of abdominal pain were probably due to the hemorrhages of the mucous membrane of the intestines.

These hemorrhages, subcutaneous and of the mucous membrane, with the other symptoms were undoubtedly due to some abnormal systemic condition. It could not be placed under the head of the symtomatic purpura, as there is no clearly assignable cause for it. Therefore, it must come under the caption of primary purpura of the hemorrhagic type. The attacks of the abdominal pain are more suggestive of Henoch's purpura, but associated as it is in this case, only goes to show that there are common etiological factors in the production of the different types of purpura.

The treatment is entirely symtomatic. Our efforts in the treatment should be directed toward the relief of the toxemia which produces changes in the blood and in the blood vessel walls. Inasmuch as we do not at the present time know the nature of this poison, we cannot hope to furnish any specific treatment for it.

We have a treatment for the hemorrhagic condition, almost specific, in the use of whole blood or serums—human or animal. In the moribund cases, direct transfusion is indicated and, if possible, should be resorted to. This should be regarded a major operation and undertaken only by one familiar with the technique. The external jugular is the vein of choice in transfusion in infants and children. The small size of the veins of children make it very difficult to get into them, for any purpose. Transfusion is not necessary in this condition except in the extreme cases.

Whole blood injected subcutaneously or intramuscularly is very efficacious in controlling the hemorrhages. The safety and simplicity of the procedure make it very available for the practitioner into whose hands these cases properly fall. The very best results are reported by careful observers in these cases from this therapeutic measure. 30 c.c. (thirty) should be given and repeated in six to eight hours, as the case demands.

If the donor is a parent or one of the immediate family, there is practically no danger of hemolysis. There seems to be no difference practically whether whole blood or the serum from the human blood is used. Equally good results are reported from both.

Horse serum is of the same value in this condition but of less value than human. Diphtheria antitoxin has been suggested and used in the absence of other available sera. Fruit juices should have a place amongst the therapeutic remedies suggested. Calcium salts, while seemingly of no service in promoting the coagulability of the blood, are generally prescribed; the lactate preferably. Adrenalin is of no value.

Bibliography: Holt's Diseases of Children; Dunn: Diseases of Children; Kerr: Archives of Pediatrics; Morse: Case Histories.

HEMORRHOIDS.

H. J. Spencer, New York (Journal A. M. A., Jan. 26, 1918), calls attention to the danger of the injection treatment of hemorrhoids. The rectal mucosa cannot be freed from pathogenic organisms which may be carried deeper by hypodermic needle. If an anesthetic is used, defensive reflexes are abolished and the mechanical spread of the infection is unretarded. Walking, jolting in cars, etc., helps spread the infection and outpatients are subjected to double perils. He reports a case in which hemorrhoids were injected with quinin and urea hydrochloride, and which ended fatally, the necropsy showing infection by gas bacillus. There was local necrosis and parenchymatous degeneration of the lungs, heart, liver, kidneys, etc. Emulsion from one of the pus pockets was injected into a rabbit which later died. The same organism found in the rectal mucosa of the patient appeared in the blood culture from the rabbit's heart.

EXSTROPHY OF THE BLADDER

Exstrophy of the bladder is a rare congenital malformation, says C. H. Mayo, Rochester, Minn., (Journal A. M. A., Dec. 22, 1917). It is a most distressing condition, probably due to variations of the salts in the amniotic fluid. The difficulty of protecting the protuding bladder and the constant dribbling of urine are hard to remedy. Mayo reviews the surgical methods that have been used and the reasons why they do not meet the conditions. He also reports his own technic, which he has learned from experience of thirty-seven patients seen and operated on by the plastic and Maydl-Moynihan methods and thirteen successfully operated on by the transplantation method, that is, with the ureteral outlets transplanted into the intestine. The secret of successfully performing this operation of anastomosing the ureter into the bowel is to tabularize the ureteral entrance for 1 1-4 inches. There are two methods of doing this. The writer finds Coffey's modification of the Witzel method the most efficient and gives the technic in detail. After the age of forty, he says, however, it is probable that ureteral anastomies with the skin in the back is best from the standpoint of low mortality and future length of life. The plastic operations when used by him did not afford control of the urine. Children to be operated on should be old enough to attend to their own needs. Among the patients he has operated on, there was one operative death, one died from pneumonia a few weeks after leaving the clinic, one died three years later from pulmonary tuberculosis, and one from typhoid fever. Children who have been successfully operated on were able to go to school and receive an education, and the older ones are all working.

REPORT OF A CASE OF COMPLETE BONY OBSTRUCTION OF BOTH NARES*

By W. H. RUTLAND, B. S., M. D., Altus, Okla.

The case which I desire to report is that of an infant born with complete bony obstruction of both nasal passages, a brief history of which follows:

On October 16, 1916, I was called by phone to assist a physician in a case of obstructed breathing. On arriving at this place I found a new born babe being held in the lap of a neighbor lady while the attending physician, Dr. G., was studiously busy performing the duty of keeping the babe's mouth open, its tongue depressed, and the angles of its jaws held up and forward. Whenever the infant was deprived of this assistance, its tongue would immediately force itself upward and backward and obstruct the oropharynx and would immediately begin to struggle for breath and become cyanosed.

After a careful examination I found that the lungs, trachea, and larynx appeared to be free and open and that the source of obstruction must be located higher up than the epiglottis.

I then observed that the uvula, soft palate, and nasopharnyx seemed to be practically normal. On examining the nose I found the anterior two thirds to be about normal in appearance, but that it was impossible to pass the smallest size probe through either naris into the nasopharynx, and that this obstruction seemed to be confined to the posterior fourth of each nostril.

Since my efforts so far seemed to fail to be of much comfort to the patient, I began to cast about to see if I might do something to relieve the doctor who had reasons to feel forelorn over the prospects of having to remain on duty indefinitely as above mentioned. Then the thought occurred to me that if a tube were inserted into the infant's mouth to extend beyond the base of the tongue, it might enable the child to breathe when its tongue and jaw were released. Acting upon this suggestion I introduced a tracheotomy tube into the childs' mouth so that the distal end of this tube would rest near the base of the tongue and to my delight it breathed comfortably with this device which was held in place by a tape passed around the back of the neck.

With this one exception the infant seemed to be practically normal, hence I hoped that with this assistance for a short time the child might develop to the point where it could breathe comfortably without the aid of this mechanical device, but such was not the case. While the child could breathe fairly well with this device yet it seemed to be a source of annoyance to it, and it required almost constant care on the part of some one to keep it adjusted, since the infant would frequently work this tube out if its mouth and get itself into trouble.

When the child was two weeks old, with the use of a burr four m.m. in diameter I drilled through the obstruction interposed between the right naris and found this obstruction to be a mass of solid bone about three-eights of an inch thick; and about three weeks later I drilled a larger hole through the obstruction in the left nostril and enlarged the opening in the right side. After the last operation the child continued to breathe with as much comfort as that of a normal child.

Failing to obtain access to any literature of any consequense upon this class of cases, I am unable to offer anything further than the above brief clinical report.

I anticipated much pleasure in watching the progress of this case through the period of development of this child, but very unfortunately the child had to depend upon artificial feeding for its subsistence and as a result it continued in a state of lower vitality and finally succumbed to an attack of pneumonia when it was about two months old.

---

*Read at Medicine Park, Okla., May 9, 1917.

Our conclusion is that the case was one of congenital osteoma, and according to the history of such cases, no doubt the patient would have suffered a recurrence of this embarrasing obstruction in the near future.

Discussion.

Dr. D. D. McHenry, Oklahoma City: Dr. Rutland asked me to open the discussion on this subject and I began immediately to look through the literature I had on hand, and all I could find and was unable to find anything on the subject. Just about a week or ten days ago it came into my mind to look up Gould's Curiosities of Medicine, and I found that in 1863 a case was reported of complete bone obstruction of both nares, and in about 1875 Jarvis reported in the *New York Medical Journal* a similar case, and in 1880 Ronaldson, in the *Edinburg Medical Journal*, reported a case, and these were the only things I was able to find. I never saw a case myself so I don't know what I can possibly add.

The doctor's method of preserving the passage for breathing was certainly unique—in using his tool to hold the tongue down so the air could be gotten through the child's mouth. It simply shows that a physician must use a little horse-sense along with his knowledge. It would certainly have been interesting if the case had lived and the doctor could have watched it.

I have never seen a case of bony obstruction, but I am treating a case now where the whole palate is drawn up into one mass. He gets a little air through one passage, but the other is completely closed. One entry is a small opening the size of a lead pencil and the other none at all;—he came to me with a case of suppurated ear, and we discovered this. I have never seen a case like that reported. I have no ideas to offer regarding it. It seems to me that the doctor did the very most that I could have suggested, under the circumstances.

Dr. H. C. Todd, Oklahoma City: I was especially interested in this subject when I saw it on the program and I wanted to be present at the reading of this report. I had a rather unique experience, judging from what Dr. McHenry reported, not with having both nares obstructed—but I have had two cases in which there was a complete obstruction on one side. I can not say that the doctor was unfortunate in not being able to observe his case any longer, because in my opinion it would have been a pathetic case for anyone to kept under observation.

In the two cases I have had I am thoroughly convinced that there is no method which the surgeon of today knows anything about in which he could cure the trouble that would not destroy the physiognomy of the patient.

I would like to report the two cases which I had. The first was a practitioner's wife, who had a complete bony obstruction on one side. It had existed through childhood and the remarkable thing was that the development of the nares was quite good. The unpleasant part to her was that the nares continued to fill and she could not blow it out. Of course it became rancid and was very annoying. It was the first case I ever saw of the kind and I kept it under observation for a year, but with no results.

Some fellow reported a very wonderful operation for this very condition in which he removed this obstruction. He cut through and elevated the mucosa and brought it back over the margin where he had moved the bony tissue and cut the mucous membrane, and in some way, that I don't understand, kept it open.

I opened the nose with a burr and in about two months it was completely closed again. The result was that with my case I destroyed every opportunity of working on that case again.

About two years afterwards a case came from way up in Alva, identically similar—on the same side of the nose, complaining of the same unpleasant feeling of the nose. In the meantime I had done a great deal of thinking about that other case. I had a more or less turbinate, which I removed to get into the nose. I want to tell you how I did this. I have never reported it before because I regarded it as more or less an accident. I removed the membrane and cleaned it off completely, and I took a long chisel, a very sharp one, about a quarter of an inch wide. I cut through right level with the floor of the nose. Then I cut through on either side., cutting up about two widths of the chisel in cutting clear up on either side. Then I took my chisel—I had the turbinate cleaned out so I could see pretty well—and cut through less than half an inch, a quarter or an eighth above the floor, but not clear through the bone; then I just took a tool, a round iron probe, and knocked that thing back. Then with a good deal of care I went back to the naso-pharnyx.

If I had had more than one case I should probably have reported this, but as I say, I regarded it as an accident that it came out as well as it did. The flap dropped down after cutting through so I introduced a string through the nares down the throat and attached to that a piece of gauze, not big enough to pack the nose, but I had a raw surface all around up there. What I wanted was drainage to to get that stuff out of the nose, it was so offensive. I pushed the mucosa up over the bony part and I got the prettiest union you ever saw, which stopped this granulation. I got good results. I think that technique was far superior to the work of the Chicago man. I succeeded. We got some granulation above the floor of the nose, and I chiseled it away once or twice, but she was able to blow the nose on that side and would not take a great deal for the results we have gotten. We have an opening there through which you could put a good sized piece of cotton. This was done some four years ago. I have seen her in the last year and in my opinion the results are perfect.

You understand that the trouble with opening with the burr is that you get a raw surface all the way around. After my difficulties and all the troubles I met with in these two cases, I have wondered what a person would have done with an infant. The only thing I could see to do would be to make the temporary opening and that the child would breathe through its mouth all the rest of its life.

Dr. A. W. Roth, Tulsa: I had a case that I operated this fall. It became an extrusion from the sphenoid. The growth occupied the whole posterior nares completely. There was a bony growth that excluded the post nares. It is an osteo sarcoma and we did the usual operation and took out a large piece of it, we were afraid to go any farther with the work for fear of fracturing the base of the skull and possible hemorrhage. He could breathe through his nose nicely. Last week I had him come in again and the anterior surface looks very nice but the posterior surface is developing very rapidly again. The two horns are coming down all the time so that it is just a matter of time before the old condition is restored. But the hemorrhages of both nares were plugged through and when we got him through he was just a mass of blood. He fainted twice as they were bringing him to from the loss of blood. That was in December, I don't remember the exact date—it was right along at that time, we tied the *common carotid* and he has not had any bleeding since. He has gained some 27 pounds. He is a boy 17 years old and is doing finely, except that the growth is enlarging.

Dr. Rutland: I have nothing to add.

JOURNAL OF THE OKLAHOMA STATE MEDICAL ASSOCIATION

VOLUME XI   MUSKOGEE, OKLA., MARCH, 1918   NUMBER 3

PUBLISHED MONTHLY AT MUSKOGEE. OKLA.. UNDER DIRECTION OF THE COUNCIL

DR. CLAUDE A. THOMPSON, EDITOR-IN-CHIEF

ENTERED AT THE POST OFFICE AT MUSKOGEE. OKLAHOMA, AS SECOND CLASS MAIL MATTER, JULY 28, 1912

THIS IS THE OFFICIAL JOURNAL OF THE OKLAHOMA STATE MEDICAL ASSOCIATION. ALL COMMUNICATIONS SHOULD BE ADDRESSED TO THE JOURNAL OF THE OKLAHOMA STATE MEDICAL ASSSOCIATION, 307-8 SURETY BUILDING, MUSKOGEE, OKLAHOMA.

The editorial department is not responsible for the opinions expressed in the original articles of contributors.

Reprints of original articles will be supplied at actual cost, provided request for them is attached to manuscript or made in sufficient time before publication.

Articles sent this Journal for publication and all those read at the annual meetings of the State Association are the sole property of this Journal. The Journal relies on each individual contributor's strict adherence to this well-known rule of medical journalism. In the event an article sent this Journal fo publication is published before appearance in the Journal, the manuscript will be returned to the writer.

Failure to receive the Journal should call for immediate notification of the editor, 307-8 Surety Building, Muskogee, Okla

Local news of possible interest to the medical profession, notes on removals, changes in address, deaths and weddings will be gratefully received.

Advertising of articles, drugs or compounds unapproved by the Council on Pharmacy of the A. M. A. will not be accepted.

Advertising rates will be supplied on application. It is suggested that wherever possible members of the State Association should patronize our advertisers in preference to others as a matter of fair reciprocity.

EDITORIAL

THE TULSA MEETING.

This meeting will be held May 14, 15 and 16. Physicians contemplating attendance are warned now to make reservations for the meeting at a very early date. Ten days or two weeks notice will not do at all, as is the case with most conventions, but the reservation must be made far in advance. Tulsa is the most crowded city in the United States, all hotels and rooming houses, as well as apartments, are crowded to the utmost at all times and the local physicians are suggesting this warning at an early date in order that attendants may provide for themselves in time or otherwise be left without any accommodations.

Following is a list of the better hotels, but in addition to that there are others, which are good, not here listed: Alexander hotel, 219 S. Boston, $1.00 and up; Tulsa Hotel, $2.00 up; Ketchum Hotel, $2.00 up; Brady Hotel, $1.00 up; Cordova Hotel $1.00 up; Detroit, $1.00 up; Drexal, $1.00 up; Boswell, $1.00 up; Lee, $1.00 up; Lahoma, $1.00 up; Majestic, $1.00 up; Marquette $2.00 up; Oxford, $1.00 up; Oklahoma, $1.50 up.

These are among the best in town. The Tulsa, Alexander, Ketchum, Marquette, Oklahoma and Brady are the best.

PRESENT CONDITION OF THE MEDICAL RESERVE.

Notwithstanding considerable misinformation to the contrary the Medical Reserve Corps of the army is in splendid condition from the numerical standpoint. Late reports indicate that we now have more than 19,500 men engaged in the service and that figure does not include those in the Regular Army.

The men throughout the country are rapidly becoming familiar with military forms and usages and the especially difficult paper work so necessary in the handling of an immense work. Promotions are coming to many of the men and there is general satisfaction as a rule among them. The "Gasoline Board"—the title is unofficial of course, is busy in the camps and cantonments and when a man gets lazy or neglectful of his duties he is soon sent home to ruminate again over the pleasures of civil life, where the 5:30 reville and "Taps" disturb him not. The special work given many of the officers is especially fine. They are sent to various medical centers for special training in that branch they feel most qualified to handle and as one officer very aptly puts it: "We get splendid postgraduate work with all expenses paid". There is a growing idea, not confined to the physician, that the rank and corresponding pay of Medical Department should be raised. We have none, excepting the Surgeon General, holding the rank of Brigadier General, yet there are scores of Brigadiers in other branches of the service, who have nothing like the responsibility placed on men of lower rank in the Medical Department.

A few men have not yet accepted the commissions sent them from the Surgeon General's office after completion of their examination, but as a rule this is due to altered circumstances of the applicant and not to a disposition to evade duty.

A VOLUNTEER MEDICAL SERVICE CORPS.

The Council of National Defense authorizes the following statement:

For the purpose of completing the mobilization of the entire medical and surgical resources of the country, the Council of National Defense has authorized and directed the organization of a "Volunteer Medical Service Corps", which is aimed to enlist in the general war-winning program all reputable physicians and surgeons who are not eligible to membership in the Medical Officers' Reserve Corps.

It has been recognized always that the medical profession is made up of men whose patriotism is unquestioned and who are eager to serve their country in every way. Slight physical infirmities or the fact that one is beyond the age limit, fifty-five years, or the fact that one is needed for essential public or institutional service, while precluding active work in camp or field or hospital in the war zone, should not prevent these patriotic physicians from close relations with governmental needs at this time.

It was in Philadelphia that the idea of such an organization was first put forward, Dr. William Duffield Robinson having initiated the movement resulting in the formation last summer of the Senior Military Medical Association with Dr. W. W. Keen as president—a society which now has 271 members.

Through the Committee on State Activities of the General Medical Board the matter of forming such a nation-wide organization was taken up last October in Chicago at a meeting attended by delegates from forty-six states and the District of Columbia. This committee, of which Dr. Edward Martin and Dr. John D. McLean—both Philadelphians—are respectively chairman and secretary, unanimously endorse the project. A smaller committee, with Dr. Edward P. Davis, of Philadelphia as chairman, was appointed to draft conditions of membership, the general Medical Board unanimously endorsed the Committee's report, the executive Committee —including Surgeons General Gorgas of the Army, Braisted of the Navy, and Blue of the Public Health Service—heartily approved and passed it to the Council of National Defense for final action, and the machinery of the new body has been started by the sending of a letter to the State and County Committees urging interest and the enrollment of eligible physicians.

It is intended that this new Corps shall be an instrument able directly to meet such civil and military needs as are not already provided for. The General Medical Board holds it as axiomatic that the health of the people at home must be maintained as efficiently as in times of peace. The medical service in hospitals, medical colleges and laboratories must be up to standard; the demands incident to examination of drafted soldiers, including the reclamation of men rejected because of comparatively slight physical defects; the need of conserving the health of the families and dependents of enlisted men and the preservation of sanitary conditions—all these needs must be fully met in time of war as in time of peace.

They must be met in spite of the great and unusual depletion of the medical talent due to the demands of field and hospital service.

In fact, and in view of the prospective losses in men with which every community is confronted, the general Medical Board believes that the needs at home should be even better met now than ever. The carrying of this double burden will fall heavily upon the physicians, but the medical fraternity is confident that it will acquit itself fully in this regard, its members accepting the tremendous responsibility in the highest spirit of patriotism. It will mean, doubtless, that much service must be gratuitous, but the medical men can be relied upon to do their share of giving freely, and it is certain that inability to pay a fee will never deny needy persons the attention required.

It is proposed that the services rendered by the Volunteer Medical Service Corps shall be in response to a request from the Surgeon General of the Army, the Surgeon General of the Navy, the Surgeon General of the Public Health Service, or other duly authorized departments or associations, the general administration of the Corps to be vested in a Central Governing Board, which is to be a committee of the General Medical Board of the Council of National Defense. The State Committee of the Medical Section of the Council of National Defense constitutes the Governing Board in each State.

Conditions of membership are not onerous and are such as any qualified practitioner can readily meet. It is proposed that physicians intending to join shall apply by letter to the Secretary of the Central Governing Board, who will send the applicant a printed form, the filling out of which will permit ready calssification according to training and experience. The name and data of the applicants will be submitted to an Executive Committee of the State Governing Board, and the final acceptance to membership will be by the national governing body. An appropriate button or badge is to be adopted as official insignia.

The General Medical Board of the Council of National Defense is confident that there will be ready response from the physicians of the country. The Executive Committee of the General Medical Board comprises: Dr. Franklin Martin, Chairman; Dr. F. F. Simpson, Vice-chairman; Dr. William F. Snow, Secretary; Surgeon General Gorgas, U. S. Army; Surgeon General Braisted, U. S. Navy; Surgeon General Rupert Blue, Public Health Service; Dr. Cary T. Grayson; Dr. Charles H. Mayo; Dr. Victor C. Vaughan; Dr. William H. Welch.

CURRENT MEDICAL LITERATURE
Conducted by
DRS. CURT von WEDEL, Jr., and L. J. MOORMAN, Oklahoma City
and FRED J. WILKIEMEYER, Muskogee

GASTRODUODENOSTOMY—ITS INDICATIONS AND TECHNIC.
By Donald C. Balfour.
(*Annals of Surgery*, January, 1918.)

Balfour takes up the indications for a modified pyloroplasty, the indications of which are as follows: When the stomach and duodenum are not so highly adherent as to make it very difficult; when pylorectomy is not indicated; when the ulcer is small and on the upper anterior surface of the duodenum; or when the ulcer can be either excised or invaginated.

Briefly, indications are: (1). A pyloric lesion with marked obstruction with associated ballooning of the duodenum. (2). Whenever it is too difficult or for any reason not feasible, to perform a gastrojejunostomy. (3). When for any reason, as jejunal ulcer, it is necessary to excise an old gastrojejunostomy.

His technic is simple, using first interrupted silk, then No. 1 chromic, no clamp, ligating all bleeding points, then inner suture of chromic No. 2. He completes anterior sutures as posterior, with chromic and interrupted silk.   C. von Wedel, Jr.

TREATMENT OF WAR WOUNDS.

By Major F. Besley, M. R. C.

(*Surgery, Gynecology and Obstetrics,* January, 1918.)

Wounds are serious directly in proportion to the amount of the circulation destroyed and the amount and character of extraneous foreign material carried into the tissues.

The all important factor to consider is, how far must one go in attempting to destroy the bacteria and how much must one promote the resisting power of the cell? The author believes that the promotion of the resisting power of the cell is paramount.

As pus under pressure and not surface pus, is the damaging agent, free incision and removal of all devitalized tissue and foreign bodies are the main factors.

It has been shown by the French that wounds well taken care of within the first nine hours, can, in most instances, be cleaned out, and sutured—primary union resulting in a large majority of cases.

He is much opposed to the bismuth-iodin-paraffin treatment, and believes that the chief benefits to the Dakin-Carrel solution are the heat and adequate drainage. Aseptic and open air treatment he believes to be the best procedure. -   C. von Wedel, Jr.

REPAIR OF TENDONS IN FINGER.

By Sterling Bunnell.

(*Surgery, Gynecology and Obstetrics,* January, 1918.)

Bunnell takes up this phase of plastic surgery in a very interesting article. He states that most failures following attempted tendon repair are due to the sheath and the loose elastic tissue around the tendon being destroyed, and the tendon becoming imbedded in firm scar tissue.

The tendons move by slipping within the sheath, and by the movement of the sheath itself. He gives the following as the chief causes of failure: (1) Traumatizing tenchic; (2) medium incision; (3) obliteration of pulleys; (4) using methods which replace gliding mechanism by adhesions; (5) too much or too little post operative movement; (6) crude suturing of tendons.

1. Traumatizing technic. Obviously great care should be taken as to asepsis and to prevent injury to the smooth tendon or sheath.

2. Medium incision, causes contracture and places scar on pulley surface. Best is lateral or combined lateral and transverse.

3. Obliteration of the pulleys. If the pulleys are cut, the tendon will naturally span the joint and not slip through. One should avoid cutting them and try to slip the tendon through them.

4. Obliteration of the gliding mechanism by adhesions. It is best to entirely replace the injured tendon and sheath if too much is destroyed or too raw a surface is left. All severed tendons should be repaired as early as possible. It is usually best to draw the whole tendon from its sheath and replace it with a new tendon, making the tendon suture at the insertion and at the palm where adhessions are less detrimental.

Movement should be instituted with much care and judgment. The tension of the tendon is a very interesting phase nicely worked out by Mayer.

Great care should be taken in suturing the tendons, as any exposed suture or very ragged joint tends to adhesions.

Bunnell has devised three very useful instruments to aid him in his work.   C. von Wedel, Jr.

PERSONAL AND GENERAL NEWS

Dr. R. D. Rector, Anadarko, is convalescing from typhoid.

Dr. E. R. Askew, Hugo, is doing special work in New Orleans.

Dr. J. S. Rollins, Paden, is doing special work in Kansas City.

Dr. W. W. Kerley, Anadarko, visited the Rochester clinics in February.

Dr. William R. Barry, M. R. C., Bradley, has been promoted to a captaincy.

Dr. J. L. Day, M. R. C., formerly of Norman, has been promoted to a captaincy.

Dr. John W. Pendleton, Kingfisher, has received his commission in the M. R. C.

Dr. M. H. Newman, Shamrock, is moving to 947 West 13th street, Oklahoma City.

Dr. M. L. Lewis, M. R. C., Ada, has been ordered to report at San Antonia for duty.

Dr. J. W. Bone, Sapulpa, announces that he will be a candidate for mayor of that city.

Dr. J. A. Cheek, Sallisaw, has been ordered to duty at Ft. Sill with the Medical Reserve.

Dr. Carl Puckett, M. R. C., Pryor, has been promoted to a captaincy in the Aviation Section.

Dr. A. P. Gearheart, M. R. C., Blackwell, has been ordered to active service at Ft. Riley, Kansas.

Dr. Geo. E. Kerr, M. R. C., Chattanooga, has received orders to report for duty at Ft. Oglethorpe.

Dr. V. Berry, Captain M.'R. C., Okmulgee, has been ordered to report at Ft. Riley for active service.

Dr. R. K. Goddard, Supply, has been ordered to a Texas cantonment for duty with the Medical Reserve.

Dr. H. M. Reeder, Asher, has removed to Shawnee, having his office now in the Monmouth building.

Dr. Louis Bagby, M. R. C., Vinita, had hardly received his commission before he was ordered to report for duty.

Dr. G. P. McNaughton, Miami, has been ordered to report for active service with the medical Reserve Corps.

Dr. G. H. Sanborn, Shawnee, has been a patient in the General Hospital for several weeks with an unresolved pneumonia.

Dr. J. E. Gallagher, of St. Louis, is assisting Dr. D. A. Myers, Lawton, during the pendency of his call into the service.

Dr. D. Y. McCary, Holdenville, spent a few days in the Henryetta Hospital recently after unsuccessfully meeting a Ford.

Dr. Thos. L. Lauderdale, Oklahoma City, has been called to the colors at San Antonio. He will be attached to the Signal Corps.

Dr. E. L. Dawson, City Superintendent of Health, Chickasha, closed one room of the city schools recently, the closing due to smallpox.

Dr. J. F. Duckworth, Tahlequah, has been ordered to active duty at Ft. Sill. Dr. Duckworth formerly saw service in the Philippines.

Dr. G. S. Barber, Lawton, has been ordered to active duty at Kelley Field. He had been commissioned in the M. R. C. just one month.

Dr. M. H. Edens, Anadarko, has been commissioned in the Medical Reserve Corps and ordered to Kelley Field for duty with the aviation section.

Dr. W. E. Lamerton, Enid, is the latest physician sufferer from Ford theft. He offers $450.00 reward for its recovery; the car contained a valuable case of surgical instruments.

The Medical Section, Oklahoma State Council of Defense, has ordered a census of Oklahoma physicians. The census is to take into consideration their specialties, physical, moral and mental fitness and their loyalty.

Dr. H. V. L. Sapper, of the State Health Department, recently visited the Miami mining district and there conferred with Federal officials of the Public Health Service relative to the control of infectious diseases. It is said typhoid has been unusually prevalent.

Shawnee officers recently uncovered what is believed to be a system for illicit sale of narcotics when two men were arrested with more than $250.00 worth of cocaine and morphine which they had just taken from the express office. The shipment was addressed to a Purcell physician.

Dr. Ralph R. Mavity, Tonkawa, and Miss Ethel Lancaster were married in Brownsville, Texas, January 27th. Dr. Mavity is First Lieut M. R. C., 111th Sanitary Train, a graduate of Oklahoma University, and Mrs. Mavity is a graduate of the Nurses' Training School of the University.

Dr. Porter Norton, formerly of Mangum, died recently in Louisville, Ky. The cause of his death is said to be accidental poisoning. Dr. Norton was serving in the Naval Reserve, but some months ago became ill, the illness necessitated his going to Louisville for treatment, where he died.

Dr. J. H. Scott, County Superintendent of Health, and Dr. G. S. Baxter, City Health Officer, are investigating the water supply of Shawnee. They contend that the water is not what it should be. The water is taken from the North Canadian river and smells very much like packingtown sewer contamination.

The Pottowatome County Medical Society have amended their resolution regarding their members in the Medical Reserve Corps. Hereafter the family of a married doctor will receive from the Society fifty dollars per month. The family of unmarried doctors shall receive twenty-five dollars per month, all during the continuance of the war.

The Pottawatome County Medical Society has appointed the following Hospital Committee to work out plans to secure more adequate hospital facilities in Shawnee: Dr. G. S. Baxter, Dr. J. M. Byrum, Dr. J. E. Hughes. Failing to get the city authorities to enlarge the Municipal Hospital to meet the demands of the Medical Society, the society will endeavor to erect its own hospital.

Medical Officers of Local and Advisory Boards very generally attended meetings at several central points over the State in February to hear the ideas and suggestions of Major Van Kirk and Lieutenant Barron of the Medical Reserve Corps, who were detailed from the 90th Division for the purpose of discussing generally the points and stumbling blocks usually encountered at cantonments as to physical rejections. It is generally conceded that the meetings will do much good to uniformize physical examinations hereafter made in Oklahoma.

The Chiropractic petition, after months of waiting and legal skirmishing, has been declared by the Secretary of State, J. L. Lyon, to have a sufficient number of signatures to warrant the matter going to the people at the next election, however the Supreme Court of the State will finally pass on the matter before the Chiros will be called on to get out and hustle votes to set aside the act of the Legislature which declared they must go to school awhile and pass an examination before they could "practice" their wonderful science on the people.

MISCELLANEOUS

TRANSFUSION OF UNMODIFIED BLOOD.

Since the publication of his former paper in the *Journal A. M. A.*, of Feb. 13, 1915, in which he described his technic, L. J. Unger, New York, has performed 165 transfusions by this method giving an analysis of it in *The Journal A. M. A.*, Dec 29, 1917. He reviews the conditions under which it was used and the indications for which it was employed. His summary and conclusions are as follows: 1. The best results of transfusion were obtained in hemorrhage, diseases of the blood, toxemias and shock. In 88 per cent. of the cases of acute hemorrhage, bleeding was stopped by one trans fusion. In pernicious anemias, remissions can be iniatiated. Repeated transfusions, he declared, frequently bring on repeated remissions. Transfusion should be performed before all the effects of the preceding transfusion have been lost. If no remission results, transfusion with a different donor should be repeated. For the hemorrhage of hemophilia, transfusion is practically a specific. It is dangerous to delay too long with palliative measures if active bleeding is present. In purpura, transfusion gives only moderately good results. In the severe cases, it would seem advisable to carry out the suggestion of splenectomy with preliminary transfusions. All attempts to influence acute leukemia failed. In bleeding of the new-born, transfusion is a specific. Especially in cases of melena, temporizing by using other methods is contraindicated. The median basilic vein can be used regardless of the baby's age, and is the route of choice. Transfusion has yielded encouraging results in toxemia, associated with acute infections (pneumonia, typhoid fever), toxemia of pregnancy, scurvy and shock. Transfusion seems to overcome shock if employed at the onset of the symptoms. Since the number of transfusions for these conditions was comparatively small, further attempts must be made in order definitely to settle the questions involved. 2. Transfusion is often of assistance in overcoming intractable suppurative processes and causing a marked increase in the vitality of the patient. In bacteremias, transfusion has had practically no success. It is possible however, that if immune donors were used the results might be better. Transfusion given preliminary to an operation will often so improve the patients condition that the surgeon is justified in risking an operation. It will prolong the life of a patient suffering with a debilitating condition. 3. The syringe cannula method (requiring only one syringe) has proved a simple, efficient and dependable one for giving whole unmodified blood. The giving of unmodified blood is the method of choice when blood is required as a tissue (as in various anemias). When it is required to replenish impoverished circulation, citrated blood may serve as a substitute.

CANCER.

J. W. Vaughan, Detroit (*Journal A. M. A.*, Dec. 8, 1917), briefly notices his former work on cancer and its corroboration by other observers. He adds that while these investigations have not added much of decided value to the solution of the cancer problem, they have contributed to what might be called its intelligent treatment and given us an exact knowledge as to when operative treatment is indicated and when it will shorten life rather than prolong it. Metchnikoff was the first to show that tissue cells introduced into the animal body were ingested by the large mononuclear leukocyte, but he himself never associated this cell with any protective function in malignancy. The next work calling attention to blood cells of splenic origin, and associating it, for the first time, with the protective apparatus against malignancy, was that done by the writer's assistants and himself. They have done more than 30,000 differential blood counts and have ascertained that there is invariably an increase in large mononuclear leukocytes following the injection of cancer protein into normal persons or animals. The percentage of increase is dependent on certain factors, chief of which is the number of body cells with which protein comes in contact. A subcutaneous injection is followed by a slight increase, an intravenous injection by a greater increase and the intraperitoneal method by a still larger increase. Another important factor is that the sensitizing dose should not be too large. From three to ten minims of 0.5 or 1 per cent solution or suspension of either residue or vaccine is sufficient. The increased percentage of large lymphocytes is of short duration, lasting from four to twenty-four hours, during which time the animal is sensitized to large intravenous doses of the protein. But such sensitization is lost when the increase in large mononuclear cells again recedes. The writer thought, at first, that this reaction was a specific for cancer tissue but Fischer's work had helped to show him that this was incorrect. The writer immediately started blood counts following injections of fetal autolysate, percental residue and tissue vaccines from all sources, and he obtained results of decided interest. Chief among these was the fact that the more the tissue used reverted to the embryologic type, the greater was the increase in the large lymphocytes following its injection. This forced him to conclude that we had not here a specific ferment, but were dealing with a specific proteolytic ferment produced by the large mononuclear leukocytes, which is specific only to a limited degree. It also explained why some forms of cancer gave but a slight increase in large mononuclear cells after injection, while others gave an increase from 200 to 300 per cent. Careful study of many tumors indicated that the more the tumor reverted to the embryologic type the greater was the resulting increase. It was, therefore, thought best to use a tissue invariably giving an increase, and a residue made from normal placental tissue was found to answer the requirements most satisfactorily. It is now always used in the writer's tests for the activity of the malignant immune mechanism, unless they have been especially fortunate in obtaining an extremely malignant sarcoma. It can now be definitely stated that the immune mechanism in malignancy is a ferment which is formed in the large mononuclear leukocytes and is usually of splenic origin. The study of blood findings in all stages of malignancy was next undertaken and, in general, it may be said that cases of early malignancy usually showed a decided decrease in the total number of polymorphonuclears with a corresponding increase in mononuclears, resembling that in exophthalmic goiter, syphilis, and tuberculosis. When a tumor is growing rapidly, and always after metastasis has occurred, the percentage of polymophonuclears runs above seventy and is usually higher. A differential count in early malignancy frequently varies from day to day, retrogressing with a high percentage of mononuclears. Also, the reverse occurs with an increase of polymorphonuclears. The study of this large series of blood counts has given one fact of decided clinical importance, namely, that metastasis does not usually occur until the percentage of polymorphonuclear cells becomes high and remains so. In other words, metastasis is an indication of failure of the immune mechanism. From this it can be seen that the first differential count in any case of malignant disease shows whether metastasis has occurred, and whether the case is operable. Operation, the writer says, is best performed when the percentage of mononuclears is high, as metastasis is less liable to occur than from the operative handling. The immune mechanism may be lost when the tumor is yet small, after which the progress of the disease becomes rapid, and operation usually aggravates it. In other cases, apparently much more advanced, the immune mechanism can still be stimulated. Such patients are likely to live longer than the physician expects, and temporary benefits they enjoy from Nature's efforts form the basis of many claims of charlatans who assume the credit.

COUNCIL ON PHARMACY AND CHEMISTRY.

Articles Accepted.

During January the following articles have been accepted by the Council on Pharmacy and Chemistry for inclusion with new and Non-official Remedies:

Chlorazene Surgical Powder: The Abbott Laboratories.

Betanaphthyl Salicylate (Calco): Calco Chemical Company.

Acetylsalicylic Acid-Merck: Merck and Company.

NEW AND NONOFFICIAL REMEDIES

Sterile Solution Coagulen-Ciba (3 per cent.) 1.5 cc. Ampoules. Each ampule contains 1.5 cc of a 3 per cent. solution of coagulen-Ciba. A. Klipstein and Co., New York City.

Sterile Solution Coagulen-Ciba (3 per cent.) 20 cc. Ampoules. Each ampule contains 20 cc. of a 3 per cent. solution of coagulen-Ciba. A. Klipstein and Co., New York City.

Tablets Coagulen-Ciba 0.5 gm. Each compressed tablet contains 0.5 gm. coagulen-Ciba and 0.46 gm. sodium chloride. A. Klipstein and Co., New York City.

Dichloramine-T (Calco).—Paratoluenesulphonedichloramide. This is said to act much like Chloramine-T, but is capable of being used in a solution of eucalyptol and liquid petrolatum, thus securing the gradual and sustained antiseptic action. Like Chloramine-T, Dichloramine-T (Calco) is said to act essentially like the hypochlorites, but to be less irritating to the tissues. Dichloramine-T (Calco) is said to be useful in the prevention and treatment of diseases of the nose and throat. It has been used with success as an application to wounds, dissolved in chlorinated eucalyptol and chlorinated paraffin oil. Manufactured by the Calco Chemical Co., Boundbrook, N. J.

Halazone-Calco.—Parasulphonedichloramidobenzoic acid. It is said to act like chlorine and to have the advantage of being stable in solid form. In the presence of alkali carbonate, borate and phosphate it is reported that halazone in the proportion of from 1,200,000 to 1,500,000 sterilizes polluted water. Manufactured by the Calco Chemical Co., Bound Brook, N. J.

Chloramine-B (Calco).—Sodium Benzenesulphochloramine. It contains from 13 to 15 per cent. available chlorine. The actions, uses and dosage for Chloramine-B (Calco) are claimed to be essentially similar to those given in New and Nonofficial Remedies, 1917, for Chlorazene. This compound was introduced into medicine by Dakin. Its physical and chemical properties are similar to those of Chloramine-T. Manufactured by the Calco Chemical Co., Bound Brook, N. J. (*Journal A. M. A.*, January 12, 1918, p. 91).

PROPAGANDA FOR REFORM.

The Carrel-Dakin Wound Treatment. William H. Welch writes that he was most favorably impressed with the Carrel treatment of wounds, and believes that Carrel should receive credit for calling attention to the possibility of the sterilization of infected wounds by chemical means. He holds that while undoubtedly the tenchic of the Carrel treatment is elaborate and requires an intelligence and skill on the part of the surgeon which cannot be counted on for the average surgeon, and that while the preparation of the neutral solution of sodium hypochlorite also requires chemical skill, surgeons should acquaint themselves with the principles and technic, and try to overcome the difficulties of applying the treatment (*Journal A. M. A.*, December 8, 1917, p. 1994).

Hemo-Therapin. The Council on Pharmacy and Chemistry reports that, according to the Hemo-Therapin Laboratories, New York, Hemo-Therapin is a "combination of highly refined creosols and phenols (which have been detoxicated by special processes) with salts of iron, potassium, sodium, phosphorus and calcium in minute but physiologic proportions—the solution as a whole being designed to approximate closely in various fundamental details the chemistry of the blood." No statement is made, however, as to the quantities of the several ingredients, nor is any information given as to the identity of the "creosols" and "phenols", or as to the nature of the processes whereby these are "detoxicated". The Council explains that the Hemo-Therapin Laboratories ask physicians to believe that the occasional intravenous administration of this liquid will benefit or cure a long list of ailments, including erysipelas, septicemia, pyemia, puerperal infection, malaria, pneumonia, typhoid fever, diabetes, chronic Bright's disease, goiter, arteriosclerosis and locomotor ataxia. The testimonials which are presented for the claims bear a striking likeness to those found in "patent medicine" almanacs. One of the cases is a woman who was bitten by a snake seventeen years ago and who, on the anniversary of the bite, suffers severely from the original bite (*Journal A. M. A.*, January 5, 1917, p. 48).

Venosal. The Council on Pharmacy and Chemistry reports that Venosal, sold by the Intravenous Products Company, Denver, Colo., is inadmissible to New and Nonofficial Remedies because its chemical composition is indefinite; because the therapuetic claims are exaggerated, and because the composition is unscientific. Venosal is a solution of sodium salicylate containing also colchicum and an insignificant amount of iron. Since it is possible to obtain the salicylate effects promptly and certainly by oral administration, the inherent dangers of intravenous medication render its routine employment unwarranted. At this time, when economy is the national policy, a further objection to the use of Venosal is the unnecessarily high expense of Venosal itself and the administration (*Journal A. M. A.*, January 5, 1917, p 48).

Our Archaic Patent Laws. The reports of the Council on Pharmacy and Chemistry on Secretin-Beveridge and the Need for Patent Law Revision are opportune. At the request of the National Research Council the "Patent Office Society", an association of employees of the U. S. Patent Office, has created a committee to study the U. S. Patent Office and its service to science and to arts. There is no question that one of two things is needed: either a radical change in the patent law itself or the application of more brains in its administration. Now the United States Patent Law is too often used to obtain an unfair monopoly of a medicament or to abet quackery (*Journal A. M. A.*, January 12, 1918, p. 95).

Secretin-Beveridge and the U. S. Patent Law. In 1916, A. J. Carlson and his co-workers demonstrated that commercial secretin preparations contained no secretin, and that secretin administered by mouth or even into the intestine was inert. Yet a U. S. patent was subsequently issued to James Wallace Beveridge, for a process of preparing secretin preparations which would contain secretin when they reached the consumer, and in a form resisting destruction in its passage through the stomach. At the request of the Council on Pharmacy and Chemistry, A. J. Carlson and his associates studied the stability of the secretin made according to the Beveridge patent. The investigation shows that the patent gives no process for the manufacture of commercially stable secretin preparations, nor any means for preventing the destruction of secretin by the gastric juice when administered orally (*Journal A. M. A.*, January 12, 1918, p. 115).

Need for Patent Law Revision. The Council on Pharmacy and Chemistry publishes a report prepared by its Committee on the patent law revision, which is an appeal for an amendment of the patent law which governs the issuance of patents on medicinal preparations, and more particularly for a revision on the procedure under which such patents are issued. The report points out that to increase our national efficiency, the government must protect and stimulate science, art and industry, and at the same time curb waste of the country's resources; and that, to this end, the patent office should encourage discoveries which go to increase national efficiency, and refuse patent protection when such protection is not in the interest of national efficiency, conservation of energy and material resources. The report presents a considerable number of specific instances which demonstrate that patent protection has been given where it was not deserved and not in the interest of the public. The report concludes with a reference to the investigation of a patent granted for a preparation of secretin, apparently without any attempt to confirm the highly improbable claims of the patent applicant (*Journal A. M. A.*, January 12, 1918, p. 118).

Arsphenamine. No this is not a new chemical, it is simply the name adopted by the Federal Trade Commission for the Hydrochloride of 3-diamino-4-dihydroxy-1-arsenobenzene in other words, salvarsan. The three firms which have been licensed to manufacture this drug are permitted to have their own trade names for it, but the official name "arsphenmine" must be the prominent one on the label of all brands. Hence physicians should at once make it a point to learn and use the name "arsphenamine". (*Journal A. M. A.*, January 19, 1918, p. 167).

Cactina Pillets. According to the manufacturer of Cactina Pillets (The Sultan Drug Co.), "cactina" is "invaluable in all functional cardiac disorders such as trachycardia, palpitation, arrhythmia, and whenever the heart's action needs regulating or support." The manufacturer gives no information as to the mode of action of "cactina", but states that it is totally unlike that of digitalis. An examination of the literature indicates that *cactus grandiflorus* is therapeutically inert, and no one except Mr. Sultan of the Sultan Drug Company claims to have isolated an active principle of it. The Council on Pharmacy and Chemistry examined the literature relating to cactus and certain proprietary preparations, including Cactina Pillets, alleged to be made from cactus, and reported that the literature does not afford a single piece of careful, painstaking work which lends support to the claims made for Cactina Pillets. Since then, Hatcher and Bailey examined genuine *cactus grandiflorus*, and also found that the drug was pharmacologically inert (*Journal A. M. A.*, January 19, 1918, p. 185).

Surgodine. The A. M. A. Chemical Laboratory having found Surgodine (Sharp and Dohme) to contain 2.51 gm. free iodin (instead of 2.25 per cent. as claimed) and 1.78 gm. combined iodin (probably chiefly hydrogen iodin), the Council on Pharmacy and Chemistry reports that it is essentially similar to the official tincture of iodin, except that it is considerably weaker and, instead of pota3sium idid, it presumably contains hydrogen iodid and probably ethyl iodid to render the iodin water soluble. Its composition, however, is secret. The Council held Surgodine inadmissible to New and Nonofficial Remedies because its composition is secret; because the therapeutic claims made for it are exaggerated and unwarranted, and because it is an unessential modification of the official tincture of iodin. Surgodine is a good illustration of the economic waste inseparable from most proprietary medicines. While the free-iodin strength of Surgodine is only about one third that of the official tincture, its price is between two and three times as high (*Journal A. M. A.*, January 26, 1918, p. 257).

Dionol. If the physicians take the word of the Dionol Company, the therapeutic possibilities of Dionol are apparently limited only by the blue sky. Even the company admits that "the unprecedented range of action" of this marvel "may come as a surprise". A glance over the published case reports confirms the inference. Dionol is furnished in two forms: as an ointment and as an emulsion. Dionol itself is a sort of glorified petrolatum, the use of which is said to prevent the leakage of energy from the nerve cells, and by overcoming the short circuiting always said to be present in inflammations, is asserted to accomplish its wonders (*Journal A. M. A.*, January 26, 1918, p.257).

LOCAL ANESTHESIA.

Torald Sollmann, Cleveland (*Journal A. M. A.*, Jan. 26, 1918), questions the desirability of testing systemic toxicity of local anesthetics on rodents as they are quite different from human beings in their response to certain poisons. He does not, however, go into this aspect of the subject, but confines himself to the subject of anesthetic efficiency. The methods and their respective merits are discussed, and the results are presented in the form of diagrams which cannot well be reproduced in an abstract. For testing anesthesia of mucous membranes, the writer finds cocain, beta-eucain, alypin, and tropacocain the most useful. Quininurea hydrochlorid is fairly active. Apothesin, novocain and potassium chlorid are relatively ineffective. Alkalization increases the efficiency from two to four times. The solution of the anesthetic salts may be mixed with an equal volume of 0.5 per cent. sodium bicarbonate, without loss of efficiency, and with a saving of one-half of the anesthetic. The mixture, however, does not keep well and should be freshly made. Epinephrin added to the anesthetic does not increase its efficiency, and is probably useless. For infiltration and injection anesthesia, cocain, novocain, tropacocain and alypin are about equally efficient. Betaeucain and quinin-urea hydrochlorid are intermediate, and apothesin and potassium sulphate or chlorid are relatively ineffective. The effectiveness is not increased by alkalization. Epinephrin greatly prolongs the anesthesia and should always be added, except to tropacocain. An isotonic solution would be equivalent to about 0.125 per cent. of cocain or novocain. It may well be used in place of sodium chloride for making anesthetic solutions. Several of the synthetic anesthetics can completely displace cocain. In view of this fact, it would be possible to prohibit entirely the importation, manufacture, sale and use of the habit-forming drug, except for scientific purposes.

OFFICERS OF COUNTY SOCIETIES, 1918

County	President	Secretary
Adair	A. J. Sands, Watts	A. J. Patton, Stilwell
Alfalfa	H. A. Lile, Aline	W. H. Dersch, Carmen
Atoka		
Beaver		
Beckham		
Blaine	J. B. Leisure, Watonga	J. A. Norris, Okeene
Bryan	J. L. Reynolds, Durant	D. Armstrong, Durant
Caddo	A. H. Taylor, Anadarko	Chas. B. Hume, Anadarko
Canadian	P. F. Herod, El Reno	W. J. Muzzy, El Reno
Choctaw	V. L. McPherson, Boswell	E. R. Askew, Hugo
Carter	F. W. Boadway, Ardmore	Robt. H. Henry, Ardmore
Cleveland	J. J. Gable, Norman	Gayfree Ellison, Norman
Cherokee		
Custer	J. Matt Gordon, Weatherford	C. H. McBurney, Clinton
Comanche	E. R. Dunlap, Lawton	General Pinnell, Lawton
Coal		
Cotton		
Craig		
Creek		
Dewey		
Ellis		
Garfield	H. B. McKenzie, Enid	A. Boutrous, Enid
Garvin		
Grady	D. S. Downey, Chickasha	Martha Bledsoe, Chickasha
Grant		
Greer	Nay Neel, Mangum	Thos. J. Horsley, Mangum
Harmon	W. T. Ray, Gould	R. L. Pendergraft, Hollis
Haskell		
Jackson	T. H. Hardin, Olustee	W. H. Rutland, Altus
Jefferson		
Johnson		
Kay		
Kingfisher		
Kiowa		
Latimer	E. B. Hamilton, Wilburton	E. L. Evins, Wilburton
Le Flore	E. E. Shippey, Wister	Harrell Hardy, Bokoshe
Lincoln		
Logan		
Love		
Mayes	J. L. Adams, Pryor	L. C. White, Adair
Major		
Marshall		
McClain	J. W. West, Purcell	O. O. Dawson, Wayne
McCurtain		
McIntosh	B. J. Vance, Checotah	W. A. Tolleson, Eufaula
Murray		
Muskogee	J. G. Noble, Muskogee	A. L. Stocks, Muskogee
Noble		
Nowata		
Okfuskee	J. S. Rollins, Paden	A. O. Meredith, Bearden
Oklahoma	John A. Reck, Oklahoma City	H. H. Cloudman, Oklahoma City
Okmulgee	W. C. Mitehner, Okmulgee	Harry E. Breese, Henryetta
Ottawa	A. M. Cooter, Miami	Blair Points, Miami
Osage	G. W. Goss, Pawhuska	Benj. Skinner, Pawhuska
Pawnee		E. T. Robinson, Cleveland
Payne	E. M. Harris, Cushing	J. B. Murphy, Stillwater
Pittsburg	T. H. McCarley, McAlester	J. A. Smith, McAlester
Pottawatomie	R. M. Anderson, Shawnee	G. S. Baxter, Shawnee
Pontotoc	B. F. Sullivan, Ada	Catherine Threlkeld, Ada
Pushmataha		
Rogers		
Roger Mills		
Seminole		
Sequoyah		
Stephens	D. M. Montgamery, Marlow	H. C. Frie, Duncan
Texas	W. H. Langston, Guymon	R. B. Hays, Guymon
Tulsa	H. D. Murdock, Tulsa	W. J. Trainor, Tulsa
Tillman		
Wagoner	C. E. Hayward, Wagoner	S. R. Bates, Wagoner
Washita	D. W. Bennett, Sentinel	A. S. Neal, Cordell
Washington	G. F. Woodring, Bartlesville	J. G. Smith, Bartlesville
Woodward	R. A. Workman, Woodward	C. W. Tedrowe, Woodward
Woods	G. M. Bilby, Alva	D. B. Ensor, Hopeton

OFFICERS OF OKLAHOMA STATE MEDICAL ASSOCIATION.

Meeting Place—Tulsa, May 14-15-16, 1918.
President, 1917-18—Dr. W. Albert Cook, Tulsa.
President-elect, 1918-19—Dr. L. S. Willour, McAlester.
1st Vice-President—Dr. McLain Rogers, Clinton.
2nd Vice-President—Dr. G. F. Border, Mangum.
3rd Vice-President—Dr. Horace Reed, Oklahoma City.
Secretary-Treasurer-Editor—Dr. C. A. Thompson, Muskogee.
Delegate to the A. M. A., 1918-19—Dr. Chas. R. Hume, Anadarko.
Delegate to the A. M. A. 1917-18—Dr. M. A. Kelso, Enid.

CHAIRMEN OF SCIENTIFIC SECTIONS.

Surgery and Gynecology—Dr. LeRoy Long, Oklahoma City.
Pediatrics and Obstetrics—Dr. T. C. Sanders, Shawnee.
Eye, Ear, Nose and Throat—Dr. L. A. Newton, Oklahoma City.
General Medicine, Nervous and Mental Diseases—Dr. A. B. Leeds, Chickasha.
Genitourinary, Skin and Radiology—Dr. W. J. Wallace, Oklahoma City.
Legislative Committee—Dr. Millington Smith, Oklahoma City; Dr. J. M. Byrum, Shawnee; Dr. W. T. Salmon, Oklahoma City.
For the Study and Control of Cancer—Drs. LeRoy Long, Oklahoma City; Gayfree Ellison, Norman; D. A. Myers, Lawton.
For the Study and Control of Pellagra—Drs. A. A. Thurlow, Norman; L. A. Mitchell, Frederick; J. C. Watkins, Checotah.
For the Study of Venereal Diseases—Drs. Wm. J. Wallace, Oklahoma City; Ross Grosshart, Tulsa; J. E. Bercaw, Okmulgee.
Necrology—Drs. Martha Bledsoe, Chickasha; J. W. Pollard, Bartlesville.
Tuberculosis—Drs. L. J. Moorman, Oklahoma City; C. W. Heitzman, Muskogee; Leila E. Andrews, Oklahoma City.
Conservation of Vision—Drs. L. A. Newton, Oklanoma City; L. Haynes Buxton, Oklahoma City; G. E. Hartshorne, Shawnee.
First Aid Committee—Drs. G. S. Baxter, Shawnee; Jas. C. Johnston, McAlester.
Committee on Medical Education—Drs. A. L. Blesh; A. K. West; A. W. White, Oklahoma City.
State Commissioner of Health—Dr. John W. Duke, Guthrie, Oklahoma.

COUNCILOR DISTRICTS.

1. Cimarron, Texas, Beaver, Harper, Ellis, Woods and Woodward; Councilor, Dr. J. M. Workman, Woodward. Term expires 1919.
2. Roger Mills, Beckham, Dewey, Custer, Washita and Blaine; Councilor, Dr. Ellis Lamb, Clinton. Term expires 1920.
3. Harmon, Greer, Jackson, Kiowa, Tillman, Comanche and Cotton; Councilor, Dr. G. P. Cherry, Mangum. Term expires 1918.
4. Major, Alfalfa, Grant, Garfield, Noble and Kay; Councilor, Dr. G. A. Boyle, Enid. Term expires 1919.
5. Kingfisher, Canadian, Oklahoma and Logan; Councilor, Dr. Fred Y. Cronk, Guthrie. Term expires 1918.
6. Caddo, Grady, McClain, Garvin, Stephens and Jefferson; Councilor, Dr. C. M. Maupin, Waurika. Term expires 1919.
7. Osage, Pawnee, Creek, Okfuskee, Okmulgee and Tulsa; Councilor, Dr. N. W. Mayginnes, Tulsa. Term expires 1920.
8. Payne, Lincoln, Cleveland, Pottawatomie and Seminole; Councilor, Dr. H. M. Williams, Wellston. Term expires 1920.
9. Pontotoc, Murray, Carter, Love, Marshall, Johnston and Coal; Councilor, Dr. J. T. Slover, Sulphur. Term expires 1918.
10. Washington, Nowata, Rogers, Craig, Ottawa, Mayes and Delaware; Councilor, Dr. R. L. Mitchell, Vinita. Term expires 1918.
11. Wagoner, Muskogee, McIntosh, Haskell, Cherokee and Adair; Councilor, Dr. J. Hutchings White, Muskogee. Term expires 1920.
12. Hughes, Pittsburg, Latimer, LeFlore and Sequoyah; Councilor, Dr. Ed. D. James, Haileyville. Term expires 1920.
13. Atoka, Pushmataha, Bryan, Choctaw and McCurtain; Councilor, Dr. J. L. Austin, Durant. Term expires 1920.

STATE BOARD OF MEDICAL EXAMINERS.

Melvin Gray, M. D., Durant, President; B. L. Denison, M. D., Garvin, Vice-President; J. J. Williams, M. D., Weatherford, Secretary; O. R. Gregg, M. D., Waynoka, Treasurer; E. B. Dunlap, M. D., Lawton; Ralph V. Smith, M. D., Tulsa; W. LeRoy Bonnell, M. D., Chickasha; Wm. T. Ray, M. D., Gould; H. C. Montague, D. O., Muskogee.

Reciprocity with Georgia, Kentucky, Mississippi, Nevada, North Carolina, Wisconsin, Kansas, Arkansas, Virginia, West Virginia, Nebraska, New Mexico, Tennessee, Iowa, Ohio, California, Colorado, Indiana, Missouri, New Jersey, Vermont, Texas, Michigan.

Meetings held second Tuesday of January, April, July and October, Oklahoma City.
Address all communications to the Secretary, Dr. J. J. Williams, Weatherford.

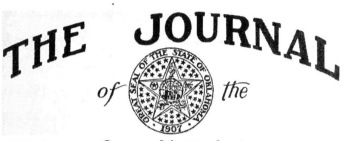

THE JOURNAL

of the

Oklahoma State Medical Association

VOLUME XI   MUSKOGEE, OKLA., APRIL, 1918   NUMBER 4

INFLAMMATION OF THE ABDOMINAL TONSIL.

The Importance of Early Diagnosis.

By G. A. WALL, M. D., Tulsa, Oklahoma.

A few years ago Robt. T. Morris wrote an article on Perineal Repair, and gave it the title of "The Office Boy Operation". This was done, I presume, to call attention to its simplicity, and to attract the reader to an old and much written about condition. In this connection I felt that so much has been written on appendicitis, that the subject is becoming rather stale, and many who should read it, would fail to do so hence, I adopted the above title, taken from Morris' Human Anatomy[1], in which he says "The appendix is essentially a lymph gland and has been called the abdominal tonsil." The writer feels that most men think that enough has been said on this subject, and that further discussion is not only useless but superfluous. In order to show that enough has not been said along this line I desire to quote rather fully from the works of the late lamented Murphy[2]. Just a few years ago he published in his clinics a picture of a gangrenous appendix, with one of his admirable talks. A few weeks later he was taken to task by another for doing so, saying that it was ancient history. Here is his answer, "Just recently a critic took a Chicago surgeon to task in the columns of a medical journal because the latter had published a colored picture of a gangrenous appendix. The writer intimated that appendicitis was ancient history. It IS ancient history; but does that mean that all practitioners are master of the situation or that the disease is efficiently handled at the present? If you will look up the statistics on the results of operations for appendicitis, you will find the average mortality rate in hospitals to be a little over 10 per cent. These are not individual surgeon's statistics, but the statistics of hospitals where the leaders of the profession operate. They include the statistics of all cases of this disease brought to the hospital. Is it time to stop talking about appendicitis? No, it is just time to begin, and talk most seriously and emphatically about it". Since the mortality is much too great, there must be a good reason for it, and that reason is delay in diagnosis, or procrastination after the diagnosis is made. Every case of appendicitis allowed to go on to suppuration with its high mortality rate is an indictment of the physician, if called in early, or of the patient if he refuses operation. It is the opinion of the writer that the great majority of acute cases present a very constant clinical syndrome, and one which can hardly mislead. It is better to be mistaken in the diagnosis than to mistake the disease, so when in doubt call consultation, *don't delay.*

---

(1) Morris Human Anatomy, page 1378.
(2) Clinics, June, 1915.

The attack of acute appendicitis usually begins with a more or less severe epigastric pain, following six or eight hours after a heavy and, usually, very indigestible meal. The writer has found this to be true in practically all of his cases seen in the past two years. Following this pain, nausea ensues, with vomiting in the great majority of cases, but not all. The pain finally localizes over the right lower abdominal quadrant, the rectus becomes rigid, tenderness over McBurney's point is pronounced, and the patient has a *rise of temperature*. Without the rise of temperature, we should hesitate to pronounce it appendicitis; but with all of the above symptoms combined with even the slightest rise in temperature, we could without much fear of error call it an acute attack. The position of the organ intra-abdominally will often mask some of the signs and may lead one into error. For instance, some very severely inflamed appendices which are situated retrocecally may fail to give muscle rigidity or tenderness over McBurney's point, but deep pressure in the lumbar region will elicit tenderness: this with the history should place you on your guard. At this time a blood count will be of value, but the count must be a differential, instead of the absolute only. In a very exhaustive article by Hewitt[3], he draws the following conclusions as to the relative value of the blood count in this disease.

"First: The absolute count, when taken alone, is of questionable value.

"Second: The polynuclear count alone is, in the majority of instances, a reliable index of diagnosis.

"Third: That the correlated absolute and polynuclear are of greater value than either count taken alone, especially as regards prognosis.

"A high absolute count with a high polynuclear count usually means a good prognosis (e. g., absolute 35000, polynuclear 95 per cent.) A high absolute (30000) with a moderately low polynuclear (80 per cent.) usually means a very good prognosis. A low absolute (7000) with a high polynuclear (95 per cent.) indicates a grave prognosis (generally speaking). A low absolute count (7000) with a low polynuclear (65 per cent.) usually indicates no infection, or that the infection, if one be present, has not stimulated the resisting powers of the body sufficiently to produce a leucocytosis.

"Fourth: Normal or subnormal figures do not necessarily indicate the absence of suppuration or its sequels.

"Fifth: Catarrhal cases, fulminating cases, moribund cases and walled off abscesses frequently do not stimulate leukocytosis".

Hewitt further says: "The surgeon who attempts to use the blood count in appendicitis as a definite diagnostic sign will soon run afoul of diagnostic disasters, but he who regards it only as a symptom invariably to be correlated with equally, if not more important clinical manifestations, cannot fail to find this method of inquiry of signal value in routine clinical surgery." The question of appendicitis, as a complication of other diseases and as mistaken diagnosis is one of importance. In the female right side salpingitis is frequently mistaken for appendicitis: if the appendix lies in the usual anatomic position in the abdomen, it is in close apposition to the right ovary and tube and any inflammation of these can and does involve this organ very frequently, but this is a secondary condition and not a primary one, and the symptoms will not be those of an acute attack, as outlined before. It is surprising how many cases of salpingitis are diagnosed appendicitis when there is involvement of the tube only. Most of these secondary appendix involvements take on the character of a chronic inflammation. On the diagnosis in this condition Morris[4] says, "About an inch and a half to the right of the navel and a trifle caudad, one will find on deep pressure a hypersensitive point in cases of one of four kinds. This tender point does not belong to cases of acute appendicitis. It does not belong to cases of pelvic irritation or infection, except in company with a similar tender point to the left of the navel. This tender point to the right of the

(3) Annals of Surgery, August, 1917, page 143.

JOURNAL OF THE OKLAHOMA STATE MEDICAL ASSOCIATION   113

navel will serve to give differential diagnosis between cases of chronic appendicitis and various pelvic irritations or infections." His conclusions are fully given in the article quoted. From a frequent use of this sign, the writer can concur in the findings of Morris.

It is surprising how often right renal colic is mistaken for appendicitis. It does not seem to the writer as though this mistake should be made as frequently as it is, since the signs are to his mind very unsimilar. The pain is of an excruciatingly severe character, cutting, spasmodic usually, passes down from the kidney region, into the vulva or scrotum as the case may be, and there is generally some bladder irritation. There is seldom, if ever, any nausea or vomiting, epigastric distress as a prodrome is very generally absent, and there is in the early stages, *no rise of temperature*. There might or might not be any leukocytosis, but the irritation might cause an increased absolute count, and here the differential would solve the riddle. There is at times tenderness on deep palpation over the ureter in the region of McBurney's point.

Appendicitis in children may be mistaken for pneumonia and vice versa. It is a most serious disease in childhood, because of the anatomical fact that the omentum in the child is small and not fully developed, hence, does not afford any protection to the general pelvic cavity, during the attack, and a diffuse peritonitis very promptly ensues upon rupture, unless the appendix is situated retrocecally, in which instance the abscess may localize post-cecal and thereby be shut off from the general cavity. Because the child is very young is no reason why it will not have appendicitis. There has recently appeared in the literature a case of operation on a child six weeks old. The writer has recently operated on a boy six years old, in which the only symptoms were pain in the stomach and tenderness over McBurney's point. This was a case in which the question of a pneumonia arose. The writer urges the general practitioner to keep the fact in mind that appendicitis in infancy and childhood does occur with no great infrequency.

The matter of appendicitis complicating typhoid fever, or mistaken for it, is one of great concern. It has been no infrequent occurrence for a typhoid case, in its early stages, to have been subjected to an unnecessary and very dangerous operation, because of a mistaken diagnosis. The writer must confess that he does not know how to avoid this mistake. It would seem that only by the most careful and painstaking analysis of the clinical symptoms and history in these cases can we avoid error, and even then it will occur, as shown by the fact that at Johns Hopkins the mistake has been made more than once.

Finally, there is one other condition in which a *very* early diagnosis is of the greatest importance, and that is, in pregnancy: Pregnancy with appendicitis, says Murphy[6], "Is one of the most dangerous conditions that occurs in the lower abdomen. With appendicitis in pregnancy, there is a colossal mortality percentage when one does not operate, and only a slightly lower one when one does operate, except in the cases which are operated on in the first few hours of the attack, before the disease has become a constitutional infection; that is, before the pus has been absorbed into the circulation, and the microorganisms are circulating in the blood. If a local abscess forms, the danger of a general peritonitis is very great. In the third and fourth months of pregnancy the intestines and omentum have been pushed out of the field by the growing uterus, where they protect the caput coli, and so cannot care for the inflamed appendix, (the writer does not believe that the uterus is high enough in the pelvis at these months to raise the intestines or omentum out of the field), consequently there is a marked tendency to the development of a fulminant peritonitis. The mortality of cases not operated upon has been shown by Wagner to be 77 per cent.; while in cases operated during the first 48 hours, the mortality is only 6 per cent. The mortality can certainly be reduced if operated on within the first 24 hours of the attack. From this you

(4) Journal A. M. A., December 15, 1917, page 2036.
(5) Clinics J. B. M., December, 1914.

you will see how very necessary it' is to be on the lookout for the disease in your pregnant patients. Early diagnosis means a life saved, perhaps we had better say two lives: The *least* delay spells for an awful catastrophy.

There has been nothing new said in this hastily written article, but the writer is sure that some good may come from it, if perchance it might save just one life, which otherwise might have been sacrificed. I may in conclusion quote this little bit:

"I have gathered a posie of other men's flowers
And nothing but the thread that binds them is mine."

TUBERCULOSIS OF THE KIDNEY.

By DANIEL N. EISENDRATH, A. B., M. D., Chicago, Illinois.

LIST OF ILLUSTRATIONS.

Fig. 1. Advanced stage. Nephrectomy in the sixth month of pregnancy.
Fig. 2. Section of advanced tuberculous pyonephrosis.
Fig. 3. Tuberculosis of kidney.
Fig. 4. Typical appearance of bladder in tuberculosis of kidney,

The object of this paper is primarily to direct the attention of the general practitioner to a disease for which he, as a rule, is first consulted. If I can succeed in showing that a more careful examination should be made of every patient who has symptoms of cystitis and does not improve after treatment, I will feel that this paper will not have been written in vain. It will be my object to show that tuberculosis of the urinary tract begins almost without exception in one kidney, the organism being carried there through the blood supply of that kidney. If we can educate the men who first *see* these cases to consult some one who is trained in the special methods *essential* to making a diagnosis of a surgical lesion of the kidney, I feel confident that the sad story told us almost daily, of the existence of typical symptoms for months and years, will be greatly changed.

Let us take up the subject in a somewhat systematic manner. First, consider the pathological changes which the kidney undergoes as a result of its invasion by the tubercle bacilli.

Pathology. By tuberculosis of the kidney the surgeon invariably refers to that form in which one or more foci are present in a chronic form in the kidney. We exclude from consideration those forms of tuberculosis of the kidney which are, as a rule, an accompaniment of a generalized miliary tuberculosis in which both kidneys are the seat of hundreds of miliary tubercles whose presence does not give rise to symptoms which can be differentiated from those due to the involvement of other organs such as the lung, spleen, liver, brain, etc., the clinical picture of which is familiar to every internist. This form of tuberculosis of the kidney in which we are interested is, as a rule, of gradual development. Occasionally one encounters cases (as I shall mention under the heads of the various groups of clinical pictures which one encounters) which apparently have an acute onset with chills and fever; with the symptoms resembling those of an acute non-tuberculous affection of the kidney. I have seen three such cases in which the infection with the tubercle bacilli was complicated by one due to the ordinary pyogenic organisms such as the bacillus coli and the staphylococcus pyogenes aureus picture to such an extent as to give rise to the impression that the disease had an acute onset. I have found but few references in the literature to the possibility of certain cases of tuberculosis of the kidney appearing in an acute form such as these cases just referred to.

Aside from these apparently acute cases practically every invasion of the kid-

A

B

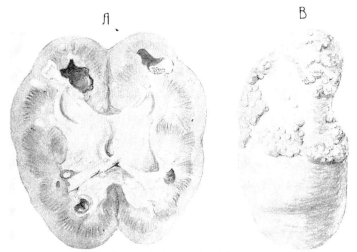

Fig. 1. Appearance of kidney in a case of early tuberculosis of the organ.
   (A). Section of kidney showing ulcer of papilla (tuberculous papillitis) and formation of a
        small cavity adjacent thereto in parenchyma of the upper pole. At the lower pole one
        sees a still earlier stage of ulcer of the papilla. Note also the miliary tubercles scattered
        over mucous membrane of renal pelvis.
   (B). Appearance of exterior of same kidney showing a large number of groups of tubercles
        scattered over its surface.

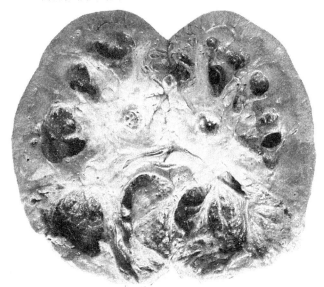

Fig. 2. Intermediate stage of tuberculosis of the kidney. Note how lower half of parenchyma has
        been destroyed and also a large portion of the upper half.

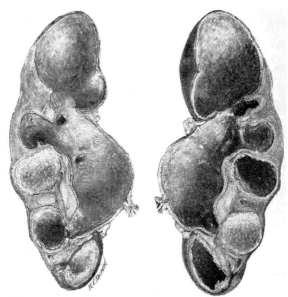

Fig. 3. End stage of tuberculosis of the kidney. Note how entire parenchyma is replaced by a series of cavities which were filled with caseous detritus.

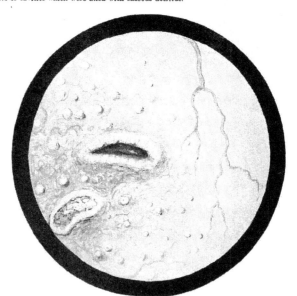

Fig. 4. Typical appearance of bladder in a case of tuberculosis of the kidney. Note gaping character with raised edematous edges of the ureteral orifice giving it somewhat the appearance of a golf hole. In the vicinity of the ureteral opening are a number of miliary turbercles, and to the left and below is a typical tuberculous ulceration.

ncy by the tubercle bacillus which is amenable to surgical treatment, is one in which the changes are of such a gradual, insidious nature that the entire kidney may be destroyed before clinical symptoms result. This is especially true if the ureter becomes closed at an early stage or the foci do not communicate with the renal pelvis so that no pus from the involved organ escapes into the bladder and causes a secondary change here.

There has been considerable discussion as to which portion of the kidney is the primary area of localization of the tubercle bacilli. The work of Wildbolz has shown conclusively, however, that the first evidence of disease manifests itself near the base of the papilla where one of the divisions of the renal pelvis is reflected upon the surface of the papilla. Here the urinary stream is slowest and all conditions are favorable to lodgement and growth of the organism. The changes incident to such lodgement of the tubercle bacilli do not differ from those characteristic of tuberculosis in other portions of the body. The formation of tubercles, caseation, and resultant cavity formation produces a more or less extensive erosion of the papilla (Fig. 1). From this focus the entire kidney is invaded by way of the intrarenal lymphatics or blood vessels so that at a comparatively early stage it is extremely difficult to say which was the primary area of localization. The entire parenchyma shows typical tuberculous cavities which vary in size so that in the early cases there is still considerable tissue left between the individual cavities, while in the later stages the entire parenchyma has disappeared and is replaced by a series of cavities (Figs. 2 and 3) filled with a caseous detritus and separated from each other by connective tissue septa. This advanced stage is sometimes referred to as the tuberculous pyonephrosis or putty kidney, and is really a form of autonephrectomy. The latter condition is no doubt the one found in practically every tuberculous kidney which has been treated medically and in which the physician in charge boasts of a nonoperative cure. There being no longer any tissue to destroy and no communication with the renal pelvis, in the majority of such cases symptoms cease and an apparent cure is boasted of. Even under these conditions the presence of such a caseous kidney or tuberculous pyonephrosis, as it is sometimes spoken of, is a constant menace to the individual and I have encountered cases in which the opposite kidney was the seat of an advanced interstitial nephritis and there was a generalized miliary tuberculosis which had resulted from such an apparently dead kidney.

I have described the most frequent form of pathological change in the tuberculous kidney, but it is necessary to take into consideration the effects of such tuberculous invasion upon other portions of the urinary tract in order to get a clear idea of the importance of clinical symptoms.

As a result of the tuberculous ulceration of the papilla, the bacilli are discharged into the urinary stream and cause typical tuberculous changes in the renal pelvis, ureter and bladder. The changes characteristic of tuberculosis of the mucous membranes in other parts of the body take place wherever urine ladened with tubercle bacilli touches, and varies from simple invasion with submucous miliary tubercles to more or less extensive ulcerations. If such an ulceration happens to occur at the point where the ureter empties into the renal pelvis or further down in the ureter, secondary cicatricial changes may occur resulting in strictures at any point along the course of the ureter from its opening into the bladder to its junction with the renal pelvis. The sequel of such a stricture varies as elsewhere in the body with its degree of permeability, but not infrequently one encounters cases in which the entire ureter and renal pelvis are greatly dilated as the result of the back pressure above the point of stricture, or as in one of my cases, a typically large hydronephrosis is found, the tuberculous nature of which is not discovered except after most careful examination of the specimen.

The secondary changes in the bladder are, as a rule, most marked around the ureteral orifice of the side affected, and if operative relief does not come at an early period of the disease the tuberculous ulcerations may be found over the entire bladder. Soon the opposite ureter becomes involved and the tubercle bacilli begin to ascend toward the healthy kidney by way of the lymphatics in the wall of the ureter, as Bauerisen has so clearly shown. The changes in the opposite kidney are exactly those described for the primarily invaded kidney, except that the pathological changes are at first most marked in the pelvis, and then invade the parenchyma. The second or healthy kidney is not invaded in the majority of cases by the mode of ascending infection which I have just described until a comparatively late period, and it is this one fact in the pathology of tuberculosis of the kidney to which I wish to especially direct attention because this is the foundation stone of our modern treatment of tuberculosis of the kidney. If we can make a diagnosis before the opposite kidney is involved, we can promise complete recovery in seventy-five per cent. of the cases. If, however, the diagnosis is not made and the second kidney is already involved, the case is an absolutely hopeless one.

The less important and infrequent changes in tuberculosis of the kidney are a massive invasion of the organ similar in its widespread involvement to the diffuse acute caseous infiltration of a single lobe or even of the entire lung which one occasionally observes. Another peculiar but rare feature of renal tuberculosis is the tendency of the perinephritic tissue to become enormously thickened as the result of the same type of fibrous hyperplasia which is seen in the hyperplastic forms of tuberculosis of the cecum. In children, but less often in adults, the first clinical evidence of a tuberculosis of the kidneys may be the presence of a perinephritic abscess with or without external fistula, which is at times very difficult to differentiate from a psoas abscess of spinal origin. The ureter becomes greatly enlarged as the result of a diffuse infiltration of all of its coats and is often so thick that it can be felt through a thin abdominal wall or through the vagina.

That chronic tuberculosis of the kidney is invariably secondary to a primary focus elsewhere in the body there is no longer any doubt, but in the majority of cases the primary localization presents no symptoms. Pulmonary tuberculosis of the chronic type is very often complicated by a unilateral tuberculosis of the kidney and such a pulmonary condition is one of the contra-indications to removal of the kidney. To sum up, we are dealing with a very slowly progressive invasion of the kidney, the bacilli being carried by way of the blood stream as a rule to only one kidney and the invasion of the remainder of the urinary tract, including the opposite kidney, being secondary. If we can only eradicate the old notion that tuberculosis of the urinary tract begins in the bladder and spreads upward and that the symptoms of cystitis which the majority of the patients present as the predominating feature of the clinical picture, are the effect and not the cause, much will be accomplished toward securing a clearer idea of what we can do for these otherwise hopeless cases by early removal of the only kidney which is involved.

(To be continued in May Journal)

DETECTION OF GALL-STONES.

G. L. McWhorter, Chicago (*Journal A. M. A.*, March 6, 1918), advises the use of a waxed tipped filiform bougie for probing the bile ducts for stones that might otherwise be overlooked. The wax tip consists of from one-half to one part olive oil and one part dental wax, both thoroughly sterilized. The wax tip has been used in probing for ureteral stones and has been recommended by Harris as late as 1912, but its use in the bile ducts has not been previously described. The wax tip should be examined under a lens before using as well as after. If while passing the wax tip a decided jump should be felt, such as might be caused by a partly ensacculated stone, the chances of obtaining a definite scratch are improved by moving it back and forth several times.

RECENT ADVANCES IN THE DIAGNOSIS AND TREATMENT OF PNEUMONIA.*

By O. J. WALKER, M. D., Oklahoma City, Oklahoma.

The important place that pneumonia occupies among our infectious·diseases and the crying need of effective treatment is now generally recognized. Pneumonia as the cause of death ranks next to tuberculosis and even surpasses the latter disease in many of the larger centers of population. Our interest in this disease is further increased by the important part it plays in the non-combatant casualities in armies. During the Civil War pneumonia was next to typhoid and dysentery as the cause of death. Reports from our cantonments show that pneumonia ranks next to venereal diseases and measles as a cause of sickness. Contrary to the former teaching that pneumonia is a disease of infancy and old age, recent statistics show that over one-half of the cases occur between the ages of 20 and 50 years. Excepting erysipelas, probably there is no infectious disease for which more vaunted forms of treatment and so-called cures have been proposed than for pneumonia. Without exception there is no infectious disease in which treatment has accomplished less. Multiplicity of forms of treatment of any disease is one of the surest proofs that all are unsatisfactory and without avail.

The treatments commonly employed are the results of argument and refutation rather than the results of controlled observation and trial. Judgment as to their efficacy has been based upon theory and speculation rather than on critical scientific analysis of facts and figures. Recently accumulated knowledge of this disease and its various phenomena has been carefully and scientifically studied so that now the physician is able to employ at least a few measures based on critical study.

Lobar pneumonia, as is well known, is "an acute, infectious disease, characterized by a diffuse exudative inflammation of entire portions of one or more lobes of the lung". Etiologically pneumonia is not always due to any one disease germ. Probably in 85 to 90 per cent. of cases the diplococcus pneumonia of Frankel can be found. In the remaining 10 to 15 per cent. of cases the etiological agents may be Friedlander's bacillus, bacillus influenza, streptococcus pyogenes, streptococcus mucosus, staphylococcus aureus and a few others.

In 1910 Neufeld demonstrated that all races of the pneumococcus are identical insofar as their immunologic reactions are concerned, i. e. agglutination and precipitation. Following this suggestion Avery, Chickering, Cole and Dochez working at the Rockerfeller Institute have studied for the past few years the agglutination and precipitin reactions of a large number of different strains of pneumococcus and have tested the power of immune serum to protect mice. As a result of their work the pneumococcus has been divided into four main types, i. e. I, II, III, and IV. Type III consists of the pneumococcus mucosus capsulatus, readily recognized by its morphologic and staining characteristics. Type IV includes a heterogenuous group which does not give the immunologic reactions common to the members of any of the other groups. Fortunately this latter group represents only about 25 per cent. of all strains isolated and is the type most frequently encountered in the mouth secretions of normal individuals. Reference to table I, taken from the reprints of Rockefeller Institute, will show the incidents of these various types and their relation to mortality. From a prognostic standpoint it will be seen that Type III, although the least common, is the most virulent. Type IV is the least virulent. Types I and II together are responsible for 64 per cent. of all cases, and are of relatively high virulence in man, causing approximately 62 per cent. of all deaths from pneumonia. Infections from Types I and II are obtained from contact with patients infected with these types. Types III and IV are found frequently in the mouth of normal individuals. A person may harbor in his mouth and throat organisms of Type IV and be infected from without by Types I, II, or III. A reference to table II suggests that the

---

*Read before St. Anthony Hospital Clinical Society, Dec. 17, 1917.

presence of the pneumococcus in the blood stream indicates a severe infection and a consequent unfavorable prognosis. Table III shows relation of total leukocyte count to mortality and emphasizes the importance from a prognostic standpoint of daily white blood counts.

The following may be noted from a study of blood changes during the course of this disease: 1. A steady rise in the leukocyte count is usually of favorable import. 2. An initial low count with no tendency toward increase is of grave prognosis. 3. The total number of white blood cells falls rapidly to normal at the time of crisis. If this does not occur it is suggestive of some complication, for example, a continued leukocytosis after crisis with diminished polymorphonuclears and increased leukocytes suggest delayed resolution, or serum sickness in treated cases.

As a result of experiments and study by Cole and his co-workers on the power of immune serum to convey protection, an anti-pneumococcic serum of wonderful efficacy has been produced. Without going into details of the method of producing this serum, a very good idea will be obtained by the reader when I refer him to the well known method employed in the production of diphtheria antitoxin. Anti-pneumococcic serum is produced by immunization of the horse after the same principles employed in the latter method. However, the serum

TABLE I[1]
Incidence of the Various Types of the Pneumococcus and Resulting Mortality.

Type of Pneumococcus	Incidence Per Cent.	Mortality Per Cent.
I	33	25
II	31	32
III	12	45
IV	24	16

TABLE II[1]
Relation of Blood Cultures to Mortality in Pneumonia.

Types	No. of Cases	Blood Cultures				Mortality			
		Positive		Negative		Cases with Positive Culture		Cases with Negative Culture	
		No.	%	No.	%	No.	%	No.	%
I	145	50	34.5	95	65.5	13	26	3	3.1
II	148	49	33.1	99	66.9	36	73.4	9	9
III	55	16	29	39	71	16	100	11	28.2
IV	100	21	21	79	79	11	52.3	3	3.8
Total	488	136	30.3	312	69.7	76	55.8	26	8.3

TABLE III[1]
Relation of Total Leukocytes to Mortality.

Leukocytes	No. of Cases	Mortality %
Under 10,000	29	65.5
10,000 to 20,000	143	23.7
20,000 to 30,000	177	18.0
30,000 to 40,000	76	14.4
40,000 to 50,000	29	24.1
Above 50,000	9	11.0
Total	463	

·has been found to be protective and curative only when homologous with the type of organism causing the infection. Furthermore, the serum of Type I is not only the most effective but is the only one recommended by the Rockefeller workers as dependable for therapeutic purposes. Serums for Types II and III are only slightly effective, while obviously it is impossible to prepare a serum for the heterogeneous strains composing Type IV.

Treatment.

Treatment of pneumonia must begin with the diagnosis, and it is important not only that the diagnosis be made as early as possible but that the specific etiologic agent be determined in each case, when the history and physical findings indicate we are dealing with pneumonia. The treatment thereafter may be outlined as follows:

1. Determination of type of pneumococcus. (a) Obtain specimen of sputum. (b) Take blood culture. (c) Obtain specimen of urine. ⟨d⟩ Test patient for sensitization to horse serum.

2. Intravenous administration of serum.

3. Additional measures of treatment.

Obviously to make an etiologic diagnosis requires the facilities of a laboratory equipped to do this work. As a detailed account of the technique of the laboratory methods employed is hardly within the scope of this paper, the reader is referred to "The Monographs of Rockefeller Institute of Medical Research," No. VII. In order that the laboratory manipulations be carried out with success, however, it is very important that a specimen of sputum be obtained early in the disease, and care be taken that this sputum be coughed up from the lung and not simply consist of the saliva which the patient has expectorated. In addition, the blood culture should be taken because of its confirmatory value when positive, in determining the type, and also because of its prognostic value as noted in table II. Furthermore, it has been found that the urine of pneumonia patients frequently contains a substance which gives a precipitin reaction with immune serum, so that when this substance is present the early determination of the type may often be facilitated, or it is at least of confirmatory value. This precipitin substance is also found in pleural and spinal fluid and may be utilized for diagnosis of type in these substances.

Owing to the high susceptibility of the white mouse to pneumococcus infection, this animal is made use of in isolating a pure culture of the organism in the shortest possible time. By reason of the high invasive power of these organisms for the mouse, a pure culture may usually be obtained in from 8 to 16 hours following the injection intraperitoneally of a small quantity of emulsified sputum. The culture of pneumococci thus obtained from the peritoneal exudate is mixed with small quantities of immune serum of the various types and gives an agglutination reaction with its homologous serum. Owing to the great demand for white mice to carry out this technique in the army camps and large cities of the country, breeders have been unable to supply the demand. At the Bierce Memorial Laboratory we have been for some time running tests with the ordinary brown house mouse. Although our series is yet small, so far we have found the wild mouse just as susceptible and as applicable for the test as the white mouse. The brown mouse may be readily obtained in any community at little or no cost by trapping them in the miniature wire cages for sale in any hardware store. They may be handled without danger from biting if the worker simply wears a pair of heavy gloves. I make this preliminary report of our work, in the hope that the use of the wild mouse may serve to tide over the present deficiency in the supply of white mice.

If serum treatment of pneumonia is being contemplated, steps should be taken at once to determine whether or not the patient is sensitive to horse serum. Questioning the patient and his friends as to previous administration of serum will occasionally elicit this history. Nevertheless, even though this history is negative, it is always advisable to perform the cutaneous test for sensitization to horse serum. This is usually best performed at the time of taking the blood culture, blood count, etc., and consists of injection intra-cutaneously of .002 of 1 c.c. of horse serum, and controlling it with a similar amount of salt solution. If the patient be sensitive, there will appear at the site of injection of horse serum a definite urticarial wheal within an hour. In case of sensitization there is time, while the laboratory is working out the type, to desensitize the patient and so prepare him for the administration of the anti-pneumococcic serum if necessary. The reader is referred to the above-mentioned monograph for the details of this procedure. If the patient has a pneumococcic infection of type I, serum treatment is indicated. This is administered intravenously by means of a salvarsan outfit. The doasge varies with the individual case, but usually is given in large quantities—75 to 100 c.c. This dose is repeated every 8 hours, unless contra-indications arise, until a permanent fall of temperature results. The average dosage per case has been found to be about 250 c.c. Usually from 20 minutes to one hour after the administration of the serum there is noted a rise in temperature, followed immediately by a marked fall. This is known as the thermal reaction. If the temperature continues low from this on, a good result has been obtained. The temperature is taken every two hours and if there is a rise to 102 degrees F. in the succeeding twenty-four hours, the dose is repeated. If there is no temperature drop after eight hours following the treatment, a second·dose is to be given.

A small number of cases may be expected to obtain relief following the first injection. The majority, however, require a second, third, or even more administrations. In almost all cases the patient's condition has been found to improve subjectively and objectively. He is better mentally, shows less cyanosis, and there is a decided diminution of the pulse rate. At all events the progress of the disease has been stopped, because: 1. In practically all cases treated with serum, there has been found to be no further extension of the process in the lung. 2. Invasion of the blood streams by the pneumococcus is prevented. In cases where septicemia is already present the blood has become sterile. 3. There is an appearance of immune bodies which ordinarily appear only at time of crisis. This may be due largely to the immune bodies present in the serum· injected. 4. There is a disappearance of the precipitin substance from the urine if it has been previously present.

Resolution has not been found to be hastened following administration of serum. However, neither has it been interferred with or delayed. Complications are not prevented by the administration of serum. In fact it is a well known principle that infection is apt to become focal in partly immunized animals. Nevertheless there has been found no increase in complications following serum treatment.

The final test of the efficacy of this treatment depends upon its effect on mortality. Of the 107 cases treated at Rockefeller Hospital, eight died with a resulting mortality of 7.5 per cent. Peter Bent Brigham Hospital, Boston, reports ten cases treated with 9.1 per cent. mortality. When these results are contrasted with the twenty-five to thirty per cent mortality for type I in cases treated by former methods, the value of this procedure is evident.

The following measures of treatment should not be neglected as a supplement to the above procedure:

1. If the case is detected early, it is always best treated in a hospital if such facilities are in easy reach. If the patient is to be treated at home, every effort should be made to provide every means possible for the carrying out of the treatment.

2. When once a patient is found to have pneumonia, he should not be allowed to exert himself in any manner whatsoever. He should not be allowed to

sit up in bed, even for physical examinations. Only such physical examinations should be made as are necessary to follow the course of the disease. ·

. 3. Open air treatment is undoubtedly a great aid in the treatment of most patients, particularly as it adds to their comfort, relieving the short, rapid, labored respirations, and quieting the restlessness and distress. However, some patients will be found on whom the open air seems to exert the exact opposite effect. Obviously these are best treated indoors.

4. The diet is not of great importance in this disease, owing to its short duration. It should consist of simple, easily digested·nourishing food which is pleasing to the patient. The patient should ingest plenty of water, as much as 3000 c.c. or more per day

5. Little good is derived by active purgation of these patients, in fact harm may be done by the consequent disturbance. A better procedure is to insure a daily bowel movement by use of a mild laxative or enema.

6. Few, if any, drugs are ever indicated in this disease. Cole recommends the early administration of digitalis in dosage sufficient to obtain the cumulative action of the drugs so that in case the heart needs support at the time of crisis the physiological effect is quickly attained. This object is accomplished most easily by the administration of one gram of digipuratum by mouth over a period of two days. At the end of this time, if the patient's condition does not indicate its further use, the drug is discontinued. Digipuratum is used because of its accurate standardization and ease of administration, and is given by mouth in preference to the intravenous method because of the no small danger attendant with the latter procedure.

7. A persistent and tenacious cough accompanied by pain in the chest is probably best treated by small doses of morphine subcutaneously. No local measures can be relied upon in all cases. Poultices and applications of cold frequently give relief. Creosote inhalations often prove of value in relieving the cough. Alcohol may be given to alcoholics.

8. Abdominal distention is frequently quite a disturbing accompaniment, but may usually be relieved by use of hot turpentine stupes, enema, or pituitrin hypodermically.

It is not possible at this time to discuss the various complications that may arise, but obviously it is one of the chief duties of the physician to keep a sharp lookout for them and to meet them when danger signals appear.

Prophylactic immunization has proven successful in animals and is theoretically possible in man. However, there is a considerable variation in the amount of natural susceptibility and immunity in different individuals. Cole has suggested that this might be detected by a method similar to the Schick test. We will all watch with interest work that is being done along this line in the armies at the present time.

References:

1. Acute Lobar Pneumonia: Prevention and Serum Treatment. Oswald T. Avery, H. T. Chickering, Rufus Cole, and A. R. Dochez, Monograph No. 7, Rockefeller Institute.

2. The Treatment of Lobar Pneumonia. Rufus I. Cole, Medical Clinics of North America, Vol. 1, No. 3, p. 545, Nov., 1917.

3. Pneumonia Among Soldiers in Camps, Cantonments and at the Front. S. Aldolphus Knopf, *New York Medical Journal*, Jan. 26, 1918, p. 165.

4. Observation at the Peter Bent Brigham Hospital on Cases of Pneumonia in Relation to Types of Pneumococci and the Serum Treatment of Type 1 Cases. H. L. Alexander, *Boston Medical & Surgical Journal*, CLXXVII-25, p. 874.

TUBERCLE BACILLI IN THE BLOOD OF TUBERCULOUS ANIMALS AND MAN.*

By HOWARD S. BROWNE, B. A.; Ph. C., M. S.

Dean of the School of Pharmacy, Oklahoma University, Norman, Oklahoma.

A study of the literature on the subject of the presence of tubercle bacilli in the blood of tuberculous patients reveals much conflict in opinion and experimental evidence.

That turbercle bacilli enter the blood vessels and are generalized by means of the circulatory blood is of course unquestioned, but to what extent this generalization takes place is still unsettled. The question has been raised, is the bacillemia in tuberculosis enough or so marked that it can be demonstrated and utilized as a means of diagnosis? In acute miliary tuberculosis the bacilli are particularly likely to be found in the circulatory blood, according to Wilson[1]. In this case the demonstration of their presence would be of practical importance in the early diagnosis of doubtful cases.

Wilson shows that tubercle bacilli can be demonstrated in stained sections of blood and clots obtained at autopsy from the heart and great vessels of a case of acute miliary tuberculosis but that the number of bacilli in the circulatory blood at any given moment is too small to be of any practical diagnostic value.

The case which Dr. Wilson reports, has a history as follows: A housewife, aged 52 years, with negative family history as regards tuberculosis, became ill about October 21, 1914, with a feeling of unusual fatigue, fever and slight chilly sensations, increasing toxemia, rapidly progressing anemia, weakness and dyspnea without any signs of localized disease. Death occurred one month later, November 29, 1914.

Autoposy showed primary miliary tuberculosis in the bronchial nodes, lungs, liver, spleen, bone marrow, kidney amd myocardium. The case certainly appears very favorable for the presence of tubercle bacilli in the blood. The large white clots and blood found in the right side of the heart were imbedded, cut and stained for tubercle bacilli. In all, about one-tenth of the entire large clot was searched carefully for the bacilli and only four typical slender acid fast bacilli were found. Sections of the tubercular lesions of the organs stained in the same manner showed the presence of enormous numbers of bacilli. The above illustrates in a measure the difficulty of detecting the organisms in the blood.

Dieterle[2] claims that the tubercle bacilli entering the blood stream quickly disappear from the circulatory blood. He maintains that it is possible that in an ordinary case all the tubercle bacilli entering the pulmonary veins from a primary bronchial gland focus, and passing into the arterial blood, might disappear from the venous blood by the time it reached the right heart.

Dieterle took 60 c.c. of blood clot from the right auricle and ventricle of a case of primary tuberculosis of the cervical lymph nodes, cut it into 60 sections and spent 60 hours searching for bacilli. He found 4 typical tubercle bacilli and 15 suspicious fragments which he disregarded. He thinks that the blood drawn from the living patient will probably give results more frequently in cases in which the primary focus is in the lungs or bronchial nodes.

Brandies[3] reports on the examination of blood from 400 cases of surgical tuberculosis with positive results in 45 per cent of these cases using 5 c. c. of blood treated by the Schnitter-Uhlenhart antiformin method. This strengthens the belief that the attempt may not be as difficult as it seems.

J. L. Berry[4] of the Department of Health, New York City, has a very interesting report in which she stated that the first investigation in this field seems to have been by Villemin, who in 1868 obtained inoculative results with the blood in miliary tuberculosis. Weichselbaum in 1884 found tubercle bacilli microscopically in otherwise sterile blood from miliary tuberculosis. Next followed Ludke[5]

---

*Read before the Cleveland County Medical Society, Norman, Oklahoma.

who demonstrated the presence of tubercle bacilli in the blood in a varying percentage of cases. Bergeron in 1904 stated that tubercle bacilli are found in the blood in miliary tuberculosis in relatively rare cases and that in non-miliary tuberculosis, even of a rapid type, bacillemia does not exist.

In 1909 the Staubli-Schnitter method of identifying the bacilli in the blood was introduced. The method is briefly as follows: 10-15 c.c. of blood from a vein are added to a like amount of 2-3 per cent. citric acid or a double the amount of acetic acid, then carefully shaken and allowed to stand for one-half hour. The fluid is centrifuged and pipetted off and 1 c.c. of water is added to the sediment Then 2 to 5 times the amount of 15 per cent. antiformin is added and the mixture is shaken. As soon as solution is complete, which happens very quickly, the mixture is again centrifuged, the fluid pipetted off and the slight deposit is washed and examined by the Ziehl-Nielson stain.

Schnitter[6] found acid fast bacilli in 31.6 per cent. of 38 cases of tuberculosis and concludes that tubercle bacilli are probably regularly present in the blood in organic tuberculosis.

Just previous to this Rosenberger[7] published a report of 100 per cent positive microscopic results in 49 cases of tuberculosis of all stages, 5 miliary. On the contrary, Schroeder and Cotton,[8] Burvill-Holmes,[9] and other American workers attempted to repeat Rosenberger's work, using the same method, but utterly failed to reach the same conclusions. A like result was reached by the English investigators, Hewatt and Sutherland,[10] working with cattle. In contradiction, Forsythe[11] with the same method reported 100 per cent positive results in ten open cases of tuberculosis and negative results in two closed cases.

Anderson[12] in repeating Rosenberger's work used inoculation and culture tests on guinea pigs. He found all direct microscopic examinations of blood were negative and that of 83 guinea pigs inoculated intraperitoneally with human blood, none developed tuberculosis. However, the blood of thirteen tuberculous guinea pigs gave no positive results when injected into other guinea pigs and with 8 infected rabbits the blood of 7 produced tuberculosis in guinea pigs. In three cases rabbit blood specimens gave cultures of tuberculosis, this being the first time, according to Anderson, that successful cultures have been reported from rabbit blood.

Lippmann[13] using the Staubli-Schnitter method found 44 per cent. of 25 cases of pulmonary tuberculosis positive in all stages.

Berry (vide supra) gives a very exhaustive resume of the work of many investigators whose findings vary from 0 per cent in 15 cases to 100 per cent. in 155 cases, with an average from 16 workers with 1372 cases of 52 per cent. showing the presence of tubercle bacilli in the blood. With extremely careful technic and favorable conditions, Berry examined 51 specimens of blood from 51 tuberculous patients. Of these, 13 were from patients in the second stage and 38 from patients in the third stage of the disease, 4 of the latter being bed patients. A most careful search was made, from 150 to 300 microscopic fields being examined with each specimen, and in all cases the results were negative. From the above results Dr. Berry concludes that tubercle bacilli are at least very rare in the blood, if present at all.

Kessel[14] employed five methods in search for the bacilli in the blood. He used the blood direct from tuberculous patients treated and stained as mentioned in the Staubli-Schnitter method, and secondly he inoculated guinea pigs intraperitoneally with the blood of tubercular patients. The pigs were previously tested with tuberculin to see if they were free from the disease.

Third, the blood from the turberculous patients who had previously received an injection of tuberculin was inoculated intraperitoneally into guinea pigs.

Fourth, the blood from tuberculous patients who had previously received a tuberculin injection, and after removal of the serum intraperitoneal injections were made into guinea pigs.

Fifth, the blood after removal of the serum, was planted upon culture tubes of gentian-violet media.

His results by these methods were as follows:

First method: The blood from 10 patients was examined microscopically with negative results.

Second method: In blood from 38 patients inoculated into guinea pigs and at autopsy two to three months later there was no evidence of tuberculosis.

Third method: Seven patients were used. Autopsies of the guinea pigs showed negative findings.

Fourth method: Three patients were used. One of the guinea pigs developed an extensive tuberculosis.

Fifth method: Was unsuccessful.

Kessel concludes that a bacillemia such as is present in other infectious diseases, is at least uncommon in pulmonary tuberculosis even in the advanced stages of the disease.

Watkins[15] maintains that tubercle bacilli can be detected in the fresh blood of a patient suffering with tuberculosis by means of a migraf, a specially devised attachment for a miscroscope.

Hess[16] performed some very interesting experiments upon rabbits and guinea pigs with rather interesting results. Four rabbits were injected for each test, two with the human type of bacillus and two with the bovine type. Later 16 guinea pigs were injected with blood from these rabbits and after six weeks were examined for tuberculosis.

In all twenty-four rabbits and one hundred twelve guinea pigs were used this way. The results were as follows: Of the pigs injected with bovine blood, sixty-nine per cent were found tuberculous. Of those injected with human blood, 18.5 per cent. developed tuberculosis. Hess concludes that there is a certain parallelism between the virulence of the tubercle bacillus and its persistence in the circulation of the rabbit.

In another series of tests, Hess[17] found that a feebly virulent type of bacillus was present in only nine per cent. of the tests whereas the virulent bovine bacillus persisted in the blood stream in 59 per cent. of the cases. He concludes from these tests that virulence plays an important role in bacteriemia.

McFarland[18] after demonstrating that acid fast bacilli are found in many samples of distilled water, concludes that the reports of many of the cases of acid fast bacilli are due to faulty methods and technic.

Conclusion.

(1) Tubercle bacilli are in the blood of patients suffering with acute miliary tuberculosis more frequently than in the more chronic types of tuberculosis.

(2) The bacilli are not present in great numbers and are undoubtedly more numerous at times in the blood stream.

(3) Owing to the fact that distilled and tap water have been found to contain acid fast organisms and that the stroma of red blood corpuscles, lecithin and cholesterin are acid fast and may be mistaken for tubercle bacilli, the posibility of error is considerable, therefore it is very difficult to make a positive diagnosis of tubercle bacilli in the blood.

(4) Many cases of so-called tubercle bacilli in the blood are due to the above facts coupled with faulty technic.

(5) Inoculation experiments show that guinea pigs and rabbits are more susceptible to tuberculosis when injected with bovine blood than when injected with human blood from tuberculous patients.

Bibliography.

(1). Wilson, U. F. Bacillemia in tuberculosis as shown by the examination of post mortem clots from the heart. Jr. Inf. Dis., 19-260-266.
(2). Dieterle, Robt. R. Bacillemia in tuberculosis. Jr. Inf. Diseases, 19-263-266.
(3). Brandies, Deutsch Med. Wchnsche, 1913, 39, p. 1137.
(4). Berry, J. L. Tubercle Bacilli in the Blood. Jr. Inf. Diseases, 14-162-175.
(5). Ludke, Wein Klein Wchsche, 1906, U. S., p. 949.
(6). Schnitter, Deutsche Med. Wnehnsche, 1909, 35, p. 1566.
(7). Rosenberger, Am. Jr. Med. Sc., 1909, U. S., 137, p. 267.
(8). Schroeder & Cotton–Bull. 116, Bureau of Animal Industry, U. S. Dept. Agri., 1909.
(9). Burvill–Holmes, Am. Jr. Med. Sc., 1910, 139, p. 99.
(10). Hewatt & Sutherland, Brit. Med. Jr., 1909, 1, p. 1119.
(11). Forsyth, Ibid. p.,1001.
(12). Anderson, Bull. 57-59 Hyg. Lab. U. S. Pub. Health Service, 1909, p. 7.
(13). Lippmann, Munchen Med. Wchnsche, 1909, 56, p. 2214.
(14). Kessel, Am. Jr. Med. Sc., 1915, 150, p. 377.
(15). Watkins, Medical Times, June, 1913, 14, p. 172.
(16). Hess, Proc. Soc. Exper. Biol. Med., N. Y., 1911, 12, pp. 9-75.
(17). Hess, Arch. Int. Med., Chicago, 1912, 10, p. 577.
(18). McFarland, Henry Phipps Inst. Report, 1908, 10, Vol. 6, p. 127.

THYROID IN UTERINE HEMORRHAGE.*

By O. C. KLASS, M. D., Muskogee, Oklahoma.

Because of the great numbers of women suffering with and from irregular, profuse, and persistent uterine bleedings or hemorrhages, without assignable cause, unexplainable, which are finally thrown into surgery, because of no better known means of alleviation, which in itself makes the result worse than the primary disease, especially in the very young patients, and due to the fact that my attention has been called to a series of the herein mentioned cases, of such character, where the most surprising, encouraging, satisfactory results were obtained through administration of thyroid extract, I was prompted to present this article.

There have been a great variety of pathological conditions due to faulty secretions of the thyroid gland, and while this subject may not be new to most well informed students of medicine, yet its use in the treatment of uterine hemorrhage, and allied conditions, is practically new. American and foreign literature is scarce and lacking in reports of use and experience of thyroid extract, in such cases, so that what is presented in this paper is new, limited and largely assumed, to a degree, until time and further experimentation fix its use and results more certainly and definitely.

E. Sehrt (Munch Med. Woch, May 6, 1913, LX No. 18, pp. 961-1016; Feb 10, 1914, LXI No. 6, pp. 289-344), (A. M. A Jour., June 14, 1913 (104), p. 1930, March 21, 1914 (90), p. 974), reviews the recent researches, which demonstrates anew the close relationship existing between the thyroid and genital organs. Excessive or insufficient function of the thyroid caused a change in the blood so that a relative reduction in the neutrophil-leukocytes and a relative or absolute leukocytosis occurred, yet with excessive thyroid functioning coagulability of the blood is greatly reduced, also with insufficiency of thyroid coagulation is hastened.

This effect of abnormal conditions in the thyroid, on the coagulating power of the blood, throws light on certain cases of hemorrhagic uterine disturbances, suggesting, that they might be abortive forms of myxodema. In 20 pure cases of hemorrhagic uterine disturbances, 13 patients showed pronounced signs and evidences of thyroid-hypo-functioning and the coagulating time in all but one was between eight and four minutes, in contrast to nine to ten minutes in the normal blood.

He (Sehrt) also remarks that the thyroid may be involved in the tendency to

---

*Read before Muskogee County Medical Society.

habitual abortion.   He states further that cases have been reported where women married for many years never conceived, but bore children after being placed upon thyroid extract treatment.

This shows, therefore, that syphilis is not responsible for all cases of habitual abortion.   (I trust you will pardon this digression from main topic).   Sehrt further states that since there is an intimate connection between the function of the thyroid gland and the ovaries, the former may be responsible for various ovarian conditions giving rise to uterine hemorrhages.   In 55 cases of uterine hemorrhage, without apparent local cause, thirty-eight showed signs of deficient thyroid action, and under thyroid administration not only was the hemorrhage arrested but the general health improved.

Osborne (*N. Y. Med. Jour.*, Dec. 1, 1906) states he has seen uterine hemorrhage in fleshy women with slow pulse cease under thyroid treatment, yet on the other hand underweight women with amenorrhea to be relieved and profuse menstruation induced in healthy women.

S. Salzman of Toledo (*Am. Jour. of Obstetrics*, Diseases of Women and Children, Vol. LXXIV, No. 5, Nov. 1916) has been doing a great deal of personal work, in attempting to show the relation existing between thyroid and pelvic organs, having used thyroid extract in uterine hemorrhage of unassignable cause, with very gratifying and encouraging results, being seemingly one of the pioneers in this research work.

Dudley (*Principles of Gynecology*, 1904) classifies unknown uterine hemorrhages into the hemorrhage of puberty and menopause, and it is at these periods of life that thyroid disturbances are most likely to occur.

Falta (*Diseases of Ductless Glands*, page 118) states chronic benign hypothyrodism is accompanied by disturbances of sleep, lassitude, especially in the morning, and menstrual disturbances, especially menorrhagia and amenorrhea.

Most cases of uterine hemorrhage can be assigned to such pathological conditions as incomplete abortion with retained secundines, infected endometrium, fibroids, polyps, uterine cancer, ovarian tumors or cysts, diseased tubes, etc., yet there are numerous other cases, where the real, definite cause is not ascertainable, where any and all measures have utterly failed in the treatment.

Since menstrual blood is non-coaguable and also the blood coming from the uterus in these cases, we are led to the final conclusion that there is and must be some substance or secretion that can and does control the same.   Sturmdorf (*A. M. A. Jour.*, Feb. 14, 1914) states in his article on "Functional Menorrhagia", that a protest should be made against the too frequent, routine, unnecessary, use and abuse of the curette, also removal of the pelvic organs in these cases.   He further states: "It must suffice here to state that the endometrium during menstruation and in the hemorrhagic cases receives normal coaguable blood from the general circulation and sheds this blood in a non-coaguable state.   This loss of coaguability is not due to the absence or deterioration of any element essential to the coagulation but to the presence of an inhibiting substance that is periodically secreted by the corporeal endometrium from which it may be expressed.   Such expressed endometrial juice is capable of inhibiting in any normal blood. * * The endometrium is active to the secretion of this inhibiting substance by a hormone generated in the graafian follicle.   To the present time we have not succeeded in isolating this substance, nor have we discovered its specific antagonist. We have, however, learned to circumvent it by effectual measures."   These measures he refers to are vasodilators, local application of acetone, liquor formaldehyde, D'arsonal spark, the treatment to extend over periods of several months.   This local treatment extending over prolonged periods cannot be expected to produce an anti-inhibiting substance which is a hormone produced in another part of the body.

There have and do occur, innumerable cases of intractable bleeding, in young women just entering upon the catamenial life, young women past puberty, primipara, multipara, etc., without assignable cause, where all forms and sorts of treatment, ordinarily used, both internal and local, have proven of absolutely no benefit whatsoever, so that we stand helplessly by, with only one alternative, seemingly—surgery, castration. My attention was drawn to this subject by the articles of Sehrt, Salzman, etc., and in despair begun to look up the treatment and use it with very gratifying and encouraging results.

In the cases of menorrhagia at the advent of puberty, Salzman suspicions and concludes that there is a possible relationship existing between the simple nontoxic forms of goiter and chlorosis, in these cases, since most of these young women are suffering with some form of anemia. If such relationship exists, which he (Salzman) is led to believe does, then the administration of thyroid would be of some possible benefit.

I recall several cases in my own practice, where the administration of thyroid extract, in young girls between the ages of twelve and sixteen, just entering upon the menstrual period of life, where profuse bleedings over long periods had existed, without evidences of the existence of goiter, chlorosis, etc., after all ordinary measures had been resorted to, were promptly relieved and greatly benefited by the administration of this gland extract. I have also been amazed to find two cases of fibroid degeneration of the uterus, one in particular, with the loss of great amounts of blood, and the other with a small amount of the bloody discharge, both stopping in a short time under the administration of thyroid extract, after all other medicinal measures had proven useless and without result.

I recall another case in a lady, married, forty years of age, mother of two children, youngest twelve years, always having been regular and without abnormal symptoms during menstruation, stated that she was called to the north to be at the bedside of her father, where she administered unto him for several weeks until he died, so that about a week thereafter she began to have flooding spells, which lasted several weeks and finally consulted a physician who succeeded in checking them. These spells came on about every three weeks thereafter, and continued for ten days to two weeks, causing her to be very weak and anemic. She would lie down, use cold to abdomen, upon the advice of another practitioner, and took ergot without effect. Packings and in fact all the ordinary means had been used for controlling same, without effect. I was asked to see her, and upon examination, both internal and external, could find no condition to account for same, and also after trying all the usual medication recommended therefor, finally placed her upon thyroid treatment, and to my great satisfaction had all cleared up in three days time, to remain that way. She left the city about a year ago, and up to that time had not been troubled therewith. This case was advised by her other medical attendant that panhysterectomy would be her only salvation, and happy I was to be able to spare her this tremendous shock and sacrifice. I also used by way of trial, having seen it used by Adler (Schauta Klinik, Vienna) calcium lactate in fifteen grain doses every four hours, without effect.

If you will pardon the report of a case I, by accident, was permitted to see that occurred at the other end of the body, hemorrhage following the extraction of a tooth, in which after twenty-four hours attempt to control same, the bleeding persisted, and finally when all known specific, sure-shot measures had been used, the last one, so-called panacea, consisting of iodin and chloroform, also failed, this being a case of so-called floating clot, in posterior molar tooth socket, was asked to see the case in the final treatment and advised the use of thyroid extract. The young man without history of being or coming from a family of bleeders, was getting weak from the constant oozing and after taking three tablets at two hour intervals, the hemorrhage ceased and has remained absent to date. This was an experiment but worked beautifully, yet was interesting, since it had never been used for such cases. I recently saw a young married lady, the mother of two children, age twenty-five, who reports that she only menstruates every four or five months, and then very little, is nervous, emotional, has hot and cold flashes, headaches, etc. When menstruation does occur it is very scanty and only lasts a day or two. I used every known means to relieve her, could find no evidence of strumous diathesis, etc., finally in despair placed her on thyroid extract, five grains three times daily, to be rewarded by the report that after three weeks treatment, her menstruation occurred, the most natural in color, amount and duration she had had in five years time. Her nervousness has become less, hot and cold flashes disappearing, insomnia giving way to peaceful, refreshing sleep, headache gone, and whole general condition greatly benefited.

These are only a few reports, considering the vast numbers that are seen daily by those of larger clientele, but are sufficient to cause us to direct our attentions to this line of treatment in the attempted solution of the great array of unexplainable menstrual disorders, hoping by more concerted application and experimentation therewith, our results and scope of application may be broadened, and more gratifying.

I conclude, in the identical words of Salzman, to-wit: There is a type of hemorrhage from the uterus not caused by any discernable pelvic disease or pathology, nor related to any of the so-called hemorrhage states, but due to an alteration or lack of one or more of the harmones, which control the normal flow of the blood from the uterus. This alteration is due to a deficiency in the secretion of the thyroid gland and such hemorrhage can therefore be controlled by a judicious exhibition of the dried glandular thyroid substance.

Finally, I would caution against the indiscriminate use of this substance. It must be used only when the diagnosis is assured, for bleeding may occur in cases of hyperthyroidism, where much harm might be done if given in such a case.

HERNIA.

J. C. Bloodgood, Baltimore (*Journal A. M. A.*, Feb. 23, 1918), calls attention to a small group of hernias that can be readily recognized at the first examination, but which are more liable, than others, to recur or fail to be cured by operation. They can be recognized when the patient is examined lying flat on his back. If the finger is pressed against the scrotum and pushed up into the external ring, as the index finger passes through the external ring (the hernia having been reduced) it usually meets an obstruction (the conjoined tendon) and is deflected upward and outward following the course of the so-called internal ring. In this smaller group the index finger meets no obstruction, but enters at once into the peritoneal cavity. Now and then one gets the impression that it does this in other cases, but if the patient is asked to raise his head, the noncontracting rectus muscle pulls tight the relaxed conjoined tendon and the examiner readily recognizes that it is not absent but simply relaxed. In those cases in which the examination detects the complete absence of the conjoined tendon, the ordinary operation for inguinal hernia fails to cure in about 50 per cent. of the cases, according to Bloodgood's observations. After his first observation of this in 1898, Bloodgood devised and published a description of the transplantation of the rectus muscle to take the place of the conjoined tendon, and this he found had been independently worked out by Woelfler in 1898. Later, Halsted modified the transplantation of the rectus muscle by turning down a pedunculated flap of the anterior sheath of the rectus. He calls attention to this class, thinking it may be of service to examining physicians of the large cantonments now in use.

JOURNAL OF THE OKLAHOMA STATE MEDICAL ASSOCIATION

VOLUME XI	MUSKOGEE, OKLA., APRIL, 1918	NUMBER 4

PUBLISHED MONTHLY AT MUSKOGEE, OKLA., UNDER DIRECTION OF THE COUNCIL

DR. CLAUDE A. THOMPSON, EDITOR-IN-CHIEF

ENTERED AT THE POST OFFICE AT MUSKOGEE, OKLAHOMA, AS SECOND CLASS MAIL MATTER, JULY 28, 1912

THIS IS THE OFFICIAL JOURNAL OF THE OKLAHOMA STATE MEDICAL ASSOCIATION. ALL COMMUNICATIONS SHOULD BE ADDRESSED TO THE JOURNAL OF THE OKLAHOMA STATE MEDICAL ASSSOCIATION, 307-8 SURETY BUILDING, MUSKOGEE, OKLAHOMA.

The editorial department is not responsible for the opinions expressed in the original articles of contributors.

Reprints of original articles will be supplied at actual cost, provided request for them .s attached to manuscript or made in sufficient time before publication.

Articles sent this Journal for publication and all those read at the annual meetings of the State Association are the sole property of this Journal. The Journal relies on each individual contributor's strict adherence to this well-known rule of medical journalism. In the event an article sent this Journal fo· publication is published before appearance in the Journal, the manuscript will be returned to the writer.

Failure to receive the Journal should call for immediate notification of the editor, 307-8 Surety Building, Muskogee, Okla

Local news of possible interest to the medical profession, notes on removals, changes in address, deaths and weddings will be gratefully received.

Advertising of articles, drugs or compounds unapproved by the Council on Pharmacy of the A. M. A. will not be accepted.

Advertising rates will be supplied on application. It is suggested that wherever possible members of the State Association should patronize our advertisers in preference to others as a matter of fair reciprocity.

EDITORIAL

NEW NEEDS OF THE ARMY MEDICAL DEPARTMENT.

Rapidly changing events of the War have caused our Government to issue insistent demand for an increase in the Medical Officers. Based on calculations made under conditions existing when we entered the War last April, an estimate was made that we needed approximately 20,000 men—we now have about 17,000 men. Discharges for various reasons have sent many men home. It is said our reserve supply—men commissioned, but not yet called—is now less than 2,000, certainly a small number.

It is now the plan to call out 800,000 soldiers in 1918, as rapidly as contonments can be emptied to care for them. For these men an additional 8,000 physicians—one physician to a hundred soldiers—will be needed. Of course the physicians will be forthcoming. The Medical Profession of our country will respond, but we must promptly get over the "Let John do it" idea, for this is too prevalent in the minds of many of us. There are today in Oklahoma many physicians who can and must lay aside their personal ideas of accumulating money, while hundreds of thousands of our spirited boys are going forward to the trenches, thousands to their graves on foreign soil.

Unforeseen events have placed on our citizenship the greatest burden our nation ever faced or will ever face again. It is the idlest twaddle to indulge in talk of Germany being starved or that they must conclude the war on account of internal troubles. We must face the cold fact that such internal troubles possibly are much more likely to occur among our own allies.

We who are now only called on to volunteer must not forget that every man in Germany is already a soldier, that probably less than a million and a half of them have, so far, been put out of action, that every woman, child and domestic animal is at the absolute disposal of the German war machine. Everything is subservient to the end that Germany must win the War. They have now probably seven to nine million men trained, while we must hurriedly make our army to meet them while our allies-hold their lines as best they can, with anxious eyes turned to America for aid. Thinking men largely agree that this year will be one of great punishment for the allies and we will do well to hold what we have, with great likelihood that in many places we will have to give ground.

Major Henry D. Jump is now touring the country calling attention to the crying needs of the new situation. Your country now requires that you come forward and offer your services. Every man under 55, whose family and dependents do not need him very greatly, is now expected to offer his services. The late estimates call for approximately a total of 35,000 physicians and Oklahoma must do its part as it practriotically will. The smug, meaningless statement "I am ready when they need me" can no longer go or be tolerated, for unless you are commissioned and have placed your affairs in order, the country has not your services.

Okahloma physicians must realize that nationally we face the greatest peril. If we lose this war we must at once turn a peace loving country into an armed camp, waste our great wealth in maintaining armies of appalling size we never dreamed of before or face the alternative of national disintegration, consequent vassalage to a people who are ready to and do go to War, practically on the order of one autocratic Emperor. The War is no longer a struggle between two mere peoples—it is a War between two systems: Autocracy and Democracy, so diametrically opposed in spirit that they can no longer exist in the world. The issue must be settled now and definitely, if possible, for all time.

We have entered into this discussion somewhat at length in order to assist if possible in awakening the individual physician from what may be characterized as a lethargic state. All of us know fairly well the conditions and dangers. Everyone must now do his part. Personal gain must now be forgotten, if in the future we are to be permitted to continue the pursuit of happiness as we have been allowed so long to do.

The physicians of every city and town in Oklahoma should meet without delay and discuss prompt action. Those who can go, but have heretofore hugged the delusion that they are too valuable to their communities, should have it pointed out to them that unless they do go, they may soon have neither country or community.

Doctor, wait no longer. If this applies to you, act at once. Two physicians must do the work formerly falling to three. Those who are unfortunately aged at this time or who have dependents they must remain with and provide for must prepare to do more work in order to spare the doctor the army now needs.

Application for examination should be forwarded to Lieut. L. M. Sackett, M. R. C., Oklahoma City. It is hoped that examinations may be held in the larger cities of the state, but you should indicate your readiness by writing your application at once.

THE DOCTOR'S OPPORTUNITY.

Breathes there a man with a soul so dead
Who never to himself has said:
This is my own, my native land.

In the formation of an army two main factors are necessary for efficiency. Well located sanitary camps for housing and good roads for travel. The personnel must be made up of first class sound men. It must be, therefore, apparent that the two main divisions of an army are the Engineer and the Medical Corps. Fortunately in a newly formed Army these two branches are, from their education and training, competent to at once begin their work. In other words, they are really the creators of mobilizations. To the doctor falls the better part, the health and the life of the troops. Never before has such an opportunity as the present been offered to the doctors of America. Your country calls—will you or can you allow this call to go unheeded? Besides your patrotism, which at this time must be burning out your very soul—think of the numberless advantages that this service offers to you individually. It is beyond argument that if you enter the Medical Corps and apply yourself diligently to its duties, when the war has ended and you return to your home you will have acquired such an experience that never again will fall to the lot of medical men: and in addition you will have demonstrated to yourself at least, that which you have so often prated about—man's humanity to man. Of course we know that you are one of, if not the leading man in your community. So much the better, for the men at the front need the best that is to be had. Of course, your community cannot spare you—not now, but wait until next summer when the news reaches the mother that her son perished because there were not enough doctors—do you think she will spare you then? Yes, we agree that there is a difference between living with an income of five thousand or more and two thousand—but, if you go now, there is a good chance of your making the five thousand again. If you do not go, you may be living on less than two thousand in the near future. If you have lived in luxury and slept on downy beds, the army fare will be coarse and cots will be hard. But if you do your full duty when you get there, the food will be sweet and you will not find fault with your bed.

And doctor, when you lay aside your civilian clothing, also cast aside all your ideas of personal greatness along with your small, petty jealousies. Be loyal to your superiors and do not crowd out your inferiors. Remember, you are but an atom in this great unit—slip in noiselessly and easily. Do not forget that

Honor and fame from no condition rise,
Act well your part, there all tne honor lies.

Before you begin to inoculate the men under your care against disease—first inoculate yourself with the serum of service and sacrifice.

C. W. Heitzman.

THE AMERICAN MEDICAL ASSOCIATION IN THE WAR.

Certain criticisms of alleged lack of activity of the officers of the American Medical Association, appearing in the February *Kentucky Medical Journal,* have been called to our attention. Editorially the Kentuckian says in part: "This should have been done long ago by the American Medical Association, through its splendid facilities for organization, but it has so utterly failed to realize its opportunities in this respect that it is barely consulted in Washington, and the duties and responsibilities it should have proudly and efficiently borne have been undertaken by the Medical Section of the Council of National Defense".

Honest, constructive criticism is certainly one of our Nation's present great needs. Such criticism helps the system or person criticised, spurs him to increased effort and efficiency. Constructive criticism has undoubtedly saved the British Empire up to this time from destruction. Criticism, even through the medium of isolated cases of mismanagement and almost unavoidable lack of necessary supplies in our cantonments, undoubtedly placed all officers on the alert and promptly improved conditions.

But in this particular instance, we are constrained to believe that either some measure of pique or malice, some ungenerous impulse or perhaps misconception of the actual work performed by the Association, prompted the editorial.

The Surgeon-General, certainly the best judge, acknowleged officially on February 22 "the great services rendered by the Americal Medical Association, to me personally and to the Office of the Surgeon-General, in organizing the Medical Department of the Army". Continuing, General Gorgas says, "Since April, 1917, the Board of Trustees, the Officers at the Chicago Headquarters, *The Journal* and all the machinery of the American Medical Association have been important and distinctive factors through which many thousands of physicians have been influenced to apply for commissions in the Medical Reserve Corps; medical officers have received valuable instruction by means of special articles printed in *The Journal*, etc., etc., and in other ways too great to enumerate here".

The Medical Section, Council of National Defense, has done a great work. The body is explicitly charged with certain duties, its members are Army Officers with all the power of the Government behind them, but everyone who knows anything of the situation is aware that the A. M. A. officers have spent a great deal of their time in Washington advising and assisting the Medical Section and have practically subordinated every possible force of the Chicago office to the same end. A glance at the back files of the *A. M. A. Journal* will convince the reader of the immense amount of labor expended for the National good and the tremendous energy expended to inform physicians of every phase of medical military activity. Certainly we would be in a sad state had not this work been carried on by the A. M. A.

We feel utterly out of patience with the critic who at this time unnecessarily criticises. This is no time for the exhibition of anything except the spirit to cooperate, to improve, to place shoulder to shoulder and use all our energy for the betterment of our National service.

A TUBERCULOSIS SURVEY.

The Oklahoma Association for the Prevention of Tuberculosis announces that in April Professors Murray Horowitz of the Massachusetts Institute of Technology and Gayfree Ellison of the Oklahoma University will begin a series of health surveys of Oklahoma's principal cities. Dr. Ellison will begin work June 1st. The State Department of Health and Mr. Jules Schevitz, Secretary of the Oklahoma Association, will cooperate in the work.

The war has forcibly called the attention of the people to the great handicap of tuberculosis to the soldier. Coming at this time, everything affecting our soldiers has an added interest and the Association could not have selected a better time as to the psychology for such an investigation. It is said that in France, more than any other country, tuberculosis is prone to reassert itself when the man goes to the hardships of trench warfare with its consequent overexposure. Every effort is made to detect liability to and incipiency of the disease before the soldier is sent abroad, but despite the efforts an unusually large number are incapacitated and have to be invalided home.

These facts brought to the attention of the people now will have a good effect toward enlisting their intelligent cooperation in the control and prevention of the infection at its fountain head, which is the home. Until those with susceptibility to the disease and those who live in surroundings conducive to its development can be brought to see the great danger to themselves and their neighbors, not much headway toward control is to be expected.

TULSA MEETING, MAY 14-15-16.

Committee on Arrangement for Meeting Places:—Dr. N. W. Mayginnis, Chairman; Dr. R. S. Wagner, Dr. D. W. Wadsworth.

Program Committee:—Dr. C. A. W. Pigford, Chairman; Dr. W. H. Rogers, Dr. F. Y. Cronk.

Badge and Registration Committee:—Dr. G. A. Wall, Chairman; Dr. J. F. Gorrell, Dr. Bertha Margolins.

Finance Committee:—Dr. S. DeZell Hawley, Chairman; Dr. S. G. Kennedy, Dr. M. P. Springer, Dr. C. L. Reeder. Dr. Ross Grosshart.

Publicity Committee:—Dr. F. S. Clinton, Chairman; Dr. F. M. Boso, Dr. C. D. F.O'Hern.

Executive Committee:—Dr. W. Albert Cook, Chairman; Dr. W. W. Beasley, Dr. A. V. Emerson, Dr. A. Ray Wiley, Dr. W. J. Trainor.

Hotel Committee:—Dr. W. Forest Dutton, Chairman; Dr. C. L. Reeder, Dr. F. S. Clinton.

Entertainment Committee:—Dr. S. DeZell Hawley, Chairman; Dr. A. W. Roth, Dr. W. E. Wright.

Reception Committee:—All members not connected with other committees.

THE ARMY MEDICAL DEPARTMENT ENCOURAGING A FALLACY.

The drug supplies that are being purchased by the medical department of the United States Army are commendably free from unscientific and worthless proprietary preparations. -This is progress. One's optimism, however, is tempered in looking through a long list of drugs and chemicals on which bids are asked by the General Purchasing Office of the Medical Department, U. S. A. Item No. 148 of "Post Supplies" calls for three tons (in one pound bottles) of the "Compound Syrup of Hypophosphites"! It is safe to say that there is not a physician in one of the army posts who, if the question were put to him frankly, would admit that "Compound Syrup of Hypophosphites" belonged in the armamentarium of a scientific physician. Yet, six thousand bottles of this relic of a past generation are called for, are to be paid for and are to occupy valuable freight space in shipping to the various army posts. What utter waste! And what a reflection!!—*Journal A. M. A.*, March 16, 1918.

PERSONAL AND GENERAL NEWS

Dr. Ralph Mavity, it is said, will locate in Billings.

Dr. W. B. Hudson, Yale, visited New Orleans clinics in March.

Dr. J. L. Adams, Pryor, is doing postgraduate work in Chicago.

Dr. A. R. Holmes, Henryetta, is doing special work in New Orleans.

Dr. and Mrs. W. E. Dicken, Oklahoma City, visited Colorado in March.

Dr. H. M. Reeder, Shawnee, lost his Ford, a 1918 model, by theft in March.

Dr. G. C. Bruce has located in Stillwell. His former home was De Lark, Ark.

Dr. and Mrs. E. S. Ferguson, Oklahoma City, visited New Orleans in March.

Dr. Phil Herod, M. R. C., El Reno, has been ordered to Ft. Riley for instruction.

Dr. Julian Field, Enid, is a "Ford" victim. The crank broke his arm March 6th.

Dr. N. P. Lee, Checotah, was rather seriously ill in a Muskogee hospital in March.

Dr. D. D. Howell, Nowata, visited San Antonio in March. He returned greatly benefitted.

Drs. E. Brent Mitchell and G. Pinnell, Lawton, announce the dissolution of their parternship.

Dr. Blair Points, Miami, has been appointed city health officer, succeeding Dr. T. W. Brewer, resigned.

Dr. T. J. Nunnery, M. R. C., Grandfield, has been ordered to report at Ft. Sam Houston for active duty.

Dr. F. W. Rogers, Carnegie, is able to be out after an extended illness and operation at the El Reno Sanitarium.

Dr. J. S. McFaddin, Hollis, visited Chicago clinics in February where he did special work in major surgery and head work.

Dr. A. H. Bungardt, Cordell, announces that he will devote his time solely to surgery hereafter. He will have charge of the Cordell Hospital.

Dr. J. R. Collins, Nowata, has accepted the position on the Local Board for his county created by the resignation of Dr. J. P. Sudderth.

Dr. J. B. Haggard, South Coffeyville, who was discharged from the Army on account of a fracture of the arm, it is said will locate in Miami.

The State Health Department estimates that more than 75,000 people were vaccinated over the state against smallpox in January and February.

Dr. J. B. Chastain, Broken Bow, has moved to Davis.

Dr. J. W. Nieweg, M. R. C., Duncan, has been ordered to Ft. Riley.

Dr. W. E. Simon, M. R. C., Alva, has been ordered to Ft. Riley for duty.

Dr. O. E. Templin, M. R. C., Alva, has been ordered to report April 1st for duty.

Dr. C. E. Northcutt, M. R. C., Lexington, was ordered to report for duty March 24.

Dr. E. S. Sullivan, M. R. C., Oklahoma City, has been ordered to report for duty at Ft. Riley.

Dr. J. S. McFaddin, Hollis, has returned from Chicago where he has been studying eye, ear, nose, and throat.

Drs. M. M. DeArman, Mangum, and General Pinnell, Lawton, have moved to Miami and formed a partnership.

Dr. Geo. W. Tilley of Pryor, who has been stationed at Camp Beauregard, has been ordered to Camp Greenleaf, Ft. Oglethorpe.

Dr. Commodore Farrington, Shawnee, died in that city February 22 from pneumonia. Dr. Farrington had practiced medicine in Shawnee for seventeen years.

Dr. R. I. Bond, McAlester, has announced his candidacy for the state senate. Dr. Bond was formerly a member of the house and made a good record at that time.

Dr. L. J. Moorman announces that the capacity of the Oklahoma Cottage Sanitarium for the Treatment of Tuberculosis will be increased by a tewlve bed addition.

Drs. J. Clay Williams, formerly of Stroud, and J. T. Wharton of Douthitt have formed a partnership and located at Picher. They have offices at the Picher Hospital.

Dr. Ralph V. Smith, Tulsa, Captain M. R. C., met many of his old Oklahoma friends when he was ordered to Oklahoma City to take special work in Orthopedic Surgery.

Dr. R. M. Howard, M. R. C., Oklahoma City, who has been stationed at Camp McArthur, has been ordered to the Rockefeller Institute, New York, for special instruction.

Dr. E. S. Lain, Oklahoma City, is joining the plutocratic class. He announces that his Medical Mining Company is striking it rich and that shortly the stockholders will be in clover.

Dr. Claude Thompson, Muskogee, tried to prevent a glass door from slamming recently. The door stopped after his arm went through; a friendly surgeon finished up the work with twenty-one stitches.

Dr. H. M. Stricklen, Tonkawa, recently took the position that a hurried physician did not have to literally obey the law. The court agreed with the doctor and ordered him released from the charge of violating the speed laws.

Dr. J. F. Means, Claremore, has been in Washington some time representing the Claremore Commercial Club. It is hoped that the War Department may establish at Claremore a Sanitarium for convalescent troops from the nearby cantonments.

Medical Army Officers will be detailed by the War Department to attend the annual meeting at Tulsa May 14-16, if the plans materialize. The object of their visit will be to have first hand information as to the actual conditions and further needs of the service.

D. J. J. Gable, Norman, has been ordered to active duty in the Medical Reserve Corps. The War Department extended the time for active service in his case until July 1st, but Dr. Gable waived the extension and reported for service. His departure cripples the State Hospital at Norman, leaving only two physicians to look after the large number of patients.

Dr. and Mrs. W. Albert Cook, Tulsa, entertained Major and Mrs. Henry D. Jump of Washington during Major Jump's recent visit and inspection through Oklahoma, accompanying them to Oklahoma City and Camp Doniphan. Dr. Cook became so enamoured with the military service that he took the examination at Oklahoma City and will enter the Medical Reserve Corps.

Beckham County Medical Society is meeting the H. C. L. with a general raise in prices for services rendered. We heartily agree to that proposition. The Medical Profession as a rule is receiving just about the same amount of fees for service as was in vogue ten years ago. Everything else has been elevated in price to the doctor, while he is sending out bills to the same old tune of long ago.

The Oklahoma City Times editorially suggests that doctors should volunteer at this time. The Times pays a high compliment to those who have already gone, pointing out the sacrifice involved but suggests, and rightly so, that the sacrifices at this time are not confined to any class and that all must take up the burden and enter the service of the country in the position they are best fitted to fill.

Central Oklahoma Medical Society met in Enid February 27th. The following officers were elected for the ensuing year: President, Dr. W. L. Kendall, Enid; first vice-president, Dr. W. J. Wallace, Oklahoma City; second vice-president, H. A. Lile, Aline; secretary-treasurer, C. J. Fishman, Oklahoma City. Clinics were held in the Enid hospitals in the forenoon, followed by lunch at the Oxford and the scientific meeting in the afternoon.

"Dr." Willard Carver, "Big Chief," "Fountain Head," etc., etc., of the Chiropractic fraternity, is again in the limelight by reason of divorce proceedings. The editor had the nauseauting privilege of reading some of the depositions in the case, which were of such a nature that the newspapers of Oklahoma City dared not even hint at the contents. They bear out generally the writer's vaguely formed opinion of some time past that Carver was either a bad actor or had something radically wrong with his Fountain "Head."

Dr. Chas. W. Heitzman, Captain, M. R. C., Muskogee, has been ordered to active duty at Ft. Riley.

The Medical Section, State Council of Defense, met in Oklahoma City March 23, Dr. L. Haynes Buxton, Chairman, presiding. The meeting was well attended and plans formulated to make the work as effective as possible. Dr. Buxton, who we all know as a forcible speaker, stated the situation well and patriotically at the committee meeting and the evening meeting as well. Addresses were also made by Drs. Le Roy Long, A. K. West and John W. Duke. The principal address of the evening was made by Dr. Henry D. Jump, Major, M. R. C., who is in service with the National Medical Section at Washington.

Major Henry D. Jump, Philadelphia, member of the Medical Section, Council of National Defense, visited Oklahoma late in March, speaking to physicians and the public at Tulsa and Oklahoma City for the purpose of calling attention to the coming needs of the Medical Department. The visit was productive of much good, as explaining many points of interest to the profession in connection with the medical service and incidentally stimulated many physicians to apply for commissions in the Medical Reserve Corps. Major Jump created a most favorable impression wherever he went. The general verdict of the doctors was that he "is a regular fellow", and they regretted that his time with us was so limited. He will make a flying visit to many parts of the west, including Pacific coast points, before his return to Washington to resume his duties.

CORRESPONDENCE

London, Eng., Feb. 12, 1918.

Dr. Claude Thompson,
    Muskogee, Okla.

Dear Dr. Thompson: I have never had the pleasure of meeting you although I have often heard my partner speak of you in glowing terms. For your information, will say that I became a citizen of your State in the fall of 1915, when I formed a partnership with Dr. Fowler Border of Mangum, and where I enjoyed a lucrative surgical practice, being half interested in the surgical practice of the Border Hospital at that place. I came to Oklahoma from New York where I had spent three years in the P. G. study and practice of surgery, being resident surgeon of Bayonne Hospital in 1915. And since going to Oklahoma I have not had the privilege of attending State Association, because my partner claimed the right by seniority, and as it was impossible for us both to be away from hospital at same time, I have been unfortunate in not making yours and many others of our colleagues acquaintance. However, I think you will be able to place me from the above data. I have been in London four months (left Mangum Sept. 9, 1917), on staff of Bermoudsey Military Hospital, where I have gotten some splendid work and am really beginning to feel like an "old army surgeon." But my greatest sorrow has been my inability to receive the Journal. So will you kindly send it to me monthly, address in care American Express Co., No. 6 Haymarket St., London, as they will always have my forwarding address.

In conjunction with my regular work I have been doing some special work at the Royal Army Medical College, principally in amputation and artificial limb fitting. Will be glad when the war is over and I can get back to dear old Oklahoma and my hospital.

Hoping you had a jolly Xmas and Happy New Year, I am,

                                     Fraternally yours,
1st Lt. M. O. R. C., attached to R. A. M. C.   Frank H. McGregor.

MISCELLANEOUS

A NEW REVIEW ON WAR SURGERY.

There has just been prepared in the Office of the Surgeon General a new pamphlet Review of War Surgery and Medicine (March, 1918, vol. i, No. 1). According to the editorial note this review is to appear monthly and to be devoted to abstracts of war medicinal literature. This little pamphlet will furnish the medical personnel of the Army abstracts of original papers of importance, necessary information in a short compass, and prompt publication of reports which otherwise might not gain circulation.

In this first volume there is a splendid review of Surgery in the Zone of Advance prepared from data written by Major George de Tarnowsky, based upon his personal observations in the French army front. It is the best description that has yet appeared in American literature of the war.

This is followed by a most readable and instructive review of the most recent data on gas gangrene, trench foot and the general principles guiding the treatment of wounds of war.

Copies of this review may be obtained by addressing the Superintendent of Documents, Government Printing Office, Washington, D. C., enclosing ten cents in stamps.

This review should be in the hands of every officer of the Medical Corps and should be of interest to the entire medical profession not in the service. The reviews are very well written and make most interesting and profitable reading.

THE STATE LABORATORY MOVING.

Dear Doctor:

Our State Laboratory is today moving from Guthrie to Oklahoma City. Following the receipt of this letter please do not send any more specimens to Guthrie.

Address all specimens, correspondence and telegrams in connection therewith to: Director, State Board of Health Laboratories, Second and Stiles Sts., Oklahoma City, Oklahoma.

Hoping that you will make free use of our increased facilities,

Sincerely yours,
JOHN W. DUKE,
State Commissioner of Health.

AMERICAN MEDICAL ASSOCIATION NEWS.

THE CHICAGO SESSION.

Committee on Arrangements.

The Local Committee on Arrangements for the Annual Session of 1918 to be held in Chicago, June 10-14, is actively engaged in perfecting plans for the comfort and entertainment of the Fellows of the Association and their guests.

All correspondence with the Local Committee on Arrangements or with any of its subcommittees should be addressed to 25 East Washington Street, Chicago.

Clinics.

The chairman of the subcommittee on clinics, Dr. Charles F. Humiston, announces that there will be a series of clinics for the Fellows of the Association on Thursday, Friday and Saturday, June 6, 7, and 8, and on Monday and Tuesday, June 10 and 11. Further announcements regarding the clinics will appear in these columns from time to time.

Alumni and Section Dinners.

Alumni and section dinners will be held on Wednesday evening from 6 to 8 o'clock so as not to conflict with other events which are being planned. The chairman of the subcommittee on alumni and section entertainment, Dr. J. H. Stowell, announces that his committee is cooperating with officers of alumni associations in arranging for reunions. The committee desires, also, to assist the officers of those sections which desire to arrange for section dinners.

HOTEL HEADQUARTERS FOR THE CHICAGO SESSION.

The following hotels have been tentatively designated as general and section headquarters for the Chicago Session, June 10 to 14:

General Headquarters: Hotel Sherman, North Clark and West Randolph.
Practice of Medicine: Hotel Morrison, 83 West Madison.
Surgery, General and Abdominal: Auditorium Hotel, 430 South Michigan.
Obstetrics, Gynecology and Abdominal Surgery: Congress Hotel, South Michigan and Congress.
Ophthalmology: Hotel LaSalle, LaSalle and West Madison.
Laryngology, Otology and Rhinology: Hotel LaSalle, LaSalle and West Madison.
Diseases of Children: Congress Hotel, South Michigan and Congress.
Pharmacology and Therapeutics: Auditorium Hotel, 430 South Michigan.
Pathology and Physiology: Auditorium Hotel, 430 South Michigan.
Stomatology: Congress Hotel, South Michigan and Congress.
Nervous and Mental Diseases: Blackstone Hotel, South Michigan and East Seventh.
Dermatology: Blackstone Hotel, South Michigan and East Seventh.
Preventive Medicine and Public Health: Auditorium Hotel, 430 South Michigan.
Genito-Urinary Diseases: Auditorium Hotel, 430 South Michigan.
Orthopedic Surgery: Congress Hotel, South Michigan and Congress.
Gastro-Enterology and Proctology: Auditorium Hotel, 430 South Michigan.
Scientific Exhibit, Registration Bureau, Commercial Exhibit, Information Bureau, and Branch Postoffice: Hotel Sherman, North Clark and West Randolph.

Reprinted from *The Journal* of the American Medical Association March 9, 1918, Vol. 70, p. 715.

RELIABLE THYROID PREPARATIONS.

In the *British Medical Journal*, October 20th, 1917, Dr. Carver, M. R. C. P., London, emphasizes the necessity of specifying a reliable brand of Thyroids and Thyroid Tablets. He called attention to the way in which some manufacturers label their preparations. If the doctor will demand Armour's he will know that his patient gets a specific quantity of Thyroid tissues because we standardize our Dessicated Thyroids and Thyroid Tablets. Each Thyroid Tablet (Armour's) contains a certain quantity of standardized Thyroids and that amount of Thyroids represents five times as much fresh thyroid gland. Whenever a preparation of any of the endocrine glands is required, the physician should specify Armour's and see that his patient gets Armour's. The doctor prescribes a preparation for a certain purpose and he can expect results only from first class products.

DETECTION OF PRETENDED LOSS OF HEARING.

Detection of pretended loss of hearing with special reference to unilateral deafness, which is said by French military physicians to be a common form of malingering and one most difficult to detect, is the subject of a paper by R. R. Brownfield, Phoenix, Arizona, (*Journal A. M. A.*, March 2, 1918). He describes a method of testing cases by which he claims certain advantages over the acoumeter used by the French physicians. In his device batteries and make-and-break contact are dispensed with, and the ordinary 110 volt alternating commercial lighting current is used. The variable current is produced by a potentiometer. No vibrating iron is used, and the maximum strength of current employed depends on no factor except the ratio of the electrical resistances used. The sound producer is similar to a telephone receiver, except that the core is of soft iron and is not magnetized. This eliminates the variability due to demagnetization, and doubles the pitch. The sound producer is provided with three lugs to hold it away from the ear, so that the sound will be transmitted solely by air conduction. By simply turning the indicator from 100 to zero, one can cause the sound to increase from the point at which it is just perceptible to one of normal hearing, the threshold of audition, or 100 per cent. acuity, to a degree of intensity at which failure to perceive it indicates that the subject has no practical hearing. In addition to the variable reciever, there is a supplementary one that always operates at maximum intensity, irrespective of the loudness of the other. In the usual test for acuity of hearing, only the variable receiver is used. As the subject holds this to the ear, the pointer is gradually carried from the zero to the 100 degree point and he is directed to tell at what point the sound ceases to be heard. This is noted and the movement of the pointer continued still farther, and he is asked to note the point at which it begins again to be heard. After some repetitions, the points will be found to harmonize quite closely, except in the case of malingering. The apparatus is of course out of the patient's sight—behind him. In case of a person claiming deafness in only one ear, he is made to hold the constantly loud receiver over the alleged deaf ear and the variable receiver over the other. Starting at 100 the pointer is gradually moved toward zero and he is asked to say when he first hears the sound in his good ear. If he has complete deafness in one ear the presence of the loud receiver will not disturb him, but if he is merely pretending, it would be absolutely impossible for him to identify any sound whatever in his good ear, to which the variable receiver is applied, until a point on the scale is reached that would normally indicate very defective or almost no hearing for the good ear. The test can be repeated with the loud receiver disconnected, and a totally different reading secured in the case of malingering.

THE GOOD SAMARITAN FUNCTION OF THE MEDICAL CORPS.

Major George de Tarnowsky, M. O. R. C. (Review of Surgery and Medicine, March 1918, vol. i, No. 1, prepared in the Office of the Surgeon General), gives one of the best descriptions of the surgery in the zone of advance, from personal observations on the French front. Attention of all medical officers is directed to the following:

"In addition to hot meals which are carried to the soldiers in the trenches, the *Medical Corps* now sends hot tea, flavor with a small amount of brandy, to the front lines twice daily—a most welcome potion, which the soldiers look forward to with eagerness. The prevailing idea of the French Medical Corps is to make the fighting men feel and know that their comfort is being looked after and that everything is being done to mitigate the hardships under which they live. The French are strong believers in the personal element—the little acts of kindness, even of tenderness towards the individual soldier which have helped to keep up both his fighting spirit and his mental serenity. The '*tisaneries*' as the hot tea stations are called did not come into existence as the result of army orders; they represent a voluntary contribution to the soldier on the part of the Medical Corps. Begun in a small way, it was soon noticed that, where the *tisaneries* existed and the regimental kitchens were installed near enough to the trenches so that the food reached the soldier hot, the morale and fighting edge were of the finest."

THE NATURE OF WOUND SHOCK.

W. B. Cannon (Boston) at the front in France (*Journal A. M. A.*, March 2, 1918), reviews the theories that have been advanced as to the nature of wound shock. He finds objections to Henderson's acapnia theory and the idea of suprarenal exhaustion, as well as the nerve exhaustion theory advanced by Crile, and gives the reasons as shown in the experimental work reported by various authorities. The cardiac factor is also not a primary one as has been shown experimentally. The problem of the lost blood in the shocked individual is at least partially solved by the congestion of the capillaries and is further supported by the possibility of the concentration of the blood. There are other conditions besides a low blood pressure that are favorable to capillary stagnation of the corpuscles, such as the vicosity factor and the effects of acidosis on the circulation. There are also various vicious circles in the effects of shock on the circulation, and these are enumerated. Cannon proposes a change in the nomenclature using for wound shock the term "exemia," a word used by Hippocrates signifying "drained of blood." A general statement offered by Cannon is as follows: "There are primary wound shock with rapid lowering of arterial pressure, and secondary wound shock with toxemia and hemorrhage, and later lowering of the pressure. Sweating occurs, leading to loss of fluid and loss of heat from the body. The blood becomes stagnant and concentrated in the capillaries, and as the blood pressure falls there is loss of the alkali reserve of the blood (acidosis) roughly corresponding to the drop in pressure." The facts are fully listed in the closing paragraphs of the article, and he concludes as follows:

"This conception of the events that take place in a wounded man who passes into shock gives a reasonable account of the primary effect of wounds, the influence of cold in continuing the low blood pressure or inducing it when the circulatory apparatus is unstable, the influence of warmth in restoring him in part to a fit condition, and the slowness of a full recovery. It leaves unsettled the occasion for the primary fall of pressure, though the suggestion is offered that it may be of reflex character, similar to fainting. The conception offers a hopeful outlook for the care of the shocked man, because two of the most potent factors making his chances unfavorable, cold and acidosis, can be controlled."

COUNCIL OF PHARMACY AND CHEMISTRY.

During February the following articles have been accepted by the Council on Pharmacy and Chemistry for inclusion with New and Non-official Remedies:

The Abbott Laboratories: Chlorcosane, Barbital-Abbott, Procaine-Abbott.

Dermatological Research Laboratories, Philadelphia Polyclinic: Arsenobenzol (Dermatological Research Laboratories) 1 gm. ampules.

Eli Lilley and Company: Typhoid Vaccine, Prophylactic; Typhoid Vaccine, Therapeutic; Typhoid Mixed Vaccine, Lilly.

Merck and Company: Mercury Benzoate-Merck.

Monsanto Chemical Works: Halazone-Monsanto.

H. K. Mulford Company: Bulgarian Bacillus, Friable Tablets.

W. A. Puckner, Secretary.

NEW AND NON-OFFICIAL REMEDIES.

Barbital. Diethyl-Barbituric Acid, first introduced under the name veronal. In small doses barbital is a relatively safe hypnotic, but fatalities have followed its indiscriminate use. It is claimed to be useful in simple insomnia, as well as in that accompanying hysteria, neurasthenia and mental disturbances. From 0.3 to 1 gm. (5 to 15 grains) in hot water, tea or milk, or, if in wafers or capsules, followed by a cupful of some warm liquid.

Barbital-Abbott. A brand of barbital complying with the New and Non-official Remedies standards. The Abbott Laboratories, Chicago.

Mercury-Benzoate-Merck. A brand of mercuric benzoate complying with the New and Non-official Remedies standards. Mercuric benzoate has the properties of mercuric chloride. It has been said to be useful for hypodermic use and in gonorrhea. Merck and Company, New York.

Chlorcosane. A liquid obtained by chlorinating solid paraffin. It contains about 50 per cent. of chlorin in stable combination. Chlorcosane is used as a solvent for dichloramine-T; with it solutions containing as much as 8 per cent. may be prepared. When used in a hand atomizer, chlorcosane solutions of dichloramine-T may be made less viscous by the addition of 10 per cent. of carbon tetrachloride. The Abbott Laboratories, Chicago.

Betanaphthyl Salicylate-Calco. A brand of betanaphthyl salicylate complying with the New and Non-official Remedies standards. Betanaphthyl salicylate is believed to act as an intestinal antiseptic and, being excreted in the urine, to act in a similar way in the bladder. It is said to be useful in intestinal fermentations, catarrh of the bladder, particularly gonorrheal cystitis, rheumatism, etc. The Calco Chemical Co., Bound Brook, N. J.

Acetylsalicylic Acid-Merck. A brand of acetylsalicylic acid complying with the New and Non-official Remedies standards. Acetylsalicylic acid is employed in rheumatic conditions, and especially as an analgesic and antipyretic in colds, neuralgias, etc.

Chlorazene Surgical Powder. An impalpable powder composed of chlorazene, 1 per cent.; zinc stearate, 10 per cent., and sodium stearate, 89 per cent. Chlorazene Surgical Powder is absorbent, slightly astringent, and forms a closely adherent film when applied to the skin. It may be dusted freely over denuded or abraded areas, cuts, wounds, and skin eruptions. The Abbott Laboratories, Chicago, (*Jour. A. M. A.*, Feb. 16, 1918, p. 459).

PROPAGANDA FOR REFORM.

Phenalgin and Ammonol. At the time that synthetic chemical drugs were coming into fame and when every manufacturer who launched a new headache mixture claimed to have achieved another triumph in synthetic chemistry, Ammonol and Phenalgin were born and duly christened with chemical formulas. However, one of the first reports of the Council on Pharmacy and Chemistry showed them to be mixtures composed of acetanilid, sodium bicarbonate and ammonium carbonate. Since then the unwarranted claims made for these preparations have been exposed repeatedly, and the danger of the indiscriminate use of headache mixtures pointed out. Despite the exposure of the methods used in exploiting Ammonol and Phenalgin, one finds just as glaringly false statements made in the advertisements of Phenalgin today as were made in its unsavory past. This would seem to indicate either that physicians have short memories or that they are strangely indifferent to the welfare of their patients, to their own reputation, and to the good name of medicine (*Jour. A. M. A.*, Feb. 2, 1918, p. 337).

Absorption and Excretion of Mercury. It may be regarded as clearly established that, in addition to the kidneys, the stomach may participate in this eliminatory function quite as well as the other portions of the alimentary tract. The occurrence of severe intoxications from the use of mercuric chloride in vaginal douches is likewise recognized. The absorption of mercury through the sound skin has been in dispute. To account for the efficacy of mercurial inunction, the contention has been made that the mercury thus applied is volatilized and absorbed through the lungs in greater part if not entirely. Experiments in the dermatologic laboratories of the Philadelphia Polyclinic leaves little doubt that the skin is an important, perhaps the most important, path of absorption of mercury applied by inunction (*Jour. A. M. A.*, Feb. 9, 1918, p. 392).

Basy'Bread. This is an asserted obesity cure put out by the Doctors' Essential Food Company, Orange, N. J. The advertising claims are extravagant and typical of other obesity treatment literature. Analyses indicated that in composition Basy Bread was similar to graham bread. Basy Bread sells for $1 a loaf. Dr. Wiley well sums up the case thus: "There is one way in which Basy Bread will reduce, that is, don't eat any of it nor much of it nor much of any other kind." (*Jour. A. M. A.*, Feb. 9, 1918, p. 407).

Campho-Phenique. The Secretary of the Harvard University Medical School received, from the Campho-Phenique Company of St. Louis, a letter stating that the concern wishes to supply the senior students of all Medical Colleges with samples of Campho-Phenique and Campho-Phenique powder, and ointment and asking the number of students and the name of every student in the graduating class. The Campho-Phenique concern believes in following the old advice, "Catching them young." In 1907, the Council on Pharmacy and Chemistry reported that Campho-Phenique (liquid) was exploited under a false "formula," that it was a solution of camphor and phenol in liquid petrolatum, and that for all practical purposes Campho-Phenique Powder was essentially a camphorated talcum powder containing apparently sufficient phenol and camphor to give the powder an odor. The report of the Council further brought out that the Campho-Phenique Company was in effect one of the numerous trade names adopted by one James F. Ballard. Mr. Ballard seems to market a number of "patent medicines," for some of which Dr. Ballard has pleaded guilty in the federal courts to making false and fraudulent claims (*Jour. A. M. A.*, Feb. 9, 1918, p. 408).

Sodium Bicarbonate. Few patients will object to the taste of sodium bicarbonate if the required dose is administered dissolved in a convenient quantity of cold water. The taste may be disguised by dissolving the sodium bicarbonate in carbonated water or else by adding a little sugar and lemon juice to ordinary water. Sodium bicarbonate may also be prescribed in the form of tablets. Though it is better that these be allowed to dissolve in the mouth, in most cases they are swallowed without discomfort (*Jour. A. M. A.*, Feb. 9, 1918, p. 410).

Acetylsalicylic Acid and Phenyl Salicylate Incompatible with Alkalies. In the presence of moisture, acetylsalicylic acid is decomposed by magnesium oxide (calcined magnesia), as is also phenyl salicylate (salol). Hence these drugs should not be combined with magnesium oxide in a prescription (*Jour. A. M. A.*, Feb. 9, 1918, p. 410).

Fellows' Syrup, and other Preparations of the Hypophosphites. An advertisement for Fellows' Syrup reads: "Fellows' Syrup differs from other preparations of the hypophosphites. Leading clinicians in all parts of the world have long recognized this important fact. Have you? To insure results, prescribe the geniune recipe Syr. Hypophos. Comp. Fellows'. Reject cheap and inefficient substitutes. Reject preparations 'just as good.'" In truth, Fellows' Syrup is not like the better preparations of this type, since after standing it contains a muddy looking deposit that any pharmaceutical tyro would be ashamed of. Examination of the literature used in the exploitation of Fellows' Syrup fails to disclose any evidence to show that it has therapeutic value. Not only is there an entire absence of any evidence of its therapeutic value, but there is an abundance of evidence that the hypophosphites are devoid of any such therapeutic effects as they were formerly reputed to have, and that they are, so far as any effect based on their phosphorus content is concerned, singularly inert. As the result of its investigation of the therapeutic effects of the hypophosphites, the Council on Pharmacy and Chemistry concluded: There is no reliable evidence that they exert a physiologic effect: it has not been demonstrated that they influence any pathologic process; they are not "foods." If they are of any use, that use has never been discovered (*Jour. A. M. A.*, Feb. 16, 1918, p. 478).

Calcium Iodide in Tuberculosis. There appears to be no work to indicate that the intravenous administration of calcium iodide in tuberculosis is of value. It has not been demonstrated that tuberculosis is associated with a deficiency of calcium. On the other hand, experiments demonstrate that the administration of calcium does not change the calcium content of the blood. Furthermore, there is no evidence to warrant the intravenous administration of iodides (*Jour. A. M. A.*, Feb. 16, 1918, p. 481).

Bell-Ans (Papayans, Bell.) "Are you going to sit there and let the other folks eat up all the good things just because you are afraid to pitch in, when 2 or 3 Bell-Ans taken before and after the meal would enable you to enjoy your share of all that's coming without a bit of discomfort or distress. Bell-Ans has restored the pleasures of the table to thousands who say: 'I can now eat anything and plenty of it, too'." The New York Tribune comments that such advertisement as this is not limited to the evil effects to the misguided individual who eats lobster and ice cream at midnight and trusts to Bell-Ans to atone for his indiscretion. The most serious effect of such reckless advice is the example which the advertising sets to other advertisers (*Jour. A. M. A.*, Feb. 23, 1918, p. 557).

NEW BOOKS

DISEASES OF THE SKIN.

By Milton B. Hartzell, A. M., M. D., LLD., Professor of Dermatology, University of Penn. Price $7.00.   J. B. Lippencott Co., 1917.

This is a well arranged text with 51 excellent colored plates and 242 fairly representative illus-· trations. The type is clear and well arranged for both student and practitioner.

Reviewing this book with the eye of a critic, would say that in regard to treatment for the general practitioner it is rather brief. Also from the standpoint of the young progressive dermatologist, he has neglected the consideration of several rational theories as regards the etiology· of certain diseases. In his favorable mention of Radium for the treatment of Epitheliomas, Lupus, Angiomas, etc., he is entirely too brief.   E. S. Lain.

A TEXT-BOOK OF THE PRACTICE OF MEDICINE.

A Text-Book of the Practice of Medicine, by James M. Anders, M. D., Ph. D., LL. D., Professor of Medicine and Clinical Medicine, Medico-Chirurgical College Graduate School, University of Pennsylvania, thirteenth edition thoroughly revised with the assistance of John H. Musser, Jr., M. D., Associate in Medicine, University of Pennsylvania. Octavo of 1259 pages, fully illustrated. Philadelphia and London: W. B. Saunders Company, 1917. Cloth, $6.00 net; half Morocco, $7.50 net.

Anders' Practice, for years, has been recognized as the standard for American practitioners. Really there is no use for new editions, except to chronicle the rapid changes occurring in American Medicine, for that matter in World Medicine. Conservative and proper always, yet the worthy improvements of aid to the general practitioner are noted and their valuation stated.

Among the newer things noted in this edition are: "Treatment of Tetanus," "Acidosis (in Diabetes)"; "Treatment of Asthma"; "Functional Tests of Hepatic Insufficiency"; "Estimation of Renal Function"; and many other subjects. Many phases have been rewritten. Among these are: "Prophylactic Vaccination"; "Specific Therapy in Typhoid Fever"; and so many other matters that lack of space prohibits their notation here.

The work remains a standard for the practitioner and a reliable guide to the harried practitioner.

MILITARY WAR MANUALS.

MILITARY ORTHOPEDIC SURGERY.

Medical War Manual No. 4. Authorized by the Secretary of War and Under the Supervision of the Surgeon-General and the Council of National Defense. Prepared by the Orthopedic Council. Illustrated. Price $1.50. Lea and Febiger: Philadelphia and New York, 1918.

Orthopedic Council, Majors Elliott G. Brackett, Joel E. Goldthwait and David Silver, Medical Reserve Corps, Major Fred H. Albee, Drs. G. Gwilym Davis, Albert H. Freiberg, Robert W. Lovett and John L. Porter.

MILITARY OPHTHALMIC SURGERY.

War Manual No. 3. By Allen Greenwood, M. D., Major M. R. C., G. E. De Schweinitz, M. D., Major M. R. C., and Walter R. Parker, M. D., Major M. R. C. Illustrated.• Price $1.50. Lea and Febiger: Philadelphia and New York, 1917.

These war manuals are becoming highly prized by men in the service on account of their compact-, ness and consequent accessibility. They bear the stamp of approval of the War Department and carry the generally adopted views of their well known authors on the subjects considered.

AMERICAN ADDRESSES ON WAR SURGERY.

By Sir Berkeley Moynihan, C. B., Temporary Colônel, A. M. S., Consulting Surgeon, North Command. 12mo. of 143 pages. Philadelphia and London: W. B. Saunders Company, 1917. Cloth. $1.75 net.

Sir Berkeley Moynihan is eminently, fitted to discuss phases of the War of interest to the physician as well as to the layman. His mastery address on the "Causes of the War" ranks with the statements made by any of the great men of the world on the subject. The volume in addition to that address contains chapters dealing with "Gunshot Wounds and Their Treatment," "Wounds of the Knee-Joint," "On Injuries to the Peripheral Nerves and Their Treatment," and "Gunshot Wounds of the Lungs and Pleura."

At this time a statement from such an authority, who has had almost unlimited opportunities for observing actual conditions from the front line dressing stations to the Base Hospital at home, carries with it great interest. The book will be read by thousands of our men now engaged in the Military Service and those who are contemplating service in the future.

OFFICERS OF COUNTY SOCIETIES, 1918

County	President	Secretary
Adair	A. J. Sands, Watts	A. J. Patton, Stilwell
Alfalfa	H. A. Lile, Aline	W. H. Dersch, Carmen
Atoka-Coal		A. Cates, Tupelo
Beaver		
Beckham		V. C. Tisdal, Elk City
Blaine	J. B. Leisure, Watonga	J. A. Norris, Okeene
Bryan	J. L. Reynolds, Durant	D. Armstrong, Durant
Caddo	A. H. Taylor, Anadarko	Chas. B. Hume, Anadarko
Canadian	P. F. Herod, El Reno	W. J. Muzzy, El Reno
Choctaw	V. L. McPherson, Boswell	E. R. Askew, Hugo
Carter	F. W. Boadway, Ardmore	Robt. H. Henry, Ardmore
Cleveland	J. J. Gable, Norman	Gayfree Ellison, Norman
Cherokee	W. G. Blake, Tahlequah	G. A. Peterson, Tahlequah
Custer	J. Matt Gordon, Weatherford	C. H. McBurney, Clinton
Comanche	E. R. Dunlap, Lawton	General Pinnell, Lawton
Coal-Atoka		A. Cates, Tupelo
Cotton		G. O. Webb, Temple
Craig		R. L. Mitchell, Vinita
Creek		H. S. Garland, Sapulpa
Dewey		E. J. Hughes, Vici
Ellis		
Garfield	H. B. McKenzie, Enid	A. Boutrous, Enid
Garvin	H. P. Markham, Pauls Valley	N. H. Lindsay, Pauls Valley
Grady	D. S. Downey, Chickasha	Martha Bledsoe, Chickasha
Grant		C. H. Lockwood, Medford
Greer	Nay Neel, Mangum	Thos. J. Horsley, Mangum
Harmon	W. T. Ray, Gould	R. L. Pendergraft, Hollis
Haskell		R. F. Terrell, Stigler
Hughes		
Jackson	T. H. Hardin, Olustee	W. H. Rutland, Altus
Jefferson		L. B. Sutherland, Ringling
Johnson		
Kay		A. S. Risser, Blackwell
Kingfisher		C. W. Fisk, Kingfisher
Kiowa		A. L. Wagoner, Hobart
Latimer	E. B. Hamilton, Wilburton	E. L. Evins, Wilburton
Le Flore	E. E. Shippey, Wister	Harrell Hardy, Bokoshe
Lincoln		
Logan		E. O. Barker, Guthrie
Love		
Mayes	J. L. Adams, Pryor	L. C. White, Adair
Major		
Marshall		
McClain	J. W. West, Purcell	O. O. Dawson, Wayne
McCurtain		R. H. Sherrill, Broken Bow
McIntosh	B. J. Vance, Checotah	W. A. Tolleson, Eufaula
Murray		W. H. Powell, Sulphur
Muskogee	J. G. Noble, Muskogee	A. L. Stocks, Muskogee
Noble	L. D. Stewart, Perry	B. A. Owen, Perry
Nowata	J. E. Brookshire, Nowata	J. R. Collins, Nowata
Okfuskee	J. S. Rollins, Paden	A. O. Meredith, Bearden
Oklahoma	John A. Reck, Oklahoma City	H. H. Cloudman, Oklahoma City
Okmulgee	W. C. Mitchner, Okmulgee	Harry E. Breese, Henryetta
Ottawa	A. M. Cooter, Miami	Blair Points, Miami
Osage	G. W. Goss, Pawhuska	Benj. Skinner, Pawhuska
Pawnee		F. T. Robinson, Cleveland
Payne	E. M. Harris, Cushing	J. B. Murphy, Stillwater
Pittsburg	T. H. McCarley, McAlester	J. A. Smith, McAlester
Pottawatomie	R. M. Anderson, Shawnee	G. S. Baxter, Shawnee
Pontotoc	B. F. Sullivan, Ada	Catherine Threlkeld, Ada
Pushmataha		
Rogers	W. E. Smith, Collinsville	W. A. Howard, Chelsea
Roger Mills		Lee Dorrah, Hammon
Seminole		
Sequoyah		T. F. Wood, Sallisaw
Stephens	D. M. Montgamery, Marlow	H. C. Frie, Duncan
Texas	W. H. Langston, Guymon	R. B. Hays, Guymon
Tulsa	H. D. Murdock, Tulsa	W. J. Trainor, Tulsa
Tillman		
Wagoner	C. E. Hayward, Wagoner	S. R. Bates, Wagoner
Washita	D. W. Bennett, Sentinel	A. S. Neal, Cordell
Washington	G. F. Woodring, Bartlesville	J. G. Smith, Bartlesville
Woodward	R. A. Workman, Woodward	C. W. Tedrowe, Woodward
Woods	G. M. Bilby, Alva	D. B. Ensor, Hopeton

OFFICERS OF OKLAHOMA STATE MEDICAL ASSOCIATION:

Meeting Place—Tulsa, May 14-15-16, 1918.
President, 1917-18—Dr. W. Albert Cook, Tulsa.
President-elect, 1918-19—Dr. L. S. Willour, McAlester.
1st Vice-President—Dr. McLain Rogers, Clinton.
2nd Vice-President—Dr. G. F. Border, Mangum.
3rd Vice-President—Dr. Horace Reed, Oklahoma City.
Secretary-Treasurer-Editor—Dr. C. A. Thompson, Muskogee.
Delegate to the A. M. A., 1918-19—Dr. Chas. R. Hume, Anadarko.
Delegate to the A. M. A. 1917-18—Dr. M. A. Kelso, Enid.

CHAIRMEN OF SCIENTIFIC SECTIONS.

Surgery and Gynecology—Dr. LeRoy Long, Oklahoma City.
Pediatrics and Obstetrics—Dr. T. C. Sanders, Shawnee.
Eye, Ear, Nose and Throat—Dr. L. A. Newton, Oklahoma City.
General Medicine, Nervous and Mental Diseases—Dr. A. B. Leeds, Chickasha.
Genitourinary, Skin and Radiology—Dr. W. J. Wallace, Oklahoma City.
Legislative Committee—Dr. Millington Smith, Oklahoma City; Dr. J. M. Byrum, Shawnee;
Dr. W. T. Salmon, Oklahoma City.
For the Study and Control of Cancer—Drs. LeRoy Long, Oklahoma City; Gayfree Ellison,
Norman; D. A. Myers, Lawton.
For the Study and Control of Pellagra—Drs. A. A. Thurlow, Norman; L. A. Mitchell, Frederick;
J. C. Watkins, Checotah.
For the Study of Venereal Diseases—Drs. Wm. J. Wallace, Oklahoma City; Ross Grosshart,
Tulsa; J. E. Bercaw, Okmulgee.
Necrology—Drs. Martha Bledsoe, Chickasha; J. W. Pollard, Bartlesville.
Tuberculosis—Drs. L. J. Moorman, Oklahoma City; C. W. Heitzman, Muskogee; Leila E.
Andrews, Oklahoma City.
Conservation of Vision—Drs. L. A. Newton, Oklahoma City; L. Haynes Buxton, Oklahoma
City; G. E. Hartshorne, Shawnee.
First Aid Committee—Drs. G. S. Baxter, Shawnee; Jas. C. Johnston, McAlester.
Committee on Medical Education—Drs. A. L. Blesh; A. K. West; A. W. White, Oklahoma City.
State Commissioner of Health—Dr. John W. Duke, Guthrie, Oklahoma

COUNCILOR DISTRICTS.

1. Cimarron, Texas, Beaver, Harper, Ellis, Woods and Woodward; Councilor, Dr. J. M. Workman, Woodward. Term expires 1919.
2. Roger Mills, Beckham, Dewey, Custer, Washita and Blaine; Councilor, Dr. Ellis Lamb, Clinton. Term expires 1920.
3. Harmon, Greer, Jackson, Kiowa, Tillman, Comanche, and Cotton; Councilor, Dr. G. P Cherry, Mangum. Term expires 1918.
4. Major, Alfalfa, Grant, Garfield, Noble and Kay; Councilor, Dr. G. A. Boyle, Enid. Term expires 1919.
5. Kingfisher, Canadian, Oklahoma and Logan; Councilor, Dr. Fred Y. Cronk, Guthrie. Term expires 1918.
6. Caddo, Grady, McClain, Garvin, Stephens and Jefferson; Councilor, Dr. C. M. Maupin, Waurika. Term expires 1919.
7. Osage, Pawnee, Creek, Okfuskee, Okmulgee and Tulsa; Councilor, Dr. N. W. Mayginnes, Tulsa. Term expires 1920.
8. Payne, Lincoln, Cleveland, Pottawatomie and Seminole; Councilor, Dr. H. M. Williams, Wellston. Term expires 1920.
9. Pontotoc, Murray, Carter, Love, Marshall, Johnston and Coal; Councilor, Dr. J. T. Slover, Sulphur. Term expires 1918.
10. Washington, Nowata, Rogers, Craig, Ottawa, Mayes and Delaware; Councilor, Dr. R. L. Mitchell, Vinita. Term expires 1918.
11. Wagoner, Muskogee, McIntosh, Haskell, Cherokee and Adair; Councilor, Dr. J. Hutchings White, Muskogee. Term expires 1920.
12. Hughes, Pittsburg, Latimer, LeFlore and Sequoyah; Councilor, Dr. Ed. D. James, Haileyville. Term expires 1920.
13. Atoka, Pushmataha, Bryan, Choctaw and McCurtain; Councilor, Dr. J. L. Austin, Durant. Term expires 1920.

STATE BOARD OF MEDICAL EXAMINERS.

Melvin Gray, M. D., Durant, President; B. L. Denison, M. D., Garvin, Vice-President; J. J.
Williams, M. D., Weatherford, Secretary; O. R. Gregg, M. D., Waynoka, Treasurer; E. B. Dunlap, M.
D., Lawton; Ralph V. Smith, M. D., Tulsa; W. LeRoy Bonnell, M. D., Chickasha; Wm. T. Ray, M.
D., Gould; H. C. Montague, D. O., Muskogee.
Reciprocity with Georgia, Kentucky, Mississippi, Nevada, North Carolina, Wisconsin, Kansas,
Arkansas, Virginia, West Virginia, Nebraska, New Mexico, Tennessee, Iowa, Ohio, California, Colorado, Indiana, Missouri, New Jersey, Vermont, Texas, Michigan.
Meetings held second Tuesday of January, April, July and October, Oklahoma City.
Address all communications to the Secretary, Dr. J. J. Williams, Weatherford.

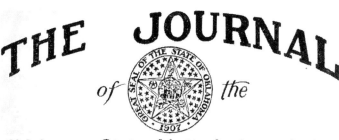

THE JOURNAL of the Oklahoma State Medical Association

VOLUME XI MUSKOGEE, OKLA., MAY, 1918 NUMBER 5

SOME FREQUENT OBSTETRIC PROCEDURES—CONSERVATIVE AND VICIOUS.*

By W. A. FOWLER, M. D., Oklahoma City

In obstetrics, as elsewhere, we are apt to allow the unusual and the spectacular to monopolize our attention and concern. Yet our conduct of the more frequent procedures determines to a much larger extent the degree of service we render our patients. It is with this fact in mind that I have chosen to discuss a few of the procedures frequently observed in obstetric practice. We might profitably strive to arrive at better methods of practice in these frequent procedures.

1. The first thing I shall mention is a closer supervision of the patient during pregnancy. In a paper read before this Association last year I tried to show the vital importance of this procedure. I consider it one of the most fertile fields for preventive medicine. Among the benefits often observed may be mentioned the following: The general health of the patient may be much improved by the proper hygiene of pregnancy. A more wholesome attitude toward the child-bearing function is often observed. Malpresentations with a mortality of from 30 to 45 per cent. can frequently be converted to the normal. Cases of tuberculosis, syphilis, gonorrhoea, pyelitis, etc., may be properly treated with great advantage to the patient. Many other dangerous abnormalities may be anticipated and prepared for. Finally, the routine careful study of these cases will do much to raise the practice of obstetrics above the plane of cheap midwifery and place it upon a scientific par with other branches of medicine. Parental care should include an early, complete written history and physical examination, with especial attention to tuberculosis, syphilis, the heart, and the genito-uninary system; full definite instructions as to the hygiene and the danger signs of pregnancy; frequent examination of the urine and estimation of the blood pressure; and, one month before term, an abdominal and pelvic examination for a complete obstetric diagnosis.

2. Close observation of the fetal heart sounds. This is decidedly a conservative practice. It is indispensable if we would conserve to the fullest fetal life, particularly in difficult or instrumental deliveries and in cases in which there is pressure on the cord. We should be exercised on account of any considerable rise or slowing or irregularity of the fetal heart rate. Some fluctuation in the rate may be expected as the head passes through the cervix. The following cases illustrate, I think, the importance of this practice in the conduct of labor:

Mrs. H., age 27, para I, confinement Nov. 20, 1915. Septate uterus and

*Read at Medicine Park, Oklahoma, May 10, 1917.

vagina. Pains rather weak, progress slow from 5:00 a. m. to 11:30 p. m. when the second stage began. Fetal heart to the right and below and constantly 126 until 3:00 a. m. when the first fluctuation was noticed. By 3:40 a. m. the fetal heart was showing very marked fluctuation, ranging from 168 between pains to 110, faint, and irregular during pains, at times being inaudible. Judging that there was pressure on the cord, (pains were not strong and frequent enough to give symptoms from cerebral pressure) an easy low forceps was quickly done and a moderately asphyxiated baby was delivered, the cord being around the neck.

Mrs. G., age 31, para III, confinement date Sept. 20, 1916. Case first seen after membranes had ruptured only a few hours before the beginning of labor. Head was found to be above, feet below. Cephalic version by abdominal manipulation. At the first vaginal examination at 10:30 p. m., the right foot was found presenting, the head being forward just above the pubis. At times the fetal heart showed marked fluctuation, due, I judged, to pressure on the cord probably by the thigh or leg against the body. Efforts to get the foot out of the pelvis and cause the head to engage by abdominal manipulation failing, the patient was given chloroform, the whole hand was introduced into the vagina, the foot pushed up, and the head partially engaged. The fetal heart continued to fluctuate from 156 to 96 and the head did not advance in spite of good pains. Cervix was fully dilated at 6:00 a. m. Pains continued until 7:30 a. m. with no progress, the fetal heart growing worse. Medium forceps at 8:00 a. m. on account of slow irregular fetal heart. Moderately asphyxiated baby delivered with the cord around the neck. Except the chloroform to relax the uterus during the manipulation mentioned above, no analgesia had been used in this case on account of the fluctuating fetal heart.

The following case illustrates the danger of neglecting this: Mrs. B., age 21, para III, confinement date Sept. 5, 1916. This patient was an incipient tuberculosis case and in order to minimize the shock I had given morphine, gr. 1-8, and atropin, gr. 1-300. This had been repeated once and the patient had been given scopolamin, 1-360, once without producing any cyanosis of the mother and without the fetal heart changing beyond the limits of 125 and 135 per minute up to the beginning of the second stage of labor. No observations of the fetal heart rate were made during the forty minutes of the second stage and an extremely asphyxiated baby was born with the cord around the neck and not pulsating. It required 25 minutes of the most active efforts at resuscitation to get the child to breathing properly. Had the second stage been prolonged in this case, the baby would undoubtedly have been still-born.

3. Anesthesia and Analgesia During Labor. Any one at all observant did not need the experiments of Crile on anoci association to be convinced that prolonged severe pain produces profound shock. If pain can be relieved or alleviated without danger to either patient it is not only humanitarian, but a scientifically proper thing to do. It is especially indicated in systemic conditions, such as tuberculosis or heart disease, and in case of very nervous patients with tedious dry labor. Generally speaking, and without going into the merits or demerits of any particular agent used for this purpose, we should hold the lives and the future health of both patients above the temporary relief of pain. Generally, analgesics and anesthetics may be safely used if we begin with small quantities and if, by constant, careful observation of both patients we limit the amount used to that degree in which there is no marked change in the rate or quality of the fetal heart sounds, no cyanosis and no marked heart or respiratory changes in the mother, and no probability of secondary relaxation of the uterine muscle with its resultant excessive loss of blood.

4. The Reckless Use of the Various Methods for Hastening Delivery. The meddlesome practice of "walking"the patient and directing bearing-down efforts in the first stage of dry labors, the clumsy and ill-advised use of forceps, and the reckless use of pituitrin are responsible for the invaliding of many mothers, and

the last two for the death of many babies. Forceps and pituitrin are often used without a careful pelvic examination in cases with faulty position of the fetus, large baby, or contracted pelvis, or before complete dilatation of the cervix, and for no other indication than that the labor is not progressing fast enough to suit the whim of the doctor. Careful observation of the fetal heart sounds during their use and the examination of both patients afterwards will cool the ardor of many men for these measures. If the condition of both patients is good; if we we have reason to believe that delivery per vaginam is possible; if the fetal heart sounds are unchanged in rate, distinctness, and regularity; and if the pains are fairly good, we would best serve the intersts of our patients by staying close to the tried and trusty policy of "watchful waiting". For my own guidance I have laid down this rule: Forceps are indicated when a rapid delivery is necessary on account of danger to either patient and when *we believe* delivery per vaginam is possible; pituitrin is indicated in cases of uterine inertia, with complete dilatation of the cervix, when we are *certain* that rapid delivery per vaginam is possible without serious injury to either patient.

THE ANTRUM.

By W. E. DIXON, M. D., F. A. C. S.
Associate Professor of Ear, Nose and Throat, University Medical College,
Oklahoma City, Okla.

In this age and time the teachings of Billings, Rosenow, and Shambaugh that at least 90 per cent. of all diseases, either acute or chronic, have their inception in a focus or foci of infection, are most generally believed by the medical profession today. The teeth and tonsils have perhaps received their just share of attention, by both the medical profession and our co-workers, the dentists.

Yet it is believed by all, that there is much work and investigation to be done by our dental friends as to the exact line of demarkation between the tooth, on the one hand, with an abscess at its roots which can be drilled, treated, the infection removed, and the tooth saved for future usefulness, and on the other hand, the tooth with a deadly infection at its roots, that must be pulled to cure the disease caused by the foci of infection.

The well informed laryngologist of today has a certain definite method by which he can not only demonstrate to his own satisfaction, but also to the patient and friends as well, that a tonsil is diseased. Thus he can say positively that this or that tonsil should be removed.

We firmly believe that our friends, the dentists, will soon work out a more exact method of diagnosis, and will soon be able to state with some degree of certainty that this tooth can be cured and saved and that that one must be pulled. I want to make a protest and in the most emphatic terms at my command; to condemn members of our own profession who ruthlessly sacrifice teeth, both good and bad, on most every patient on whom they are called to operate.

Did these men ever stop to think that if these same cases suffering, we will say, from a goitre or chronic appendicitis were referred to a good up to date dentist or nose and throat surgeon, and their case properly worked out, that the patient might be spared many teeth as well as a more serious operation? If the foci of infection be removed, many cases of goitre and appendicitis will get well without operation.

My plea then is, that we of the medical profession co-operate with the dental profession and encourage them to do the work in their line. All things being equal, they as a profession, should know better than we, what is best to be done with this tooth or that.

So much has been said and written about the teeth and tonsils as the site of foci of infections, that I am afraid lest the profession as a whole are apt to forget or overlook the fact, that there are foci of infection in the various accessory sinuses of the nose which are as important to have relieved as those either in the tonsils or teeth. The facial bones contain cavities, filled more or less with pus, which may remain for years without causing definite symptoms other than those of foci of infection, and an occasional headache or neuralgia. Especially is this so after the disease has become chronic.

While any of the accessory sinuses of the nose may be a source of foci of in-infection, the purpose of this paper is to deal only with the antrum. The antrum, or maxillary sinus as it is sometimes called, because it is developed within the maxillary bone, has been known to exist over 400 years. It was first discovered by Vesalius in 1515 who then stated that it only contained air. For the next 270 years various opinions were held about the antrum; some writers believing that it held air; others that it was a resonator for the voice; while many held the antrum had to do with the elimination of the animal spirits.

Morgagni in 1783 thought that this sinus secreted impurities from the blood and held them. Nathaniel Highmore in 1651 was the first to publish the history of a case of suppurative disease of this sinus. For the original work done by Highmore in clearing up the field his name still lives and always will, as the maxillary sinus bears his name.

Following Highmore, in those days of limited knowledge, many men, among the most conspicious of whom were Velpeau, Mabonius and Zwingler, operated on this antrum. William Cowper in 1717 operated on this sinus and it is his operation that our friends, the dentists, are still using today. We will refer to this later.

The antrum is present in the newly born infant in the form of a long slit-like cavity. It very rapidly increases in size, measuring at six months of age about a cubic centimeter. This increase in size continues until adult life, when it is the largest of the accessory cavities of the nose. This fact is important for us to remember for if the foci of infections are so important as we are taught to believe then we should ever be on the alert to detect suppurative conditions of this sinus in children.

Don't say to parents when they consult you about their child having a foul nose, that it won't amount to anything, that he will outgrow it, etc. No, never! Perhaps that very child's future will depend upon your answer. Do you realize that in your answer you may be condemning that child to an incurable heart disease, rheumatism in its various forms, tuberculosis, appendicitis, gall bladder trouble or empyemia, yes, to death itself.

Again, it is my belief that the foul smelling atrophic rhinitis which causes the sufferer to be ostracized from society on account of his or her awful nasal stench, is caused by a diseased antrum. Had this been relieved when the doctor was first consulted the patient would not have been condemned to years of mental anguish, a constitution far below par amd to a condition now incurable.

The antrum is infected in one of two ways. In this it differs from all the other sinuses of the nose. Therefore the antrum is more often diseased than any of the others. First, it is infected as all the other sinuses of the nose, by bacteria gaining entrance into them through the natural opening. Anatomically, the reason for this is that with the exception of the frontal, the natural openings are situated at the uppermost part of the sinus, which does not facilitate drainage. And where drainage is interfered with disease is bound to result.

Second, the antrum is also infected by certain teeth whose roots lie in close proximity or even pass into the sinus. These are the second bicuspid and first molar. So that an abscess at the roots of either of the above teeth will cause an extension of the infection into the antrum.

Here our friends, the dentists, sometimes discover our mistakes and have done much to clear up this once obscure disease. They locate an infected bicuspid or first molar, extract either one and discover a disease by pus flowing out of the antrum through the opening thus made. They enlarge this opening for drainage. I wish to call your attention to the fact that this is the Cowper operation devised by Wm. Cowper in 1717, just two hundred years ago, and has been discarded by rhinologists for many years because it will not cure a chronic antrum trouble.

There are no defined symptoms by which we can make a diagnosis of antrum infections. We may or may not have headache. In acute cases we usually have a severe headache which is most marked at the junction of the nose with the eyebrow, which radiates over and back of the eye. We may have pain over the antrum on the cheek bone, yet this is not constant. By pressure over the antrum we may elicit pain. We may have pain in the upper teeth or we may have pain all over one side of the head and face. This pain may be paroxysmal in character, coming on at indefinite periods, as once or twice a month. The patient may be extremely nervous or may have a severe cough which cannot be relieved. The patient may present the appearance of one suffering from a toxic condition such as bad teeth or tonsils and give a history of loss of weight, loss of appetite, loss of vigor, restlessness and complains of being tired all the time.

If we will take a careful history we will find that the trouble usually dates back to a severe cold, that when the patient stoops over she becomes dizzy and the pain is aggravated. This is an important and constant symptom. In conclusion I want to report three cases from my records, which I hope will aid us in making a diagnosis or at least cause us to become more on the alert to find these cases, as I am constrained to believe that many, many of these cases pass in and out of our offices daily without having a proper diagnosis made, let alone their suffering relieved.

Case 1. Miss E. J. L., a trained nurse, 28 years of age, referred by a surgeon with a probable diagnosis of frontal sinusitis.

Patient gave history of having had a severe cold about five or six days before she presented herself for treatment. The whole left side of the head ached but the pain was most acute at the root of the nose, at the junction of the eyebrow, and over and back of the left eye, neuralgic condition of face. Patient was weak and indifferent and upon stooping over was dizzy. For years she has spit up bloody pus in the morning.

At the beginning of the treatment, March 13th, 1917, patient weighed 115 pounds. After the third treatment she was entirely free from pain and after eight treatments was free from pus and had gained eight pounds. Case discharged well.

Case 2. J. W. R., a life insurance man, 40 years old, gave a history of an antrum infection which was treated for about a week or ten days, one year previous. When he presented himself for treatment he had been extremely nervous and suffering severe pain on both sides of face and head for about six weeks. The pain was most severe at the junction of the nasal and frontal bones. Patient had slight tenderness over both cheek bones. Both antra were affected. After twelve treatments extending over a period of fourteen days, he was free from pain and pus, was discharged cured. Two months later patient reported that he had gained 22 pounds, was over his nervousness and happy.

Case 3. Mrs. L. W., age 49 years, contracted a cold last November. Following this she had pain at the root of the nose radiating over and back of the right eye; as well as a severe cough which, though she was treated by a physician for several months it continued day and night, until the antra were treated. After ten treatments, she was relieved of pus, pain, and cough. This case is of interest on account of the constant aggravating cough, which cough medicine did not affect in the least, and might recall to mind many such cases to each one of us.

VARIED TOPICS OF SURGICAL INTEREST.

By F. L. WATSON, M. D., McAlester, Okla.

Gentlemen of Pittsburg County Medical Society:

Preliminary to any remarks I may make on the above subject, I must say that after attempting to analyze it, I find it so voluminous that any attempt to do the subject justice in the short time allotted would be futile effort.

Taking up this subject as the title reads, I have made subdividions of the same which will be taken up singly, considered briefly, and passed on. The first subdivision I have is *Firmness of Conviction*. However, before proceeding further, I wish to say that any remarks that I may make are not intended as personal, but are largely the results of errors that I have made, and I am included in the company of anyone whose toes may be stepped upon.

Under this sub-topic I wish to again take up our old time yet ever present enemies, appendicitis and cancer. True enough they have been talked about 'and written about, until we are all tired of them, yet every once in a while some great-big-hearted fellow lets his acquaintance with the family, and his sympathy for them, get the better of his otherwise good judgment and common sense, and gives some absolutely worthless (often injurious) remedy and waits to see 'if a child will not get over this attack, until at last forced to advise operation as a last resort, and the child passes on into that vague and great hereafter to remain as a thorn in some man's memory, who let his sympathy overrule his common sense. Let us not wait to see what a little sore will do, if it will not heal in three or four weeks under kindly treatment. Would you waste your time standing around to see if a baby boy would grow to manhood if he were "carefully watched". Then why let some poor soul go on to lymphatic involvement, mixed infection and death in spite of operation simply because you were watchfully, disastrously waiting, and did not have the moral courage nor firmness of conviction to say, I am right, we must act, act intelligently and promptly if we are to save your life.

In all our associations with the public we should be candid and truthful. I had a thousand times rather be truthful and wrong, and have my patient get well, than to be a careless, miserable liar and smooth over something because I wanted to injure my fellow medical man or appeal to the natural desires of the patient; only to have that same patient, a few months or possibly years later, say: "If Dock Blank had only told me the truth, I would not now be in the fix I am."

Next I want to devote a few words to the *Surgery of Children*. A man who is a successful child's surgeon is KING OF THEM ALL.

In operating for children remember that anesthetics are hard on children, those little tender growing tissues can ill afford to loose blood excessively.[1] Operations for children should be executed with as much dispatch as is consistent with good work; and *emphatically* with the minimum loss of blood possible. In the adult 8 per cent of the body weight is blood, in children it is only 5 per cent, so that oozing points, to which in the adult we would hardly notice, must be carefully watched and the hemorrhage arrested in the child. Another place besides appendicitis, where prompt and heroic action is vital to both life and limb, is osteomyelitis. I have seen altogether too many deformities because time was not taken to think that this chill in the night, high temperature, excessive pain does not mean rheumatism nor growing pains, but osteomyelitis; neither should children with crooked arms and useless legs be seen running around because they had been treated by conglomerous filtrates containing imaginary antigens that were insanely, or maliciously, represented as the treatment for an acutely inflamed bone, when a hole should have been drilled into it and the destructive tension relieved. Another feature of surgical interest is the anesthetic, no small part of which is due to the anesthetist, who should first be an observer and then be under the observation, of an experienced anesthetist, before being turned loose on a helpless public.

Next, *The Anesthetic.* While I was in Phliadelphia I heard Dr. Jopson[2] out at the Presbyterian Hospital say what I have said many times before—that the patient was the indicator of the anesthetic rather than the anesthetic being the indication for the patient. All anesthetics have their place, and the surgeon should be an anesthetist before being a surgeon, so that he may judge what anesthetic is best adapted to this patient, and then use it.

There are two or more operations to which I wish to refer before I close these remarks. One is *Cesarean Section* and the other *Gastro-enterostomy.* A whole book could be made on either of them and then enough would not have been said. Given a contracted pelvis with head above the pelvic brim, not engaged, a cleanly executed carefully staged cesarean section is preferable, both as to safety of mother (primipara especially) and child than any high forceps delivery yet devised. Again placenta previa seen early close to hospital, and certain selected cases of puerperal eclampsia, where the pathologic "hormone toxin" has not yet accomplished organic destruction of vital tissues.

Gastro-enterostomy has had its day. We used to curette a uterus for all the ills woman was heir to. Oh, reflect our consternation when we speedily recommended a curettage as a specific, and learned that our patient had had a previous hysterectomy. The Sippy treatment of gastric ulcers has so much favorable preponderance of evidence in its favor, that I do not think any man is warranted in subjecting an ulcer patient to the high mortality of gastro-enterostomy (to say nothing of the last result worse than the first), without first treating them for at least four weeks in bed, according to the rules laid down by Dr. Sippy.

One more thing, don't just in order to do something, because you have opened an abdomen, sew a section of jejunum onto some friable gastric cancerous tissue and say: "Lo, what a big gastro-enterostomist am I." You will surely have a funeral. Why not be honest and courageous enough to say, "I did nothing but make the diagnosis"—that it was too late.

Summing up, the indications to me for gastro-enterostomy are very clear, and occur in the order named. Perforation with or without hemorrhage. Pyloric stenosis. Intractable non-malignant ulcer where faithful medical treatment with rest in bed has been a failure.

Just a few words as to *Thorough Examination,*[3] and I am through. When we have not exhausted all the means obtainable by us for examination it spells inefficiency; and so rank that the general profession are going to recognize it, and ere long the laity. With our propaganda for reform, our state and national health bulletins, the wide publicity of health articles in the periodicals and magazines, the public is going to do as it should, in a comparatively short time, push aside the inherited ignorant customs and traditions of by-gone days, and become cognizant that the knowledge that the physician possesses, comes through the channels of the senses plus work and study; and not as a mysterious heredity, or divine dispensation. And the automatic rapid fire, hot air vender and superstition peddler, is going to have to give a logical explanation of his exploitation, which will be based on an exhaustive investigation employing all the resources which will augment the accuracy and acuteness of the senses, plus the application of God's grandest gift to man,—common sense.

Bibliography:
  1 Buford—Sur. Gyn. and Obsts., May, 1916.
  2 Jopson—Personal conversation, Oct., 1916.
  3 Peterkin—Interstate Med. Journal, 1916.

TUBERCULOSIS OF THE KIDNEY—(Concluded).*
Symptoms, Diagnosis and Treatment.

By DANIEL N. EISENDRATH, A. B., M. D., Chicago, Ill.

In the early history of this disease we were dependent upon the clinical history alone combined with the finding of tubercle bacilli in the urine to make a diagnosis, but this has been entirely supplanted by the following additional factors: (1) A careful clinical history combined with (2) Cystoscopy and ureteral catheterization, (3) Pyelography and ureterography, (4) Bacteriological examination of urine obtained directly from the suspected kidney.

In rare instances where such an extensive tuberculous cystitis exists that repeated attempts to catheterize the ureters are unsuccessful, it may be necessary to expose one or both ureters to secure enough urine to determine whether both kidneys are so involved as to make the case an inoperable one.

Cases of chronic renal tuberculosis present themselves under one of the following clinical pictures, in their order of frequency:

Group 1. *Those in which bladder symptoms are the first to appear and overshadow all other symptoms for a long period.* The earliest of the bladder symptoms to be complained of is an increased frequency of urination both during the day and at night. Gradually this is accompanied by pain on urination and a slight vesical tenesmus or desire to repeat the act of urination. These symptoms of bladder irritation increase in severity gradually, i. e., over a period of months. The urine contains at first only a few pus and red blood cells, but gradually both of these increase in number until a distinct pyuria is present. Examination for organisms to be of value must be made from a freshly catheterized specimen. In the male, one must first irrigate the urethra with sterile water in order to eliminate the smegma bacilli which greatly resembles tubercle bacilli in appearance and staining qualities. If examination of such urine is unsuccessful in finding the tubercle bacilli, methods which will succeed in about 80 per cent. of cases are the Forssell or the Crabtree. In the former, one collects the urine of a patient for 24 hours, then pours off the supernatant fluid and places the sediment in a high power centrifuge for two hours and strains the deposit at the bottom of the tubes. In the Crabtree method, the urine specimen is first placed in the centrifuge at low speed so as to throw down the pus cells. The fluid lying above the sediment is then again centrifuged at high speed.

The guinea pig test is not as frequently employed at present as in former years. The reasons for discarding this method are that it requires from two to three weeks and even in the modifications proposed by Bloch and Morton the minimum time is reduced to ten days. The urine at a comparatively early stage contains a large number of pus cells when stained for organisms, one is struck in the majority of cases by the fact that frequently none of the ordinary organisms producing renal or bladder infection are found. It is this absence of the organisms usually found in stained specimens of purulent urine that should attract one's attention to the possibility of a tuberculous pyuria and lead to staining of the pus for the tubercle bacillus and to the employment of the more exact methods of cystoscopy, ureteral catheterization and pyelography.

Incontinence of urine is rarely encountered as a symptom of renal tuberculosis except in children.

To sum up, we find that in fully 75 per cent. of the cases the symptoms of cystitis appear at first in an insignificant manner and gradually increase in severity until the frequency of urination accompanied by pain, tenesmus and the passage of a few drops of blood at the end of the act of urination force the patient to consult a physician. The latter finds that the case does not improve as it should

*Continued from April Journal, Oklahoma State Medical Association.

after the usual method of treatment of cystitis, in fact the use of silver preparations causes great distress. If the general practitioner will only remember that many of his cases of intractable cystitis are in reality the distant expression of tuberculosis higher up in the urinary tract, these patients will have much cause to be grateful to the conscientious progressive family physician.

Group 2. *Those complaining of a dull ache over the affected kidney.* This group is second in frequency, and a history of pain over one kidney should always lead to a thorough examination of the urinary tract or at least of the urine. In some of the cases of this group there is a further history of attacks of colicky pain due to the passage of caseous detritus or of blood clots. It is only by the use of the X-ray and of the cystoscope and ureteral catheter that the pain and pyuria can be differentiated from similar symptoms due to ordinary pyogenic infection and to calculus.

Group 3. *Those in which a sudden hematuria is the first symptom.* The frequency of this group varies according to individual experience, some authors like Pilcher estimate that 25 per cent. of the cases show hematuria as the first symptom. My own experience and that of many others is that hematuria alone does not occur in nearly as large a number of cases. When, however, a patient presents himself with such a symptomless hematuria, it is our duty at the present day to determine the source of the bleeding by cystoscopic examination at as early a period as possible.

Group 4. *Sudden onset of chills and fever accompanied by pyuria.* These are the cases of mixed infection in which there have been no symptoms due to the invasion of the kidney by the tubercle bacillus until a secondary infection by the ordinary pyogenic organisms occurs. In three such cases I had no suspicion of the mixed character of the infection until the time of operation.

Group 5. *Silent cases.* In this group there is either no communication of the foci with the renal pelvis, a condition known as a closed tuberculous pyonephrosis, or the bladder changes are so slight as to cause no symptoms. Cases in this group are very difficult to recognize and the diagnosis is only made as a rule during a routine examination of the urinary tract for other conditions.

Other methods of diagnosis. In addition to the clinical groups just described and the examination of the urine, the making of a diagnosis is greatly aided by the use of one or more of the modern methods now universally accepted as indispensable to accurate work in this field of surgery. I refer particularly to radiography of the urinary tract, cystoscopy and ureteral catheterization and the newest method termed ureterography and pyelography.

Simple radiography is of little value in this disease unless it be in very advanced cases of so-called putty kidney, a term applied to the last stages of a tuberculous pyonephrosis, and we do not need the method here.

Cystoscopy is our main reliance in the diagnosis of tuberculosis of the kidney, and the bladder changes vary from simple redness and edema of the ureteral orifice to extensive dissemination of tubercles and of typical ulcerations in all parts of the bladder. A glance at figure 4 will show some of the most typical changes which may terminate in the conversion of the ureteral orifice on the affected side into a rigid gaping opening resembling that of a golf hole. The irritability of the bladder is so great that it will either not retain any fluid at all or not sufficient to enable a satisfactory cystoscopic examination to be made without a general anesthetic being given. In advanced cases it is almost impossible to identify the ureteral orifices so as to catheterize them.

Ureteral catheterization enables one to determine to confirm the diagnosis by obtaining urine directly from the kidney and staining it for tubercle bacilli. It also is invaluable in the diagnosis of involvement of both kidneys and in securing enough evidence to determine whether the remaining healthy kidney will do the work of both after the tuberculous one has been removed.

By pyelography and ureterography we refer to a method which is based upon the fact that if solutions impervious to the X-ray are allowed to flow through a ureteral catheter you will obtain upon the X-ray plate an exact reproduction of the degree of dilatation or other changes of the ureter and renal pelvis. In doubtful cases in which not sufficient evidence has been obtained by one of the methods just referred to, this newer development of urologic diagnostic technic will enable one to differentiate a tuberculosis from other surgical lesions of the ureter and kidney.

To sum up, the modern diagnosis of tuberculosis of the kidney is based upon the proper interpretation of the clinical history combined with the use of one or all of the more exact methods now used by every surgeon with special training in this special field.

Treatment. A few years ago there was still some difference of opinion in regard to whether a case of tuberculosis of the kidney should be treated by medical methods or by the more radical procedure of removal of the kidney. At the present time the opinion that non-operative treatment should not be considered is unanimous. The only exceptions, i. e., contra-indications to operation, are, patients suffering from either advanced pulmonary tuberculosis, peritoneal tuberculosis or multiple bone foci. That bilateral renal tuberculosis is a contra-indication to operation is self evident. The reason for this unanimity of opinion in regard to the advisability of surgical measures in unilateral tuberculosis of the kidney is that statistics both from European and American clinics show that medical, i. e. non-operative treatment, are most discouraging. Of 48 non-operated cases reported by Braasch from the Mayo clinic, the mortality was 80 per cent. and in only three cases did all of the symptoms disappear.

I have already explained under the description of the pathology of the tuberculous kidney that such apparent clinical cures are due to the fact that all of the renal parenchyma has been destroyed, a process known as autonephrectomy. Such apparently cured kidneys, however, have been shown to contain active tubercle bacilli and remain a constant menace to the individual who carries them. In 316 non-operated cases collected by Wildbolz from Swiss hospitals, there was only one apparent cure, i. e. cessation of clinical evidences, and only 20 per cent. of the 316 were alive after five years. In 200 cases reported by Rovsing, 40 were found inoperable, and in 71 inoperable cases from the Mayo clinic in 48 per cent. the symptoms had existed for over five years. When such figures are compared first, with the mortality of all cases after operation, which is 75 per cent., and second, with the mortality of cases which were recognized and operated before the disease had become too advanced, it teaches that we can offer the patient a percentage of recovery of at least 75, and in course of time a much higher one as compared with a sure mortality of 80 per cent. and of permanent cure in less than one per cent. of the cases. Therefore it is incumbent upon us to try to make a diagnosis at as early a period as possible and to perform a nephrectomy if none of the contra-indications just mentioned exists and if the opposite kidney is shown to be functionally active. The question of how to deal with the ureter is far from being settled. Some advocate complete removal, others to inject carbolic acid into the stump and close the wound, and still others to suture the ureter into the end of the abdominal incision. I prefer the last named method, which was first described by Rovsing. After removal of the kidney the upper end of the ureter is sutured to the skin edges at the anterior end of the abdominal incision.

The technic of removal of a tuberculous kidney requires no special mention except that the utmost care should be exercised not to allow any of the tuberculous pus to escape into the wound because a very slow healing tuberculosis infection of the retroperitoneal tissues results. I always drain such nephrectomy wounds by the same methods as in non-tuberculous cases. The bladder symptoms disappear very slowly after nephrectomy, especially in cases where the disease has existed for years. Often a year or more passes before the benefits of the nephrectomy are manifested by a cessation of the increased frequency and painful, often bloody, urination. In one of my recent cases we obtained a most striking amelioration of symptoms and disappearance of all cystoscopic findings characteristic of tuberculosis by the use of mesothorium kept in the bladder for 24 hours in the manner in which it is employed in cancer of the bladder, and I can warmly recommend its use in this most disagreeable sequel of renal tuberculosis.

EUGENICS.

By J. W. LYNES, M. D., Byron, Okla.

In common parlance, eugenics means the bettering of our physical, mental and social conditions, an improvement on every generation, in brain and brawn. A standardization of human lives is bringing the cost of a perfect body within the reach of all.

The progress of the human race is measured by the enforcement of its laws, and there is no law in our human understanding that has appealed to the human family, as the one of legalizing birth-control. It has revealed to us, as doctors, and friends of the human race, some remarkable and heart searching views of life.

Public sentiment requires that all up-to-date medical men be able to give sound advice on all subjects, but this "one thing thou lackest". Freedom of speech is denied us on this vital question, and sometimes legislation ceases to be remedial.

The proper control of reproduction is surely one of the most vital problems in intelligent concern for the betterment of the human race. Race conservation has been so impressed upon the majority of people that they lose sight of the necessity of guarding the lives of those already produced. Some are so concerned by the problem of race suicide that they have considered it necessary to prohibit the imparting of imformation in regard to prevention of conception, holding it as a duty of each individual family, regardless of fitness, to bring into the world as many children as nature enables them to bear.

In England, the question of birth control has been more thoroughly investigated than in any other country. The first investigation made developed the fact that of the forty millions of inhabitants, twelve millions, or nearly 33 per cent., are paupers. Some connection was thought to exist between birth-control and pauperism. It was concluded that large families was one of the main causes of poverty, and of all countries authorized to testify on poverty, England is entitled to the first place as a witness. As a direct result of these investigations, there was organized in London a society whose function it is to give advice to the married persons and those contemplating marriage, on hygienic methods of birth-control; known as the Malthusian society, in honor of that learned economist, who first asserted that population increases more rapidly than the food supply, hence causing the population to live in constant want and misery, if not downright semi-starvation.

Thanks to the law makers of England, they have enacted a statutory law indirectly imposing poverty on a large portion of the living population and children yet unborn. My information is, that some years ago, in order to prevent young men and boys in colleges from getting hold of obscene pictures and literature, the late Mr. Anthony Comstock, of New York, was instrumental in having passed by congress an act prohibiting the transmission of such matter through the U. S. mails and by express companies. He is to be commended for that noble piece of legislation. Later, as a result of his activity, congress passed a law making it a crime to circulate information, either written or by word of mouth, on the prevention of conception, or contra-ception, as it is now called. Here, we think, Mr. Comstock erred, that law has brought unhappiness to thouasnds of

American homes, where joy and prosperity reigned before. We question the truth of the much vaunted statement to the effect that a child owes so much to the state. Large families, with few exceptions, have at their heads poor fathers. It is manifestly better for the state that a few children be born, who are healthy, mentally and physically strong, than so many who are weak intellectually and physically unfit. Weaklings are prolific, having no sense of restraint, they are easily swayed by the force of their passions, and add burdens of helpless beings, unfit for society.

Rapid birth rate goes hand in hand with infant mortality and low income. When the family income is just sufficient to provide wholesome food for four, what of necessity must be the chances for physical and mental development when that family is increased to eight? The physically strong, who are capable of producing strong children, and whose income is sufficient to support them, are usually instructed in the manner of prevention of conception. The law withholding knowledge of prevention of conception from those unfit, is an injustice, first to the state, which must provide for defective children; second, to innocent, unborn children, who are forced into conditions of poverty, disease, and crime. Third, to the over-burdened parents, who, work as they may, cannot provide for a constantly increasing family.

We are spending large sums, every year, upon our juvenile courts, our reformatory homes, and the insane. Would it not be better and nobler if a little of this money and scientific knowledge was used to alleviate the suffering and poverty of men and women who are bowed down with the burden of large families?

It is a well known fact a large percentage of the boys and girls who go wrong, especially in cities, are from homes of large families. Our government spends through the Department of Agriculture, thousands of dollars and sends thousands of phamplets to our farmers yearly, telling them how to breed cattle and swine, that it is better to have a few head of healthy well-bred cattle and swine than to have a large herd of inferior stock. Are cattle and hogs more valuable than children?

In conclusion, let me say, that I probably have not introduced one new thought on this intensely vital question. I have only skimmed over the surface, and the horizon is enlarging. I have not touched on the question of social purity, nor the toll of unborn generations exacted of humanity, nor the laws governing eugenics, marriages lacking in power of enforcement. A vital necessity in settling this matter is the education of the people to their duty, then the education of the unfit to restraint. When we have successfully and legally solved the problem of birth-control, then all these other perplexing questions will fold their tents, like the Arabs, and silently steal away.

URETHRAL SEALING MEDICATION.

E. G. Ballinger and O. F. Elder, Alanta, Ga. (*Journal A. M. A.*, March 23, 1918), describe their method of prolonged application of suitable remedies to the urethral mucosa, which they have used for treatment and prophylaxis, by sealing urethral canal with collodion. The chief indications for such treatment, as might be expected, are fresh infection and prevention. The details of the method are given in full. As a prophylactic measure the treatment with it has been most satisfactory. They have never seen gonorrhea develop when it was applied within forty-eight hours after exposure, and when empolyed a little later it seemed to make the disease milder, and he has never seen stricture develop from the treatment or the urethritis intensified. The solution usually employed for them is arygrol, 5 per cent. Stronger solutions are unnecessary.

JOURNAL OF THE OKLAHOMA STATE MEDICAL ASSOCIATION

VOLUME XI   MUSKOGEE, OKLA., MAY, 1918   NUMBER 5

PUBLISHED MONTHLY AT MUSKOGEE. OKLA., UNDER DIRECTION OF THE COUNCIL

DR. CLAUDE A. THOMPSON, EDITOR-IN-CHIEF

ENTERED AT THE POST OFFICE AT MUSKOGEE, OKLAHOMA, AS SECOND CLASS MAIL MATTER, JULY 28, 1912

THIS IS THE OFFICIAL JOURNAL OF THE OKLAHOMA STATE MEDICAL ASSOCIATION. ALL COMMUNICATIONS SHOULD BE ADDRESSED TO THE JOURNAL OF THE OKLAHOMA STATE MEDICAL ASSSOCIATION, 308 SURETY BUILDING, MUSKOGEE, OKLAHOMA.

The editorial department is not responsible for the opinions expressed in the original articles of contributors.

Reprints of original articles will be supplied at actual cost, provided request for them s attached to manuscript or made in sufficient time before publication.

Articles sent this Journal for publication and all those read at the annual meetings of the State Association are the sole property of this Journal. The Journal relies on each individual contributor's strict adherence to this well-known rule of medical journalism. In the event an article sent this Journal for publication is published before appearance in the Journal, the manuscript will be returned to the writer.

Failure to receive the Journal should call for immediate notification of the editor, 307-8 Surety Building, Muskogee, Okla.

Local news of possible interest to the medical profession, notes on removals, changes in address, deaths and weddings will be gratefully received.

Advertising of articles, drugs or compounds unapproved by the Council on Pharmacy of the A. M. A. will not be accepted.

Advertising rates will be supplied on application. It is suggested that wherever possible members of the State Association should patronize our advertisers in preference to others as a matter of fair reciprocity.

EDITORIAL

THE OKLAHOMA DOCTOR'S DUTY TO THE ANNUAL MEETING.

Year after year we have heard excuses, reasonable and unreasonable, given as a reason for not attending the annual meeting. Usually they are from men who did not attend the year before, often on account of some fantastic idea that positively all the wheels in the neighborhood would stop revolving if they should leave the engine of the universe unattended or in the hands of some rival engineer during their absence from home.

Now ordinarily these excuses go, but this time they should be forgotten. If there was ever a time when the recluse should be rudely jarred from his self-complacent, stay-at-home, sufficient-unto-myself attitude, it is now. Men never needed the stimulating ideas of their fellow practitioners as they do now. No future medical generation will have to face the problems, so completely, we may say, of a socialistic nature, if that word means the individual's best effort for the good of all, as our profession is now facing and must solve and make the best of.

Contact with your fellow physician will reveal a world of short cuts and suggestions for improvements in the handling of your every day problems. If you know how to do something better than he does, and of course you admit you do, it is now your duty to help along the general good by telling him how to do it properly.

Drop your absorbing problems and make arrangements to attend the Tulsa meeting. Everything calls you to make this sacrifice.

THE QUESTION OF RANK.

When the war first started the writer thought he would like to be at least a Major—in fact the suggestion was made to Washington, but Washington was very busy just then trying to make a dollar buy fifty dollars worth or doing a year's work in a week. So the matter of the Majority progressed not.

Oklahoma physicians in and entering the army certainly are all qualified for high rank, they all ought to be not under the rank of Major, but we simply cannot have so many of high rank; there would be no one left to issue orders to.

Our physicians should not be deterred on account of the possible rank they may be given. We should not forget that we have splendidly equipped men in France and England, very competent surgeons and of other branches, who are still wearing the bars of a first lieutenant.

Billings, Binnie, Bloodgood and others are Majors, but they were lieutenants for a long time. It seems hardly equitable for most of us to expect to step from civil life into high rank. We should not forget, that to win the war our forces must be evenly balanced—We must have the stalwart man in the trench, the Medical lieutenant mostly, after that the higher ranks perceptably decrease as we go toward the top.

We should have the spirit to serve where we are most needed regardless of the rewards.

LEST WE FORGET.

These are piping times. Men are prone to forget the freaks of yesterday, but in order to do the people of Oklahoma some good, and we hold doing them good is a continuous act of our profession, we herewith republish the vote on the Medical Practice Act as registered by the last legislature. The men who voted for that measure should not be forgotten, but above all things physicians should not forget the representative who potentially did his constituents a grave wrong in opposing a measure, which if lost would have resulted in turning loose on Oklahoma's citizens a horde of misinformed ignoramuses with power to do damage only limited by their opportunity.

The Legislative Record on 111.   Save This.

The following members of the legislature voted for Senate Bill 111, erroneously called by many the "Medical Bill," the "Doctors' Bill," the "Anti-Chiropractic Bill," etc. As a matter of accuracy and correctness this bill, which is now law, should have been called what it really is, a bill to raise the standard of examination to those who propose hereafter to "practice medicine," without reference to the wild claims that the candidate is not proposing or does not propose to practice medicine, but cures by "conjuring," rubbing, etc.

The medical profession, sponsors of common sense and the rule of reason, should not lightly forget these men who voted to protect the people of Oklahoma against charaltanism and inefficiency:

Senate—Yeas: Beauman, Board, Buckner, Burns, Carpenter, Chase of Nowata; Cordell, Davidson of Tulsa; Davidson of Haskell; Edmondson, Ferguson, Hall, Hogg, Kerr, Knie, Logan, McAlister, McIntosh, Rider, Risen, Snyder, Thomas, Vaughan, Wilson of Greer. Total 24.

House—Ayes: Acton, Adams, Baker, Barry, Beatte, Beck, Berry, Blackard, Bobo, Bond, Butler, Campbell, Cartwright, Cahapman, Collums, Condon, Craver, Dickinson, Disney, Dolan, Draughon, Durant, Eakins, Elder, Fitzgerald (Kiowa), Fitzgerald (Pittsburg), Fox, Gibson, Gish, Haile, Hamilton, Harper, Harris, Harvey, Hartenbower, Headley, Hensley, Hicks, Hinds, Hodges, Hughes, Hultsman, Humble, Hurst, Jackson, Johnson, Kelly, Marsh, Mayfield, Meacham, Miller, Neff, Newman, Northcutt, Norvell, Pardoe, Petry, Powell, Riley, Robertson, Rogers, Sheegog, Shirley, Shores, Speer, Thomas, Ticer, Treadway, Vaden, Waldrep, West, Wheeler, Wimbish, Wismeyer, Woodard, Woods, Mr. Speaker Nesbitt. Total 77.

From a physicians' standpoint the following should be relegated to exactly the same status as a certain insignificant minority of the United States Senate, who recently voted to tie the hands of the President in the great emergency confronting the Nation.   Certainly they, who forgot the plight of a helpless people as to public health protection, deserve the same execration at the hands of intelligent people:

Senators Voting "No"

Name	Address
Cline	Newkirk
Clarence Davis	Sapulpa
John Golobie	Guthrie
R. A. Keller	Marietta
O. W. Killam	Grove
Thos. J. O'Neill	Chickasha
M. M. Ryan	Poteau
J. J. Smith	Afton
Tom Testerman	Morrison
Fred E. Tucker	Ardmore
Geo. E. Wilson	Cestos

Representatives Voting "No"

County	Name	Address
Alfalfa	J. C. Smith	Cherokee
Atoka	Jas. A Thurmond	Tushka
Beckham	Algernon Mansur	Elk City, R. No. 4, Bx 57
Blaine	L. A. Everhart	Bickford
Canadian	Jack Barker	El Reno
Cimarron-Texas	M. W. Pugh	Boise City
Comanche-Cotton	Lewis Hunter	Lawton
Creek	J. M. Morgan	Bristow, R. No. 1, Box 7
Creek	Will Cheatham	Bristow
Dewey	M. L. Jones	Trail
Ellis	Bert E. Hill	Gage
Garvin	Alfred Stephenson	Stratford
Greer	J. O. McCollister	Mangum
Jackson	R. J. Morgan	Altus
Logan	Amos A. Ewing	Guthrie
Major	S. J. Beardsley	Fairview
Oklahoma	S. S. Butterfield	Oklahoma City
Pawnee	Millard F. Grubb	Maramec
Washita	W. T. Graves	Sentinel, R. No 2.
Woods	W. H. Olmsted	Waynoka

Senate—Excused: Bickel, Brown, Chase of Seminole, Edwards, Johnson, Knight, Watrous. Total 7. Absent: Hickman, Leach. Total 2.

House—Absent: Christopher, Garrett, Hendrickson, Houston, Keegan, Neal Nicholson, Platt. Rowland, Scott, Walden, Warren, Welch. Total, 15.

Mr. Graves offered in explanation of his vote on Senate Bill No. 111, that the bill was too drastic in form.

THE SUCCESS AT CAMP GREENLEAF.

Washington medical authorities are proud of the showing made at Camp Greenleaf when the Warden McLean Medical Auditorium was dedicated March 10th. The information then disclosed is official and should be borne in mind by all medical men who are daily asked questions, wise, foolish and perplexing, as to the part the doctor is playing in the War. On account of much silly misinformation written in daily papers, for a time there was an impression among the thoughtless and misinformed that we were not doing our part, that an impossible thing—a draft of medical men solely—would be resorted to to fill the needs only in the imagination of the idle.

Practically all the General Medical Board attended as well as the Surgeon General and his staff and many men distinguished in civil and military medical life.

Dr. William H. Welch stated that 21,824 men had been recommended for commission, of which 17,313 had accepted. 5,378 dentists were recommended, 5,086 had accepted. Of 1,067 for the Sanitary Corps, 865 had accepted. 138 out of 152 had accepted for the Ambulance Service. There are 844 officers in the Naval Corps and 103 in the Dental Corps; 827 medical and 199 dental officers in the Naval Reserve. Chief pharmacists, pharmacists, hospital corpsmen, run into many thousands.

From 8:30 to 10:30 each morning Admiral Braisted receives telegraphic and telephonic reports from all Naval Stations and is accurately in touch with the situation everywhere.

Restaurants, barber shops, in fact every place in a wide zone around each camp is given the same thorough sanitary inspection as prevails in the camps and insistence is made that bad conditions be corrected.

Dr. William D. Haggard, Nashville, for the Red Cross reported that there are 20 base hospitals on active duty abroad, 14 mobilized and 19 certified ready for immediate service.

Dr. William J. Mayo reported that 21,000 physicians have been indexed as to particular qualifications and suggestions as to selection made. This index is in the hands of the Surgeon General, and a duplicate is in France. He closed with a plea for increased rank for the medical officer, stating that they are not doing work to which they are unaccustomed and untried, but are engaged in the work of their lives.

The Committee on Nursing have enrolled 18,344, of which 10,000 have enrolled with the Red Cross since April 6, 1917. This organization has supplied the Army with 6,220 up to March 1 and 1,000 to the Public Health and Navy Service. It was shown that a deficiency in nurses in December was due to lack of housing facilities in some and to a larger quota not being called for others.

Dr. Arthur Dean Bevan for the American Medical Association expressed the opinion that whether the War lasts three years or five, requires 3,000,000 men or 5,000,000 men, the medical profession will continue to "stand by until the job is finished"; that the one job of the Association was to educate the profession to realize the extent of the work to be done.

General Gorgas said that notwithstanding handicaps the American Army has established a sanitary world's record never before equalled, the nearest approach being by the Japanese whose death rate was 20 per thousand while ours was 10, that the work was only begun and would improve.

Victor C. Vaughn related an interesting conversation with Wassermann in Berlin in 1907, who then expressed the fear that the 50,000 soldiers quartered in Berlin and other like units in other cities indicated that "some day" Germany's military leaders would plunge the country in War which might mean the dismemberment of the empire. Dr. Vaughn hoped that some day he would again walk the streets of Berlin and see flying not the flags of the Allies, but of the German republic.   He contrasted present conditions with those of Chickamauga in 1898 when there was not a single microscope or test tube in the camp, observing that the line officer of today had the work-together spirit.

Since organization of the camp 4,000 officers and 20,000 enlisted men have been trained and sent abroad or to instruct other camps.

WHAT MANNER OF DOCTORS ARE THESE?

A letter to the State Council is printed in full below.   Comment is unnecessary.

To the State Committee of National Defense,
      Medical Section.

Gentlemen:

Last year three of our best men who were all past middle life left their business, which they had been years in building up, and entered active service.   These men lived in _____ and _____ (small towns), and had arranged with men who could not, because of age or physical disability, get into the army to take care of their work.

But now comes the grafter.   These men had not been gone six weeks until four young able-bodied slackers moved onto their fields and began to absorb the patronage of the men who had sacrificed so much to go.

We older men have gone after them; but do you think they will volunteer for service?   Not one of them! ·

I am past age, but, Doctor, I am going to make a break to get into service of some kind and let those _____ cowards stay.   I don't want to live in the same country with them.   Buying Liberty Bonds may salve the conscience of these men of proper age and ability, who can do active service, but every town should make them wear yellow or go.

Don't write me any more letters, but come out and hang some of the blood-suckers.   It may be you need all your rope at home; if you do, use it.

                Yours,

PERSONAL AND GENERAL NEWS

Dr. W. T. Hill, Tamaha, has moved to Stigler.

Dr. J. A. Pryor, Avard, has moved to Dilworth.

Dr. O. E. Templim, Alva, has joined the colors at Ft. Riley.

Dr. C. E. Thompson, M. R. C., Enid, has sailed for France.

Dr. Albert A. Stoll, Arnett, has moved to Longton, Kansas.

Dr. S. N. Stone, Edmond, has been called to the colors at Ft. Rilry.

Dr. J. L. McIlwain, Lonewolf, has entered Army service at Ft. Riley.

Dr. J. J. Caviness, M. R. C., Altus, has been ordered to Camp Beauregard.

Dr. E. P. Miles, formerly of Duke, has moved to Hobart and will open a hospital.

Dr. R. W. Williams, M. R. C., Anadarko, has been ordered to Ft. Riley for duty.

Dr. A. E. Martin, Marietta, has been ordered to Army service at Ft. Sam Houston.

Dr. C. E. Northcutt, Lexington, has been ordered to duty with the Medical Reserve at Washington.

Dr. O. J. Street, Louis, has been ordred to active service in the Medical Reserve at Ft. Riley.

Dr. S. E. Cummings, Ravia, has announced his candidacy for the legislature for Johnson county.

Dr. R. L. Mitchell, Vinita, has been commissioned in the Medical Reserve and is awaiting orders.

Dr. J. E. Davis, McAlester, attended the meeting of the Tennessee State Medical Association in April.

Dr. J. R. McLaughlin, Norman, Succeeded Dr. Gable as assistant physician to the State Hospital, taking up the work April 15.

Dr. McClain Rogers, Clinton, is receiving the congratulations of his friends on recovering from a dangerous attack of pneumonia.

Dr. and Mrs. A. Ray Wiley, Tulsa, have returned from an extended residence in New York City where Dr. Wiley was House Surgeon in the Polyclinic for more than a year.

Drs. F. B. Fite and C. A. Thompson, Muskogee, visited Ft. Worth and witnessed the Review of the 36th Division April 11th. The show was splendid and worth going many miles to witness.

Dr. C. M. Pratt, for may years at Maysville, has moved to Pauls Valley and formed a partnership with Drs. Lindsay and Callaway, taking the place created by Dr. G. L. Johnson's entering Army service.

Dr. W. T. Huddleston, Konowa, according to press dispatches, was required by the Seminole County Council of Defense to apologize for making alleged seditious and disloyal utterances. The matter is one of regret to his friends.

Dr. Newton Rector, Hennessey, suffered the greatest bereavement when Mrs. Rector died at their home in Hennessey April 7th. They have lived in Hennessey since its founding and Dr. Rector has the sympathy of hosts of friends on his loss.

Dr. Wm. T. Howell, located at Duncan for many years, died at his home March 24 after a long illness. Dr. Howell was a member of the Masonic fraternity, a native of Texas and was highly respected by the people of Duncan and vicinity. He was 61 years of age.

Dr. F. E. Rushing, Coalgate, who was recently ordered to report for Army duty at Washington, was tendered a banquet by Coal County physicians on his departure, who expressed their regret on his absence, but applauded the motive and wished him god-speed and a safe return.

Physicians Generally are responding to the call now issued for an increase in the Medical Reserve to fill the demand made by increase in the army. Many prominent men who heretofore have refrained on account of the press of practice at home are applying and Oklahoma bids fair to make a remarkably good showing within the next few weeks.

The Annual Meeting promises just some more than any other meeting ever offered visitors, as was to be expected from Tulsa. A real President's reception and ball, a smoker or "War Banquet," a visit to one of the largest refineries in the United States and an automobile tour of one of the really wonderful cities of the country is only a part of the things in store for the visitors.

Dr. W. C. Mitchell, Commerce, is said to have accidentally dropped an amputated finger in a street of that city. The authorities made a horrible example of the doctor and fined him. The dispatches do not indicate that the incident spurred the city fathers to renewed efforts to clean up unsanitary alleys or abolish the good old fashioned back houses, so prolific in their midst.

Dr. H. C. Montague, Muskogee, our good personal osteopathic friend and member of the State Board of Examiners, according to report recently suffered from an attack of smallpox. Really our very good feeling for the doctor personally is the only thing that prevents us from "lambasting" him proper. The opportunity is certainly at hand and he owes us a treat for not using it.

Dr. L. Haynes Buxton, Oklahoma City, Chairman Medical Section, State Council of Defense, is doing most effective work in stimulating Medical Reserve Corps applications. He has secured a very complete roster of Oklahoma physicians with their abilities and disabilities noted. His special bete noir is the physician financially and physically able to go to War, having no dependents to hold him, yet who hesitates.

Dr. D. U. Wadsworth, Tulsa, died April 11th from pneumonia. He was one of the best known physicians of the city, having held many important positions. He was born in Copiah County Miss., January 16, 1874, educated at Centenary College, receiving his medical degree from the University of the South, an Elk and Mason of high standing. Served Tulsa as Superintendent of Health two terms. He is survived by a wife and one son five years of age.

Oklahoma Pharmaceutical Association meeting in Oklahoma City in April went on record as opposed to the lowering of the standard of examination requirements on account of the war. This is proper and to be expected. The War's demands simply mean that the druggist, as well as all of us, must work harder and accomplish more, but the work must by no means be inferior; if it is, both the profession and the people will eventually suffer from the low standard.

Women Physicians, according to Washington opinion, will not be commissioned in the Medical Department. This determination is certainly debatable. We have no particular delusions as to Woman's Suffrage, but undoubtedly there are many highly competent women physicians in the country who are extremely anxious and able to render good service to the country. They would fit well into laboratory work, in many executive positions and as internists as well.

Dr. A. W. Nieweger, dentist, Oklahoma City, was twice called before the County Council of Defense and his alleged utterances as to sedition and disloyalty inquired into. Shortly after the inquiry, which resulted in an admonition from the Chairman, Judge C. B. Ames, the office of Dr. Neiweger was entered in the night, according to the police, by parties "unknown" and completely demolished. It is said the charges were based on his circulating to soldiers a book laudatory of the trip of the Deutsch--land. He has left Oklahoma.

Dr. S. B. Mayfield, Eufaula, has announced his candidacy for the State Senate, the District comprising McIntosh, Muskogee and Haskell Counties. Well; we are for Dr. Mayfield. We believe the State would be better off if the legislature was composed of more doctors and our unqualified opinion, based on first hand observation at the legislature, is that he made a splendid representative, voting for all measures strictly on the question of their merit, taking orders from no one and going home with the ability to look all men in the face in the knowledge that he performed his duty to the best of his ability, which is by no means of mediocre character.

1918 Graduates of the Medical Department of the State University who were recently examined by the State Board of Examiners, it is said to a man, will seek entry into the Medical Reserve Corps.

The Blacksmith as a pioneer pointing the way to improvements in chiropractic manipulations was much in evidence in a suit brought in the Federal Court at Oklahoma City by "Dr." David A. Reisland, Duluth, Minn, against "Dr." A. A. Gregory. Reisland admitted that he had never practiced, but was a machinist before he invented a mechanism for "stretching" the human infections out of our frames. He wants Gregory to pay him for using his discovery for the purpose of jimmying, lock-nutting and otherwise applying the principles of the Spanish Inquisition to his patients. It seems that every time these gentry fall out we get a better insight into their "science".

Fee Splitting is assuming importance enough to be given editorial notice (see Oklahoman reproduction this issue), incidentally "professional ethics", a thing, state or being often scoffed at by our newspaper brothers, is hinted at as the probable means of eradication of the practice. Well, it will take more than "ethics" to curb the matter. The remedy will be found in merciless publicity and in the realization by the offenders that they are betraying a noble profession from which they should be scourged. Just why a physician should reduce himself to the level of a boot-black, with his hand out for a cheap reward, is beyond our psychological interpretation. No physician should have a transaction with another physician about his patient which he would object to any other physician and especially the patient interested in knowing all about. We favor fee-splitting, unqualifiedly, provided the man paying the bills is fully aware of split, otherwise it is downright dishonesty.

Church and Denominational inclinations and affiliations of our soldiers now in cantonment is strikingly set forth in figures taken from an official investigation recently made. As these men are mostly young, in the prime of life, as a rule normal from a mental standpoint, some of the results as shown at Camp Doniphan are worth remembering. The investigation at Camp Doniphan was the most thorough made and covered more detail than that of any other camp.

137th Infantry, 3527 men, shows: Methodists, 1181; Christian, 617; Baptists, 452; *Christian Scientists*, 13.

128th Machine Gun Battallion, 637 men, contains 3 Christian Scientists. Division Headquarters, 73 men, showed up with 2 of the cult, who believe, instead of administering antitoxin, antitetanus serum, vaccines to prevent typhoid, smallpox and paratyphoid, that "there's nothing to it", "purely imagination", "state of mind", et cetera, therefore just ignore such small matters. It is indeed fortunate that the Government takes an obsolete and "erroneous" view of the matter and insists on "poisoning" the men with prophylactic vaccines.

MISCELLANEOUS

MEDICAL OFFICERS MUST SUBMIT PAPERS BEFORE PUBLICATION.

1. Attention of medical officers is directed to the provisions of paragraph 423, M. M. D.— "Medical Officers will not publish professional papers requiring reference to official records or to experience gained in the discharge of their duties without the previous authority of the Surgeon General."

2. Numerous scientific papers written by officers of the medical department have recently appeared in the medical press without specific authority from this office. This practice will be discontinued, and the above regulation will be strictly complied with.

3. Officers desiring publication of professional papers will submit two copies to the Surgeon General with request for permission to publish same. Upon approval, a copy will be forwarded to the journal designated by the officer for publication.

By direction of the Surgeon General:

C. L. FURBUSH
Lieutenant Colonel Medical Corps, N. A.

THE BULGARIAN BACILLUS AS A REMEDIAL AGENT.

A simple and effective remedy for the summer diarrheas and other common ailments of the intestinal canal is the Bulgarian bacillus. This was popularized a few years ago by the late Professor Metchnikoff, who pointed out that this organism, in the form of buttermilk, is extensively used by the Bulgarians, who have the reputation of being the longest lived people in Eurpoe. While this lactic acid organism is not, of course, a panacea for senility, it is a remedy of very great value for many intestinal affections. Clock and others have shown that by its use summer diarrheas of children can be controlled more quickly, and with less disturbance of the child's regular food than with any other remedy. It has also been recommended for intestinal indigestion, autotoxemia of intestinal origin, and even for such serious diseases as diabetes.

It is important to use a culture of the Bulgarian Bacillus which you can depend upon. Galactenzyme (Abbott) is such a culture. This product is made from the type A organisms, of established virility, under the most careful, aseptic precautions. It is available both in tablet form and in bouillon. For ordinary use the tablets are generally preferred. We recommend a careful trial of Galactenzyme in cases of summer diarrhea. Now is the time to secure a supply.

MEDICAL RESERVE APPOINTMENTS FOR OKLAHOMA.

Supplementary List, December 16 to March 31, inclusive.

William W. D. Akers ....Ada
Carl Rudolph Williams (colored)..Bristow
Robert Edward Lee Thacker..Lexington
William Lewis Haywood (colored), 203 E. 1st. St...............................Oklahoma City
Merle Quest Howard, 2228 W. 11th...Oklahoma City
John William Riley, 119 W. 5th..Oklahóma City
Frederick Charles Brown...Sparks
Alba Jesse Whittey (colored), 505 E. Archer...................................Tulsa
Louis Bagby...Vinita
Powell Lambert Hayes..Vinita
Ralph E. Workman...Woodward
James Jackness, 709 N. Brdy...Altus
Walter Henry Dersch...Carmen
Charles C. Conley...Frederick
William Thomas Polk...Maysville !
Roy Francis Von Cannon...Miami
James Jackson Gable...Norman
Reuben Morgan Hargrove...Norman
Robert Berry Gibson, 319 Colcord Bldg..Oklahoma City
Wann Langston...Oklahoma City
Elijah Stover Sullivan, 611 Colcord Bldg......................................Oklahoma City
William Wesley Lightfoot..Thackerville
Lawrence Heard Carleton...Tulsa
Casper A. Hicks...Wetumka
Oscar Elsworth Templin..Alva
Henry Lee Johnson...Centrahoma
Alexander Bartholomew Leeds...Chickasha
Andrew Nelson Lerskov...Claremore
Sidney Baldwin Bellinger, All Saints Hosp....................................McAlester
Jesse Monroe Pemberton...Okemah
Archie Bee, 1320 Classen Blvd..Oklahoma City
Frederick Albert Cochran, Jr., 1429 W. 21st..................................Oklahoma City
Francis Asbury DeMand, 411 State Nat. Bk.....................................Oklahoma City
Galvin Luther Johnson...Pauls Valley
Erskine D. Johnson, 515 E. Hobson St...Sapulpa
Lewis Edgar Emanuel...Chickasha
Wallace Andrew Aitken, Stephen Bldg..Enid

THE FEE-SPLITTING DOCTOR.

The American College of Surgeons in a recent bulletin denounces vigorously the practice of fee-splitting—"Division of Fees," it calls it—and asks the co-operatoin of all hospitals in stamping out this evil. It suggests the adoption of a resolution, the text of which it prints, pledging all physicians who avail themselves of hospital privileges against parciipating in such spoils. It defines fee-splitting, in any guise whatsoever, as "the buying and selling of people who are ill." A severe definition, it is true, but a correct one.

Many states have legislated against the practice. How effective such laws are is not known. It is obvious, of course, that such laws are easily evaded. And since it is to the interest of the parties engaged in it to guard the secrecy of the transaction discovery is difficult. It is an evil hardly remediable by law. Professional ethics is the force which must be depended upon to eradicate it—the professional ethics which obtain by virtue of the character of the members of the profession.

The utter eradication of this practice may not be looked for immediately. The fee-splitting doctor like the snitch lawyer, or the grafter of any other profession or trade, is likely to be with us quite a while. Yet the reputable physicians who constitute the great majority of the profession, can undoubtedly do much to minimize this trafficking in misfortune. Professional ostracism should follow hard upon proof of guilt, together with publicity, that the public, as well as the profession, may be informed. We imagine, too, that the medical profession, supported by law if necessary, will some day establish a rigorous standard of requirements for the physician who conducts a hospital. Such an institution is far too solemn a trust to be vested in a physician except he be of irrreproachable standing.—Oklahoman.

ACIDOSIS IN SHOCK.

W. S. McEllroy, Pittsburgh (*Journal A. M. A.*, March 23, 1918), reports his studies on the acidosis in shock. The methods of experimentation were those described by Guthrie in *The Journal* of Oct. 27, 1917, p.1394. Essentially, they comprise prolonged strong rhythmic stimulation of the afferent nerves of dogs, under ether anthesia. When necessary other means, such as exposure and manipulation of the abdominal viscera, were used to hasten the conditions. In later experiments peripheral nerve stimulation combined with partial cerebral anemia was found to be the most satisfactory procedure yet employed in refractory cases. Anemia was caused by temporary occlusion of arteries supplying the brain and medulla. A little blood was lost but not enough to cause a serious condition. Acidosis was studied by the indicator methods of Levy, Rowntree and Marriott for H-ion concentration, and of Marriott for reserve alkalinity, and of Van Slyke for plasma bicarbonate, the former two being used in the earlier experiments. Variations in different animals were found. The greatest variation soccurred in reserve alkalinity. In the later experiments, Van Slyke's method was followed in detail and the results showed the effects of ether administration on the plasma bicarbonate, the plasma bicarbonate in shock and the effects of injection of sodium bicarbonate in skocked animals, the effect of maintaining the reserve alkalinity during shock production, are briefly summarized as follows: "In the type of experimental shock studied there was a gradual decrease in the reserve alkalinity of the blood. The decrease varied in different animals. Anesthesia was an important factor. In some instances, the reserve alkalinity in shock was as great as in other animals before shock. This shows that acidosis was not an important causative factor. In no case was a change in reserve alkalinity sufficient to account for the condition observed. In experimental primary acidosis the alkali reserve may be lowered to a degree observed in shock without producing any marked change in the condition of the animal. The injection of sodium bicarbonate into animals reduced to a terminal state by injection of acid resulted in prompt recovery. The injection of sodium bicarbonate into animals in shock was without beneficial action, although the reserve alkali was restored. Shock may be induced while the alkali reserve is maintained by injection of sodium bicarbonate." They conclude that in the type of experimental shock studied, acidosis was only one of the many secondary changes produced.

THE ANTI-VIVISECTIONISTS.

The anti-vivisectionists have aroused the wrath of a certain congressman from Nebraska who charges them with treasonable utterances. He quotes them as saying that "thousands of deaths have been deliberately inflicted upon our soldiers and sailors who were pumped full of disease by compulsory inoculation and vaccination." It seems to us that such a charge is too silly to be dignified by congressional consideration and that, as a matter of fact, the anti-vivisectionists as a tribe should never be taken seriously.

They are a queer crowd, these anti-vivis. Their emotions have many grotesque angles. Some of them go on sprees of morbidity. They revel in anguish at the heartlessness of other folks. The brutality of science that sacrifices a guinea pig in the interest of human life flushes whole coveys of burning adjectives. They think more of brutes than they do of people. Of course, they don't think any such thing, but some of them, perhaps, think they think so.

It may be assumed, we guess, that the serum theory of healing, if it may be so called, is cursed with the usual quota of extremists that fasten themselves to every new school of endeavor. That persons have died from inoculation or vaccination is, of course, a fact. But preventive medicine has justified itself in the judgment of all rational persons. Typhoid, for example, has been all but eradicated from the armies of the world by vaccination. The number of lives saved in that one respect is a vast return for all the sacrifices enrolled by experimentation and mistake.

With the cheap, factitious grief spread about the imaginary torture chambers where calloused surgeons wax gleeful over the suffering of the noble dog—well, it's nothing but hyprocrisy. And the absurdity of the statement that soldiers have been deliberately killed by physicians is what the immortal Dana characterize as damphoolia. We needn't take all the serums that are recommended. We must make allowances for the enthusiasts of this school. But we must accept vivisection as an earnest effort on the part of medicine to grapple more successfully the grim old adversary. It is doing it, too.—Oklahoman.

CHLORETONE: SUGGESTIONS FOR DOSAGE.

For its hypnotic effect Chloretone may be administered in doses sufficient to produce the desired result without endangering the life of the patient. As one writer points out, it is useless to expect to attain that end by giving the patient small doses—5 grains—at long intervals—three times daily. In general, a single dose, of 5 to 20 grains, will have the best effect. It would be well to give about 10 grains the first night, 15 the second, and 20 grains the third. When a dose is found that produces the desired result, the same dose may be repeated until the "sleep habit" has become established, when it should be reduced gradually.

When the use of Chloretone must be continued for a protracted period, as in the treatment of epilepsy, its effects should be watched lest cumulative action manifest itself. It should not be pushed to the point of dullness and drowsiness.

As a sedative in asthma, chorea, pertussis, nausea, emesis gravidarum, and seasickness, doses of 3 to 10 grains, at stated intervals according to the effect, are generally sufficient. As a preventive of post-anesthetic nausea the administration of ether, is the usual practice.

The principal effects of Chloretone are manifested upon the central nervous system. It acts like other hypnotics, but, unlike most of the latter, it does not depress the circulatory system, nor does it disturb digestion.

Chloretone is procurable in 3-grain and 5-grain capsules, convenient for administration.

THE BRITISH ZONE OF THE ADVANCE.

George de Tarnowsky, Chicago, at the front in France (*Journal A. M. A.*, March 16, 1918), describes conditions as observed by him in the British zone of advance on the western front. The British have maintained a comparatively short front, difficult to hold, and correspondingly more difficult to advance in. The continuous fighting has increased the distance between the firing lines and the regimental aid posts, and lengthened the elapsed time between the wound reception and treatment. The evacuation hospitals or casualty clearing stations are under more or less continuous bombardment, and have frequently had to be moved from place to place. Primary closure of wounds, which is almost an axiom in the French army, is still in the experimental stage on the British front. Tarnowsky describes the topography of the land with its ruined villages and towns, and the almost universal shell holes, filled with mud and water, which render "duck board" walks necessary to transport the patients across the desolated tracts. He says one can not help feeling admiration for the bulldog tenacity, courage and spirit of self-sacrifice which have enabled the British to hold on to the difficult situation for four years and to advance their lines in the face of such gigantic topographic and climatic difficulties. The regimental aid posts are first described. They are situated about a thousand yards back of the trenches. The relay posts are about a thousand yards apart. Two or more relay posts are maintained between the regimental aid station and the advanced dressing station. The advanced dressing station represents a division field ambulance occupying a semi-permanent post, five thousand yards behind the firing line, and from its narrow gage railway could bring the wounded to the corps main dressing station. The advanced dressing station described is in the ruins of a chateau, which have been protected by corrugated iron roofing, and four layers of sand bags. In it, however, emergency operations could be performed only during periods of comparative calm. Situated one thousand yards behind the advanced dressing station was a collection post for the slightly wounded and sick. The corps main dressing station, about eight thousand yards from the extreme front, represented the first semi-permanent field ambulance where emergency operations could be performed, amid proper surroundings, though as yet no advanced surgery was performed, but de Tarnowsky received the impression that it was being considered. The British corps rest stations correspond to our hospitals for the slightly wounded. Trench foot prophylaxis stations receive the greatest single percentage of casualties. The present system of prophylaxis and active treatment has given the most satisfaction, though the ideal has not yet been reached. The regulations for the prevention of trench foot are elaborate, and are detailed in full but they can not always be carried out by the soldiers. De Tarnowsky describes the delousing stations where the men's clothes are cleaned and the vermin destroyed. It is well nigh impossible to live in the zone of the advance without becoming lousy, and this is not surprising under the conditions. The British casualty clearing stations are placed considerably more to the rear than those of the French, owing to the exposure to bombardment and the constant harrassing warfare being carried out on the British front. Many of them also are still housed in tents, and the life of a tent, thus used, is about four months according to British experience. The article is interesting and instructive, and gives a rather adequate idea of the difficulties and hardships encountered.

COUNCIL ON PHARMACY AND CHEMISTRY.

The following articles have been accepted by the Council on Pharmacy and Chemistry for inclusion with New and Nonofficial Remedies:

Calco Chemical Company: Chlorcosane (Calco).

Gilliland Laboratories: Normal Horse Serum, Concentrated and Refined Diphtheria Antitoxin, Concentrated and Refined Tetantus Antitoxin, Typhoid Vaccine, Small-pox Vaccine, Original Tuberculin, "O. T.", Tuberculin Ointment in Capsules (for the Moro Percutaneous Diagnostic Test), Bouillon Filtrate Tuberculin, "B. F.", Bouillon Emulsion Tuberculin, "B. E.", Tuberculin Residue, "T. R.", Tuberculin for the Detre Differential Diagnostic Test.

Monsanto Chemical Works: Dichloramine-T.

NEW AND NONOFFICIAL REMEDIES

Typhoid Vaccine, Prophylactic. A vaccine made from killed bacillus typhosus. The vaccine is used for the prevention of typhoid fever, for which purpose typhoid vaccines are of recognized utility. Marketed in different sized containers, containing 500 million and 1000 million killed bacillus typhosus in 1 c.c. Eli Lilly and Company, Indianapolis.

Typhoid Vaccine Therapeutic. A vaccine made from killed bacillus typhosus. The vaccine is proposed for the treatment of typhoid carriers and as a concomitant measure to the usual routine of typhoid therapy. Marketed in different sized containers, containing 100, 250, 500 and 1,000 million killed bacillus typhosus in 1 c.c. Eli Lilly and Company, Indianapolis.

Typhoid Mixed Vaccine (Typho-Bacterin Mixed). A vaccine made from killed alpha and beta bacillus paratyphosus and bacillus typhosus. The vaccine is used for the immunization against typhoid and paratyphoid fevers and in the treatment of mixed infections of the typhoid bacillus and the paratyphoid bacilli. Marketed in different sized containers, containing 250 million alpha and beta bacillus paratyphosus and 1000 million bacillus typhosus in 1 c.c., and 500 million alpha and beta bacillus paratyphosus and 1,000 million bacillus typhosus in 1 c.c. Eli Lilly and Company, Indianapolis.

Bulgarian Bacillus Tablets-Mulford. Tablets containing a practically pure culture of bacillus bulgarious. Used in the prevention and treatment of conditions due to intestinal putrefaction. Marketed in vials containing fifty tablets. An expiration date is stamped on the label. H. K. Mulford Company, Philadelphia (*Journal A. M. A.*, March 2, 1918, p. 623).

Arsenobenzol (Dermatologic Research Laboratories) 1 gm. Ampules. Each ampule contains 1 gm. arsenobenzol (Dermatologic Research Laboratories), a brand of arsphenamine complying with the New and Nonofficial Remedies standards. These ampules are prepared for use in hospitals in divided doses. Dermatological Research Laboratories, Philadelphia Polyclinic, Philadelphia.

Halazone-Monsanto. A brand of halazone complying with the New and Nonofficial Remedies standards. Halazone is parasulphonedichloramidobenzoic acid. The Monsanto Chemical Company, St. Louis, Mo.

Procaine-Abbott. A brand of procaine complying with the New and Nonofficial Remedies standards. Procaine was first introduced as "novocaine". Chemically it is the monohydrochlorid of para-aminobenzoyldiethyl-amino-ethanol. It is used as a local anesthetic as a substitute for cocaine. The Abbott Laboratories (*Journal A. M. A.*, March 16, 1918, p. 779).

PROPAGANDA FOR REFORM.

Shotgun Nostrums. As the soldier of today uses a rifle instead of a blunderbuss, so the modern physician uses single drugs rather than shotgun mixtures. There are many types of "shotgun" nostrums. Some are dangerous, as in the case of "Bromidia"; some are preposterous therapeutic monstrosities which excite the contempt of educated physicians, as in the case of "Tongaline"; some are merely useless mixtures of well known drugs sold under grotesquely exaggerated claims, as in the case of "Peacock's Bromides". It is impossible to determine from the published formulas just how much hydrated chloral and potassium bromide Bromidia contains, but it is probable that there are about 15 grains of each of these two drugs to the fluidrachm and variable amounts of Indian cannabis and a small amount of either extract or tincture of hyoscyamus. Bromidia is a distinctly dangerous mixture for indiscriminate use, particularly so if the advertising creates the impression that in it the chloral hydrate has been deprived of its untoward effects. Tongaline is said to consist of tonga, cimicifuga racemosa, sodium salicylate; colchicum and pilocarpin. This jumble of drugs would be merely ludicrous, if anything that degrades therapeutics could be considered so lightly. Peacocks' Bromides is said to consist of the bromides of sodium, potassium, ammonium, calcium and lithium. The exploiters claim superiority over extemporaneously prepared mixtures because of the absence of contaminating chlorids said to be present in commercial bromids. The truth is that the chlorids are used as antidotes in bromid poisoning. Bromidia, Tongaline and Peacock's Bromides have been the subject of reports of the Council on Pharmacy and Chemistry. (*Journal A. M. A.*, March 3, 1918 p. 642).

Hypophosphites for the Army. The purchasing department of the medical department of the U. S. Army asks for bids on three tons, in one pound bottles, of the "Compound Syrup of Hypophosphites". These six thousand bottles of a relic of past generations must be paid for and are to occupy valuable freight space in shipping to various Army posts (*Journal A. M. A.*, March 16, 1918, p. 783).

Compactibility of Phenolphthalein. It is better not to combine several laxatives, but those who believe in doing this may combine phenolphthalein with drugs that can be properly prescribed in powders or pills as, for instance, calomel. Since phenolphthalein and calomel are both tasteless, they may be prescribed in powders or enclosed dry in capsule, cachet or wafer, the amount of each ingredient being estimated according to the susceptibility of each patient (*Journal A. M. A.*, March 30, 1918, p. 950).

Barbital (Veronal) Classed as a Poison by England. Because of frequent reports of accidents and habit formation, the Privy Council of Great Britain has classified as poisons "diethylbarbituric acid, and other alkyl, aryl, or metallic derivatives of barbituric acid, whether described as veronal, proponal, medinal, or by any other trade name, mark or designation; and all poisonous urethanes and ureides". As a result veronal will seldom be dispensed except on a physician's order, and that a record of such sales will be kept in the pharmacist's poison book. (The official name for diethyl-barbituric acid of the British Pharmacopeia is barbitonel; in the United States the official designation for this product is barbital.) (*Journal A. M. A.*, March 30, p. 953).

NEW BOOKS

Under this heading books received by the Journal will be acknowledged. Publishers are advised that this shall constitute return for such publications as they may submit. Obviously all publications sent us cannot be given space for review, but from time to time books received, of possible interest to Oklahoma physicians, will be reviewed.

A TREATISE ON REGIONAL SURGERY.

By various Authors, Edited by John Fairbairn Binnie, A. M., C. M., F. A. C. S., Kansas City, Mo. Volume III, Cloth with 521 illustrations, 830 pages. Price $7.00. P. Blakiston's Sons and Company, Philadelphia.

This volume has for its contributors James P. Mitchell on Traumata of the Upper Extremity; J. W. Perkins on Fractures of the Upper Extremity; Dean Lewis on Diseases of the Upper Extremity;

E. H. Bradford and Robert Sutter on Deformities and Paralyses of the Upper Extremity; J. F. Binnie on Operations upon the Upper Extremity; and the following on the Lower Extermity: Amputation, Operations upon the Joints, W. J. Frick on Traumata (Exclusive of Fractures and Dislocations); Sir W. Arbuthnot Lane on Fractures, Charles Herbert Fagge on Dislocations, Emmet Rixford on Tumors, Stanley Stillman on Non-Traumatic Affections, Sir Robert Jones and David McRae on Deformities, and Infantile Paralysis, and Howard Lilienthal and John C. A. Gerster on Thoracic Surgery.

This volume completes the series of a remarkably splendid system on Regional Surgery. As stated before, the writer is of the opinion that Dr. Binnie is the most effective placer of facts of value and technic on surgical subjects in our country. His first volume on operative surgery issued years ago stands today a reliable guide on operative procedures then recommended, with the exception of those in which there has been a complete revolution, and they are few. It is not necessary to enter here on descriptive details of this work. Enough is said when the array of authors is noted.

TUMORS OF THE NERVUS ACUSTICUS.

Tumors of the Nervus Acusticus and the Syndrome of the Cerebellopontile Angle. By Harvey Cushing, M. D., Professor of Surgery at Harvard University. Oxtavo of 296 pages with 262 illustrations. Philadelphia and London: W. B. Saunders Company, 1917. Cloth, $5.00 net.

This work is a special study and report of the author on certain brain tumors with especial reference to meningeal growths associated with the acoustic apparatus. The subject matter is largely devoted to consideration of a series of cases, which are reported individually at length, the symptoms with the history, neurological findings, clinical diagnosis, the operation and its disclosures, postoperative notes, subsequent notes covering a variable length of time, the pathological notes, based on minute examination of the tumor substance and comments on the case make of the book, a very exact and instructive work.

Cushing stands at the head of the profession in brain work and speaks with the authority of a master in his field.

INFECTION, IMMUNITY AND SPECIFIC THERAPY.

A Practical Text-book of Infection, Immunity and Speciac Therapy with special reference to immunologic technic. By John A. Kolmer, M. D., Dr. P. H., M. Sc., Assistant Professor of Experimental Pathology, University of Pennsylvania, with an introduction by Allen J. Smith, M. D., Professor of Pathology, University of Pennsylvania. Second edition thoroughly revised. Octavo of 978 pages with 147 original illustrations. 46 in colors. Philadelphia and London: W. B. Saunders Company, 1917. Cloth, $7.00 net, Half Morocco, $8.50.

This work remains one of the very interesting productions of recent years. The questions of Infection, Immunity and Specific Therapy are of constant and ever-increasing interest to the practitioner and intelligent advantage is being taken more and more of the phenomena associated with them by the alert physician. Kolmer has given the physician a very helpful work. His deductions are not only based on the researches of others, but come from one himself a recognized authority in the intricacies and pitfalls of laboratory work.

Additions and alterations have been made in this volume throughout. Special attention has been given focal infections, the Schick reaction, complement fixation, quantitative Wassermann, Anaphylaxis. An interesting portion is that devoted to the treatment of certain infections with the serum of convalescents and normal persons. Transfusion and Chemotherapy are also considered.

CLINICAL LECTURES ON INFANT FEEDING.

By Lewis W. Hill, M. D., Children's Hospital, Boston, and Jesse R. Gerstley, M. D., Michael Reese Hospital, Chicago. 12 mo. of 377 pages, illustrated. Philadelphia and London: W. B. Saunders Company. 1917. Cloth $2.75 net.

Here is a book valuable to the physician, as it gives clearly and thouroughly, though concisely, two methods of infant feeding.

Dr. Lewis Webb Hill gives a good idea of the Boston method, while Dr. Jesse R. Gerstley gives the Chicago methods, which are those of Finkelstein and Czerny. By cooperation, they have avoided unnecessary repetition and neither has neglected the essential details of his subject which brings these two widely different methods together in a helpful manner for the physician interested in infant feeding and disturbances of nutrition.   C. V. Rice.

NEW AND NONOFFICIAL REMEDIES, 1918,

NEW AND NONOFFICIAL REMEDIES, 1918, containing descriptions of the articles which stand accepted by the Council on Pharmacy and Chemistry of the American Medical Association on January 1, 1918. Cloth. Price, postpaid, $1. Pp. 452—26. Chicago: American Medical Association, 1918.

This annual should be in the office of every physician. It lists and describes all those proprietary remedies which the Council on Pharmacy and Chemistry has examined and found worthy of the confidence of the medical profession; that is, articles the composition of which is disclosed, which are exploited truthfully and which give promise of some probable therapeutic value. The discription of each article aims to furnish a statement of its therapeutic value and uses, its dosage and method of administration as well as tests for the determination of its identity and quality.   Articles of similar composition are grouped together and in most cases each group is accompanied by a general article which compares the members of a group with each other and with the established drugs which they are intended to replace.   The description of the individual articles and the general discussions are written by experts and furnished information of a trustworthiness unsurpassed by any other publication.   The book is especially valuable to the busy physician who desires a concise and up-to-date discussion of such subjects as digitalis therapy, the newer solutions for wound sterilizations, iron therapy, food for diabetics, the value of sour milk therapy and of the bulgarian bacillus, the use of radium externally and internally, of arsphenamine (salvarsan, arsenobenzol, diarsenol) and neoarsphenamine (neosalvarsan neodiarsenol), of local anesthetics, and other advances in therapeutics.

In addition to this annual issue of the book, supplements are sent from time to time to the purchasers.   With this volume for ready reference, the physician will be able to determine which of the proprietary remedies that are brought to his notice deserve serious consideration.   At least he will be justified to subject to close scrutiny those which have not met the requirements for acceptance for New and Nonofficial Remedies.

The book is sent, postpaid, for one dollar.   Address the American Medical Association, 535 North Dearborn Street, Chicago.

ANNUAL REPRINT OF THE REPORTS OF THE COUNCIL ON PHARMACY AND CHEMISTRY OF THE AMERICAN MEDICAL ASSOCIATION FOR 1917.   Cloth.   Price, postpaid, 50 cents.   Pp. 169.   Chicago: American Medical Association, 1918.

This volume contains the reports of the Council which were adopted and authorized for Publication during 1917.   It includes reports of the Council previously published in *The Journal of the American Medical Association* and also reports which, because of their highly technical character or of their lesser importance, were not published in *The Journal.*

In this volume the Council discusses the articles which were examined and found to be in conflict with the rules for admission to New and Nonofficial Remedies.   Among these reports are discussions of such widely advertised proprietaries as Corpora Lutea (Soluble Extract), Wheeler's Tissue Phosphates, The Russell Emulsion and The Russell Prepared Green Bone, Trimethol, Eskay's Neuro Phosphates, K-Y Lubricating Jelly, Ziratol, Hepatico Tablets, Hemo-Therapin, Venosal, Surgodine and Kalak Water.   A report on Iodeol and Iodagol covers 51 pages and illustrates the exhaustive investigation which the Council is often obliged to make of proprietary articles.

Similarly illustrative of the Council's thoroughness is the clinical study of Biniodol, a solution of mercuric iodid in oil, and the investigation of Secretin-Beveridge, made for the Council by the physiologist, Professor Carlson, of the University of Chicago.   The volume also contains reports which explain why certain preparations, such as Alcresta Ipecac tablets, the German made biologic products and antistaphylococcus serum, which were described in the last edition of New and Nonofficial Remedies are not contained in the current 1918 edition.   Those who wish to be informed in regard to proprietary remedies should have both the annual Council Reports and New and Nonofficial Remedies.

IMPOTENCE AND STERILITY with Aberrations of the Sexual Function and Sex-Gland Implantation.   By G. Frank Lydston, M. D., D. C. L., Formerly Professor of the Surgical Diseases of the Genito-Uninary Organs and Syphilology in the Medical Department of the State University of Illinois, Member of the American Urological Association, Fellow of the American Medical Association, Member of the Society of Authors, London, England, etc.   Illustrated, Cloth, 333 pages.   Chicago: The Riverton Press, 1917.

BLOOD TRANSFUSION, Hemorrhage and The Anaemias.   By Bertram M. Bernheim, A. B., M. D., F. A. C. G., Instructor in Clinical Surgery, The Johns Hopkins University, Captain, Medical Officers Reserve Corps, U. S. A., Author of "Surgery of the Vascular System", etc.   Illustrated, Cloth, 259 pages.   Price $5.00.   J. B. Lippincott Company, Philadelphia and London, 1917.

THE SPLEEN AND ANAEMIA, Experimental and Clinical Studies.   By Richard Mills Pearce, M. D., Sc. D., Professor of Research Medicine, with the assistance of Dr. Edward Bell Krumbhaar, M. D., Ph. D., and Charles Harrison Frazier, M. D., Sc. D., Professor of Clinical Surgery, University of Pennsylvania.   16 Illustrations, Color and Black and White, Cloth, 419 pages.   Price $5.00.   J. B. Lippincott Company, Philadelphia and London.

DISEASES OF THE STOMACH, INTESTINES, AND PANCREAS.   By Robert Coleman Kemp, M. D., Professor of Gastro-intestinal Diseases at the Fordham University Medical School.   Third edition, revised and enlarged.   Octavo of 1096 pages, with 438 illustrations.   Philadelphia and London: W. B. Saunders Company, 1917.   Cloth. $7.00 net; Half Morocco, $8.50 net.

ESSENTIALS OF PRESCRIPTION WRITING.   By Cary Eggleston, M. D., Instructor in Prarmacology, Cornell University Medical College, New York City.   Second Edition.   Reset.   32 mo. of 134 pages, Philadelphia and London: W. B. Saunders Company, 1917.   Cloth, $1.25 net.

INTERNATIONAL CLINICS, Volume 1, Twenty-Eighth Series.   Cloth, illustrated, 298 pages.   Price $2.50.   J. B. Lippincott Company, Philadelphia and London, 1918.

THE SURGICAL CLINICS OF CHICAGO, Volume II, Number I (February, 1918).   Octavo of 226 pages, 73 illustrations.   Philadelphia and London: W. B Saunders Company, 1918.   Published Bi-Monthly.   Price per year: Paper $10.00   Cloth $14.00.

PROGRAMME

TWENTY-SIXTH ANNUAL MEETING, OKLAHOMA STATE MEDICAL ASSOCIATION, TULSA, MAY 14-15-16, 1918.

(Subject to addition and modification)

GENERAL INFORMATION.

MEETING PLACE. All meetings will be held, unless otherwise announced, in the Old High School Building, 4th and Boston.

REGISTRATION. Every person attending any section or meeting is expected to register by cards furnished for that purpose. You are requested to write your home and local (Tulsa) address plainly. If you are not in good standing for 1918 you cannot register without making arrangements with the Secretary or his representative. Registration will be made only from the stubs of your membership certificates. Visitors are requested to register, marking the words "Visitor, from_____" across face of registration card. Physicians resident of Oklahoma having no county society will see the Secretary.

HOTELS. Despite a letter sent out some time ago advising that it might be necessary to house visiting physicians in private residences, the Tulsa committees have succeeded in having reserved ample hotel accommodations for all who attend, **but to secure such hotel rooms it will be necessary for the member to go to the meeting place, 4th and Boston, register and secure order for room.**

TELEPHONE. The telephone number of the meeting place is 7465.

CLINICS. The Oklahoma Hospital, West Ninth and Jackson. Telephone 3990, announces that Dr. Wm. Engelbach, Professor of Medicine, St. Louis University, will present lantern slide demonstrations on "Diagnosis of Diseases of the Ductless Glands". Unless otherwise announced these will be given from 7:30 to 9:00 A. M., May 15th and 16th. Other features of the clinics will be announced at the meeting.

THE WALTER E. WRIGHT LABORATORY will present during the three days of the meeting continuous demonstrations in Roentgen Examination and Laboratory Technique. The Laboratory is located at 3rd and Cheyenne.

DELEGATES AND CREDENTIALS. Delegates will present their credentials either to the Secretary or one of the following members of the credentials committee, Drs. F. W. Ewing, J. B. Murphy, W. A. Tolleson.

YOUR PAPER prepared for this meeting is the property of this Association. If you want reprints of it, so state on the margin of first sheet. You will, however, receive proof before it is printed. **Please under no circumstances carry your paper away with you.** It only entails unnecessary correspondence and often loss of the paper.

COMMITTEE ON ENTERTAINMENT of wives of visiting physicians is: Mesdames A. W. Roth, Chairman; N. W. Mayginnes, W. E. Wright, F. S. Clinton, R. S. Wagner, H. D. Mudrock.

TUESDAY, MAY 14, 1918, 1:30 P. M.

THE COUNCIL will meet at 1:30 P. M.

HOUSE OF DELEGATES will meet at 2:30 P. M.

GENERAL MEETING, 4:00 P. M. Address by Major Homer T. Wilson (San Antonio), Medical Reserve Corps, Camp Bowie, and Captain L. S. Willour, Medical Reserve Corps, President-elect of the Association, Camp McArthur. (McAlester, Oklahoma).

GENERAL MEETING, 8:00 P. M.

Call to order by the President, Dr. W. Albert Cook, Tulsa.

Invocation, Reverend J. W. Abel, Tulsa.

Address of Welcome, Honorable Chas. Hubbard, Mayor of Tulsa.

Response, Dr. J. W. Duke, State Commissioner of Health, Guthrie.

Address by Dr. Homer T. Wilson, Major, M. R. C., Camp Bowie (San Antonio, Texas).

Address of the President, Dr. W. Albert Cook.

WEDNESDAY, MAY 15, 1918.

From 4:00 to 5:00 P. M., as announced in the different, sections, visiting physicians and their wives will be given a "Seeing Tulsa" tour by automobile, the trip to include a visit to the Cosden Refinery, the largest in the world.

9:00 P. M. The President's reception followed by an informal dance will be tendered the Association at the Elk's Club.

SCIENTIFIC SECTIONS.
9:00 A. M., May 15, 1918.

(Attendants are especially requested to be on time for the opening of the sections in order that the programs may be completed in the time allotted). All sections, unless otherwise announced by the chairmen, will start promptly at 9:00 A. M., May 15, and continue until the programs are completed.

SECTION ON OBSTETRICS AND PEDIATRICS

T. C. Sanders, M. D., Chairman, Shawnee.

1. Chairmans' Address.
2. "Rectal Examinations in Labor", Dr. C. V. Rice, Muskogee.
   Discussion opened by Dr. H. M. Reeder, Shawnee.
3. "The Prevention and Treatment of Puerperal Lacerations", Dr. W. W. Wells, Oklahoma City.
   Discussion opened by Dr. Lee W. Cotton, Enid.
4. "Some Surgical Aspects of Obstetrics", Dr. E. Forrest Hayden, Tulsa.
   Discussion opened by Dr. C. S. Bobo, Norman.
5. "Complications That May Accompany Dentition", Dr. H. M. Williams, Wellston.
   Discussion opened by Dr. J. Raymond Burdick, Tulsa.
6. "Obstetric Morbidity", Dr. W. A. Fowler, Oklahoma City.
   Discussion opened by Dr. J. A. Hatchett, El Reno.
7. "Practical Thoughts on the Care of the Pregnant Woman", Dr. Martha Bledsoe, Chickasha.
   Discussion opened by Dr. A. B. Leeds, Chickasha.
8. "Syphilis in Children", Dr. Roscoe Walker, Pawhuska.
   Discussion opened by Dr. W. M. Taylor, Oklahoma City.
9. "What Can We Do to Improve Humanity", Dr. M. A. Warhurst, Seminole.
   Discussion, General.
10. "Clinical Aspects of Endocarditis", Dr. M. P. Springer, Tulsa.
11. "Classification of Primary and Secondary Manifestations of Pulmonary Tuberculosis in Children",
    Dr. O. A. Flanagan, Tulsa.
12. "Infant Mortality," Dr. R. M. Anderson, Shawnee.

SECTION ON SURGERY

LeRoy Long, M. D., Chairman, Oklahoma City.

1. Chairman's Address.
2. "Diagnosis of Kidney and Ureteral Stone", Dr. J. Hutchings White, Muskogee.
   Discussion opened by Dr. Walter E. Wright, Tulsa.
3. "Neisserian Infection of the Uterus", Dr. J. S. Hartford, Oklahoma City.
   Discussion opened by Dr. W. E. Dicken, Oklahoma City.
4. "Surgery of the Gall-Bladder with Special Reference to Metastases—High Mortality Attending Operation with Acute Infection as Compared with Operation During Quiesence", Dr. McLain Rogers, Clinton.
   Discussion opened by Dr. Fred Y. Cronk, Tulsa.
5. "Nerve Wounds", Dr. Horace Reed, Oklahoma City.
   Discussion opened by Dr. J. Hutchings White, Muskogee.
6. "A Quarter of a Century in Emergency Surgery—Some Observations of a General Practitioner",
   Dr. J. S. Fulton, Atoka.
   Discussion opened by Dr. Claude Thompson, 1st Lieut., M. R. C., Muskogee.
7. "The Carrel-Dakin Treatment of Wounds", Dr. Millington Smith, Oklahoma City.
   Discussion opened by Dr. A. Ray Wiley, Tulsa.
8. "The Character and Quality of Base Hospital Surgery Outside the War Zone", Major A. L. Blesh, M. R. C., Base Hospital, Ft. Sam Houston (Oklahoma City).
9. "Some Observations in Connection With the Duties of the Medical Officer on This Side", Captain Ralph V. Smith, M. R. C., Base Hospital, Allentown, Pa. (Tulsa).
   Discussion on above two papers opened by Dr. William Patton Fite, 1st Lieut., M. R. C., Assistant Sanitary Inspector, Camp Bowie (Muskogee)).
10. "The Modern Treatment of Burns", Dr. Fred S. Clinton, Tulsa.
    Discussion opened by Captain Chas. W. Heitzman, M. O. T. C., Ft. Riley (Muskogee).
11. "Treatment of Fractures of the Shaft of the Femur", Dr. Robert L. Hull, Oklahoma City.
    Discussion opened by Dr. I. B. Oldham, Muskogee.
12. "Complete Avulsion of the Shoulder", Dr. G. A. Wall, Tulsa.
    Discussion opened by Dr. Ross Grosshart, Tulsa.

SECTION ON EYE, EAR, NOSE AND THROAT

L. A. Newton, M. D., Chairman, Oklahoma City.

EYE.

1. Chairman's Address: "The Early Care of Eye Diseases and Injuries", Dr. L. A. Newton, Oklahoma City.
2. "Eye Strain as a Factor in Gastric Neuroses", Dr. A. C. McFarling, Shawnee.
   Discussion opened by Dr. D. D. McHenry, Oklahoma City.
3. "Keratoconus", Dr. W. T. Salmon, Oklahoma City.
   Discussion opened by Dr. L. M. Westfall, Oklahoma City.
4. "Squint", Dr. Edw. F. Davis, Oklahoma City.
   Discussion opened by Dr. A. W. Roth, Tulsa.

EAR.

5. "The Significance of Pain in the Ear", Dr. J. H. Barnes, Enid.
   Discussion opened by Dr. E. B. Mitchell, Lawton.
6. "Carcinoma of the Mastoid", Dr. C. M. Fullenwider, Muskogee.
   Discussion opened by Dr. E. F. Stroud, Tulsa.
7. "Conservative Treatment of Acute Mastoiditis", Dr. J. Walter Beyer, Tulsa.
   Discussion opened by Dr. L. Haynes Buxton, Oklahoma City.

NOSE.

8. "Operations on the Nasal Septum", Dr. H. Coulter Todd, Oklahoma City.
   Discussion opened by Dr. W. Albert Cook, Tulsa.
9. "The Accessory Sinuses of the Nose", Dr. R. O. Early, Ardmore.
   Discussion opened by Dr. E. S. Ferguson, Oklahoma City.

SECTION ON GENITO-URINARY DISEASES, SKIN AND RADIOLOGY

W. J. Wallace, M. D., Chairman, Oklahoma City.

1. Chairman's Address: "Symptoms and Diagnosis of Syphilis of the Bladder," Dr. W. J. Wallace, Oklahoma City.
2. "Prevention of Venereal Diseases", Dr. W. B. Pigg, Henryetta.
   Discussion opened by Dr. W. C. Griffith, Weleetka.
3. "Foreign Body in the Bladder—Case Report", Dr. C. R. Day, Oklahoma City.
   Discussion opened by Dr. John W. Riley, Oklahoma City.
4. "Pyelitis", Dr. J. H. Hays, Enid.
   Discussion opened by Dr. C. P. Linn, Tulsa.
5. "Diagnosis of Rupture of Bladder in its Various Locations—Case Report", Dr. J. F. Kuhn, Oklahoma City.
6. "Pathology and Constitutional Symptoms of Stricture of the Urethra", Dr. Walter A. Howard, Chelsea.
   Discussion opened by Dr.
7. "Early Paresis", Dr. A. D. Young, Oklahoma City.
   Discussion opened by Dr. E. Forrest Hayden, Tulsa.
8. "Radium and its Application to Medicine and Surgery", Dr. E. S. Lain, Oklahoma City.
   Discussion opened by Dr. J. T. Martin Oklahoma City.
9. "Focal Infection of the Genito-Urinary Tract as a Cause of Constitutional Diseases", Dr. Julius Frisher, Kansas City, Mo.
   Discussion opened by Dr. J. H. Hays, Enid.
10. "Cystoscopy—Its Necessity in Medicine and Surgery", Dr. F. K. Camp, Oklahoma City.
    Discussion opened by Dr.
11. "The Problem of Venereal Diseases in the Army", Dr. R. M. Ilisson, Captain, M. R. C., Camp Funston, Kan. (Wichita, Kan.)
    Discussion opened by Dr. L. S. Willour, Captain, M. R. C., Camp McArthur (McAlester).

SECTION ON GENERAL MEDICINE, NERVOUS AND MENTAL DISEASES

A. B. Leeds, M. D., Chairman, Chickasha.

1. Chairman's Address.

2. "Tonsils and Teeth as Chronic Pus Foci", Dr. W. H. Livermore, Chickasha.
   Discussion opened by Dr. L. H. Murdock, Tulsa.

3. "Spastic Colitis", Dr. A. W. White, Oklahoma City.
   Discussion opened by Dr. Lea A. Riely, Oklahoma City.

4. "Significance of Abdominal Pain", Dr. J. M. Byrum, Shawnee.
   Discussion opened by Dr. G. A. Boyle, Enid.

5. "Diabetic Coma", Dr. Lea A. Riely, Oklahoma City.
   Discussion opened by Dr. O. J. Walker, Oklahoma City.

6. "Radium and Its Application in Medicine", Dr. E. S. Lain, Oklahoma City.
   Discussion opened by Dr. J. T. Martin, Oklahoma City.

7. Paper: To be supplied. Dr. L. J. Moorman, Oklahoma City.

8. "The Military Aspects of Cardiovascular Diseases", Julien E. Benjamin, Captain, M. R. C., Camp Funston, Kan.
   Discussion opened by Dr. A. E. Davenport, Captain M. R. C., Camp Funston, Kansas.

OFFICERS OF OKLAHOMA STATE MEDICAL ASSOCIATION.

Meeting Place—Tulsa, May 14-15-16, 1918.
President, 1917-18—Dr. W. Albert Cook, Tulsa.
President-elect, 1918-19—Dr. L. S. Willour, McAlester.
1st Vice-President—Dr. McLain Rogers, Clinton.
2nd Vice-President—Dr. G. F. Border, Mangum.
3rd Vice-President—Dr. Horace Reed, Oklahoma City.
Secretary-Treasurer-Editor—Dr. C. A. Thompson, Muskogee.
Delegate to the A. M. A., 1918-19—Dr. Chas. R. Hume, Anadarko
Delegate to the A. M. A. 1917-18—Dr. M. A. Kelso, Enid.

CHAIRMEN OF SCIENTIFIC SECTIONS.

Surgery and Gynecology—Dr. LeRoy Long, Oklahoma City.
Pediatrics and Obstetrics—Dr. T. C. Sanders, Shawnee.
Eye, Ear, Nose and Throat—Dr. L. A. Newton, Oklahoma City.
General Medicine, Nervous and Mental Diseases—Dr. A. B. Leeds, Chickasha.
Genitourinary, Skin and Radiology—Dr. W. J. Wallace, Oklahoma City.
Legislative Committee—Dr. Millington Smith, Oklahoma City; Dr. J. M. Byrum, Shawnee;
Dr. W. T. Salmon, Oklahoma City.
For the Study and Control of Cancer—Drs. LeRoy Long, Oklahoma City; Gayfree Ellison,
Norman; D. A. Myers, Lawton.
For the Study and Control of Pellagra—Drs. A. A. Thurlow, Norman; L. A. Mitchell, Frederick;
J. C. Watkins, Checotah.
For the Study of Venereal Diseases—Drs. Wm. J. Wallace, Oklahoma City; Ross Grosshart,
Tulsa; J. E. Bercaw, Okmulgee.
Necrology—Drs. Martha Bledsoe, Chickasha; J. W. Pollard, Bartlesville.
Tuberculosis—Drs. L. J. Moorman, Oklahoma City; C. W. Heitzman, Muskogee; Leila E.
Andrews, Oklahoma City.
Conservation of Vision—Drs. L. A. Newton, Oklanoma City; L. Haynes Buxton, Oklahoma
City; G. E. Hartshorne, Shawnee.
First Aid Committee—Drs. G. S. Baxter, Shawnee; Jas. C. Johnston, McAlester.
Committee on Medical Education—Drs.'A. L. Blesh; A. K. West; A. W. White, Oklahoma City.
State Commissioner of Health—Dr. John W. Duke, Guthrie, Oklahoma

COUNCILOR DISTRICTS.

1. Cimarron, Texas, Beaver, Harper, Ellis, Woods and Woodward; Councilor, Dr. J. M. Workman, Woodward. Term expires 1919.
2. Roger Mills, Beckham, Dewey, Custer, Washita and Blaine; Councilor, Dr. Ellis Lamb, Clinton. Term expires 1920.
3. Harmon, Greer, Jackson, Kiowa, Tillman, Comanche and Cotton; Councilor, Dr. G. P Cherry, Mangum. Term expires 1918.
4. Major, Alfalfa, Grant, Garfield, Noble and Kay; Councilor, Dr. G. A. Boyle, Enid. Term expires 1919.
5. Kingfisher, Canadian, Oklahoma and Logan; Councilor, Dr. Fred Y. Cronk, Guthrie. Term expires 1918.
6. Caddo, Grady, McClain, Garvin, Stephens and Jefferson; Councilor, Dr. C. M. Maupin, Waurika. Term expires 1919.
7. Osage, Pawnee, Creek, Okfuskee, Okmulgee and Tulsa; Councilor, Dr. N. W. Mayginnes, Tulsa. Term expires 1920.
8. Payne, Lincoln, Cleveland, Pottawatomie and Seminole; Councilor, Dr. H. M. Williams, Wellston. Term expires 1920.
9. Pontotoc, Murray, Carter, Love, Marshall, Johnston and Coal; Councilor, Dr. J. T. Slover, Sulphur. Term expires 1918.
10. Washington, Nowata, Rogers, Craig, Ottawa, Mayes and Delaware; Councilor, Dr. R. L. Mitchell, Vinita. Term expires 1918.
11. Wagoner, Muskogee, McIntosh, Haskell, Cherokee and Adair; Councilor, Dr. J. Hutchings White, Muskogee. Term expires 1920.
12. Hughes, Pittsburg, Latimer, LeFlore and Sequoyah; Councilor, Dr. Ed. D. James, Haileyville. Term expires 1920.
13. Atoka, Pushmataha, Bryan, Choctaw and McCurtain; Councilor, Dr. J. L. Austin, Durant. Term expires 1920.

STATE BOARD OF MEDICAL EXAMINERS.

Melvin Gray, M. D., Durant, President; B. L. Denison, M. D., Garvin, Vice-President; J. J. Williams, M. D., Weatherford, Secretary; O. R. Gregg, M. D., Waynoka, Treasurer; E. B. Dunlap, M. D., Lawton; Ralph V. Smith, M. D., Tulsa; W. LeRoy Bonnell, M. D., Chickasha; Wm. T. Ray, M. D., Gould; H. C. Montague, D. O., Muskogee.
Reciprocity with Georgia, Kentucky, Mississippi, Nevada, North Carolina, Wisconsin, Kansas, Arkansas, Virginia, West Virginia, Nebraska, New Mexico, Tennessee, Iowa, Ohio, California, Colorado, Indiana, Missouri, New Jersey, Vermont, Texas, Michigan.
Meetings held second Tuesday of January, April, July and October, Oklahoma City.
Address all communications to the Secretary, Dr. J. J. Williams, Weatherford.

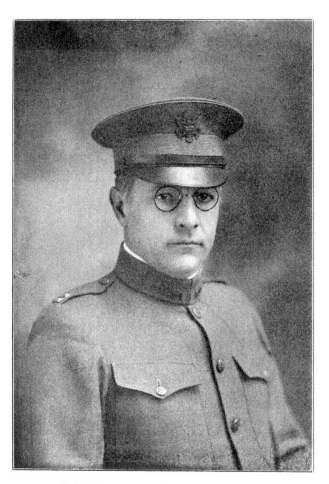

MAJOR LEONARD S. WILLOUR, M. R. C., U. S. A.
PRESIDENT, OKLAHOMA STATE MEDICAL
ASSOCIATION, 1918-1919

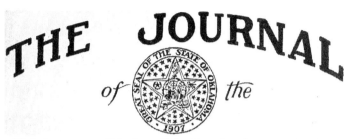

Oklahoma State Medical Association

VOLUME XI   MUSKOGEE, OKLA., JUNE, 1918   NUMBER 6

THE PRESIDENT'S ADDRESS*

By W. ALBERT COOK, M D., F. A. C. S., M. R. C.
Tulsa, Oklahoma

There never has been a time in the history of the world when the medical profession occupied as important a position as it does today, and the great struggle of democracy against barbarism could not be carried on to a successful termination if it were not for the important part being played by our chosen profession.

Uncle Sam figures on ten medical men to every one thousand soldiers and recently sent out an S. O. S. call for eight thousand more to take care of the 800,000 men called for in the new draft, who are to be sent over as soon as they can be examined and put into shape, to help stop the brutal Huns in their vain attempt to break through the western front in their mad endeavor to control the World.

The response of the profession has been very liberal and up to the time of the last call, over twenty thousand of the leading men in the profession in our land have donned the khaki and are working harder than they ever did before in their lives, and when you consider that this is about one-fourth of the regular practicing physicians of the U. S., you can see that the ones who remain at home will have added responsibilities to bear, but if this terrible War continues much longer, all of the able bodied physicians will be in the service, and the physically fit ones who remain at home will be kept busy explaining why they are not in.

Never before have the members of the medical profession demonstrated to the people of the entire universe, the ideals of duty as during the present world-wide War. This has been done, not for love of gain or prestige, not for love of country alone, but because of duty to their chosen profession.

When the War started, there were three men in the office of the surgeon general and three months ago they numbered one hundred and forty, and that number is being increased weekly. The business of the surgeon's office can be likened to a merchant in a small town being called to take charge of a business of the proportion of Wanamaker's or Field's—he is bound to make mistakes, but if the other departments of our government make no more mistakes than have the medical profession, this War would be nearer the end than it is at present. When the National Council of Medical Defense was organized, and began to make suggestions to the War department, they were not looked upon very kindly, but today is depending upon the Council of Defense and the A. 'M. A. to furnish the men for the medical corps of our army, for we are to the army what gasoline is to the motor car. They cannot succeed without us.

---

*Delivered at the Twenty-sixth Annual Meeting of the Oklahoma State Medical Association, Tulsa, May 14, 1918.

No such unsanitary conditions as existed during the Civil War where men died by the hundreds of scurvy, nor the Spanish-American War where more lives were sacrificed by disease (especially typhoid) than by Spanish bullets, prevail in the present conflict, and many camps have been moved when it was found the location was unpractical from a sanitary standpoint, after being investigated by the medical officers.

In this war the army surgeon is no longer a ministering angel who does his work in a safe place after the fighting is over—he is a soldier, sharing the hardships and the peril of the troops whom he serves. Military honors have been bestowed upon the medical officers of France and England, in proportion to the size of the medical corps, as freely as upon line officers. During three years of War, the British Medical Corps suffered 11,667 casualties with a death roll of 1,200. The first Americans to lay down their lives as part of a United States force at the front, were six medical officers and nurses who were doing their work of mercy in an Allied hospital when they were struck down by bombs from German air-raiders. It was not like this in olden Wars, for the casualty lists were much smaller, there was comparatively little field surgery, and it was much easier to get away from the firing-zone.

In the Civil War, little was done toward speeding up the treatment of the wounded, except in a few cases that came to the attention of the army surgeon as he rode about the battlefield in company with mounted staff officers. He would select a few of the less serious cases, carry them to a favorable place, and give treatment. Only in the latter part of the War, was anything like dressing stations, or field hospitals established, and then only when buildings near by offered temporary shelter.

The wounded were collected at night by both armies, instead of during the conflict, each side by mutual agreement allowing the other to carry on the work unmolested. In the present World-war, agreements of this character were attempted in its early phases, but the few truces arranged were broken by the Germans and the Turks. Many medical officers were killed by machine-gun and rifle fire, and the Red Cross—Emblem of Mercy—was proved to offer no protection to those who wore it.

An interesting incident that illustrates the German attitude toward the medical Corps, is vouched for by an Americam Red Cross worker who has just returned from the French front after several months of ambulance service near first line trenches. After an offensive stroke, a Red Cross ambulance was hurrying a German officer to a field hospital. An army surgeon was sitting behind the wounded man. While the doctor's attention was distracted, the German drew his revolver and pointed it at the surgeon's head. Fortunately the ambulance driver divined his sinister purpose, knocked the weapon from the prisoner's hand and saved the medical officer's life. This German declared that his army regarded killing a medical officer more important than to slay 500 infantrymen.

The enormous casualty lists of the present War soon convinced medical authorities that the medical corps should attend to the wounded as soon as they could be brought from the scene of battle. It was shown that the sooner a wound can be cleaned of dirt, pieces of clothing carried by the bullet, and other foreign matter, the less the danger of infection and the greater the chance for ultimate recovery. This made it necessary to send medical officers with the troops going "over the top" and to establish field dressing stations near the front line trenches.

As soon as the advancing infantry has made its way across the battlefield in the face of terrific gun-fire, the support troops are sent out of the trenches. With them go the medical officers, wearing steel hemlets for protection against shrapnel. Accompanying them on their errand of mercy are the stretcher-bearers and other enlisted men in the Medical Corps.

Theirs is no easy task. They must advance under the same hail of shells that greets the men of the line, traverse the same ground, often waist deep in mud, cross deep shell craters, and struggle through the same barriers of barbed wire entanglements. Heedless of exploding mines and dense waves of poison-gas, they must direct first-aid treatment and the transportation of wounded men.

After the battle the line troops may rest. Not so the medical officer. He must continue to work on the bleeding and broken stream of humanity which pours into the casualty clearing-station. When all have been cared for, he may seek well-earned repose.

Recognizing the necessity of physical and military training for the medical officer, that he may learn to direct the transportation of wounded, and realizing the need of stamina that he may be able to stand the fatigue of long hours, three medical officers' training camps have been established at Fort Benjamin Harrison, Indianapolis, Fort Riley, Kansas, and Fort Oglethorpe, Georgia, by direction of Surgeon-General of the Army William C. Gorgas, conquerer of diseases in Cuba and Panama and the greatest sanitarian of all time. From these Camps have been graduated many thousand officers and men, all of whom have had physical and military training which will fit them to bear the same hardships as the men of the line—they are soldiers.

There is no place at the front for the medical weakling. The army surgeon has always been given the duty of relieving suffering, conserving, reclaiming and rebuilding human life wrecked by the ravages of warfare, and has always been considered as a ministering agency who worked in safe places behind the lines.

This great War has presented to the world a new form of community life with a new combination of the various elements which are to be found in every concentration of the population of western countries.

This War is unlike any previous War in that the old idea of campaign with armies fighting and moving over large districts of territory was true in Belgium and France only for the first few weeks of the conflict. Such a conception has been realized more in the distant battlefields of Asia and Eastern Europe. The majority of the troops engaged on the west front have settled down to a permanent location and have continued more or less fixed in positions for three years while they carry on their daily and nightly tasks of combat in what is known as trench warfare, until March 21st, when the long advertised spring drive started.

Such a community has developed new medical problems and has exaggerated some older ones already well known to the army medical departments of all nations. The modern weapons with their high explosives and rapid fire and the inhumanities of asphyxiating gases and liquid fire have produced surgical conditions which are extremely infrequent as complications of the accidents of civil life. The habit of continuous warfare also has compelled the relief squads to delay their merciful tasks, and there results a high percentage of neglected infections and of the severer forms of blood poisoning and gangrene which modern aseptic surgery had eliminated from the experience of hospital practice.

At the beginning of the War an appreciable number of troops had not been protected by the modern methods of vaccination against typhoid. That disease and more particularly the closely allied condition, paratyphoid, were very prevalent. At the present time, both diseases have been controlled to a large extent by a full application of the methods which were developed and applied first in the army of the U. S.

The War has necessitated the formulation of methods to control diseases communicated by water. This has been done, and dysentery, one of the oldest foes of armies, has been made less prevalent than in former wars. The present day army physician must do more on this line, however. He must discover by quick action, any contamination of wells and other supplies of drinking water, from the addition of dead animals, sewage, and even of mineral poisons, such as arsenic, whenever the allies advance in the territory lately occupied by the modern Huns.

The War has emphasized the importance of the group of diseases·which are transmitted by the bite of vermin. One of these, known as "spotted typhus," is caused by the body louse, and is normally found in southeastern Europe. It has been controlled by a rigid application of sanitary rules, and by inoculation. Another disease of this group is known as "Trench fever" and has been discovered and introduced into Western Eurpoe by the War, probably from the Orient. It is a short, very debilitating fever of low mortality, but which incapacitates its victims for an appreciable period,

The greatest additions to the antiseptic treatment of wounds have come from the chemical studies of Dr. Dakin, who has applied in various ways, the properties of chlorine preparations to the disinfection of wounds of war. The problem which Dr. Dakin solved was to discover strong antiseptics which were able to destroy microbes without damaging normal tissues. Dr. Alexis Carrel developed a method of using antiseptics of Dr. Dakin in the severly infected wounds which came to his hospital on the French front. His method consists of putting into the wounded tissues, a system of multiple tubes and keeping the wound constantly washed with the antiseptic solution. The progress of the wound is watched by a daily bacteriological examination, and as soon as it is germ free, it is closed and healing is quite prompt if the observations have been done in a precise manner.

The War has developed two large groups of cripples, one including those who have been maimed by the loss of arms, legs and eyesight and in other physical ways. A great endeavor has been begun to re-educate these men and to fit them for new trades and for a useful and self-supporting life. The second group are those who suffer from functional disturbances of the central nervous system. These cases present paralysis and other disturbances of locomotion, which are purely hysterical, or they show mental disorders which are also functional, but which stimulate true insanity in many of its manifold varieties. One of the most characteristic cases is that known as "shell-shock" which is directly attributed to the vibration and noise of the discharge of high explosives in a person over-tired by physical work and over-wrought by mental fatigue. A great success has been achieved by systems of nerve and muscle education especially in French institutions devoted to this work. Many of the sufferers from these functional disturbances of the nervous system have been returned to a useful life and some have rejoined the fighting ranks.

Our Government is preparing hospitals in the U. S. capable of taking care of 100,000 patients who are incapacitated in the service. abroad, who are so badly wounded that they cannot again take their place in the line, and they will be brought back on the transports which are constantly taking new troops over, and unfortunately some are being brought back already, but I hope that these institutions will not be needed very long.

The Germans are now face to face with a different type of fighting men from any they have ever encountered or ever dreamed of. The American soldier who has been stalking their patrols in No-Man's-Land is an unknown quantity in the German scheme of things. The German makes a good fighting machine with all the cogs oiled and geared and the engineer on the job—the machine works smoothly enough, but smash any part of it, throw out the gears, or disable the engineer and the machine stops.

On the other hand, the American is a born fighting man, an instinctive soldier. He is a thinker and a doer, and has initiative, he has pluck, he has the things the German lacks, things the German could never have because of his environment, his system, his whole outlook on life.

The Germans will learn many things from the men they are fighting. They have already learned many things from the French, and from the English, from the Italian, but in the American they are going to find the dash of the Frenchman the bulldog tenacity of the British, the high courage of the Italian, the endurance and capacity of sacrifice of all three, and in addition the initiative, the personal element that will take great risks to gain great ends, and a sense of responsibility that will make the American Soldier the Savior of the World.

THE EARLY CARE OF EYE INJURIES AND DISEASES*

By L. A. NEWTON, M. D., Oklahoma City

The proper care or treatment of eye injuries and diseases instituted early undoubtedly saves many eyes from becoming blind. No other part of the human body succumbs to disease more rapidly than the eye. After death it is about the first part of the human body to decay. Being largely made up of fluids and very rich in blood supply, with the exception of the cornea, it is naturally very delicate and susceptible to disease and injury.

The peculiar manner in which the cornea gets its nourishment and having no real blood supply of its own, leaves it with very poor resisting power, and the eye being situated where it is constantly exposed with only the tears, eyelids and nervous reflexes to protect it from dust, dirt and many other ways of injury, it is remarkable that we do not have more eye diseases than we do, and so when we do have a disease or injury it behooves us to give it prompt and careful attention.

All of us have seen eyes that were entirely lost due to lack of treatment early in the disease or injury. The blame is on the patient many times and sometimes upon physicians who do not apparently take enough interest in the eyes to recognize and impress upon the patient the serious nature of their condition. It is a common remark among nearly all physicians, except oculists, that they do not pretend to know anything about the eye, and let it go at that. And it is my purpose in writing this paper to try to stimulate more interest, if possible, among physicians or get them to take a more careful notice of eye conditions than they do many times, so that many serious conditions will be recognized early.

Corneal ulcer is one of our most destructive eye diseases and one of the most easily recognized, especially the serpiginous ulcer of the pneumococcus infection, and it should be recognized very early and heroic treatment instituted or we will have a blind eye, as this infection spreads very rapidly and will soon involve the whole surface of the cornea. This type of ulcer is always associated with lots of pain and deep circumcorneal injection and photophobia.

Iritis is a disease that should always be recognized early and atropine instilled and the pupil thoroughly dilated before adhesions take place, which so complicates matters and is prone to help cause relapses and more or less permanently impair the vision, or possibly a complete posterior annular synechea occurs giving rise to glaucoma and total blindness of the eye.

Injuries to the eye always need prompt attention. In our own private practice and visiting large clinic centers, we see so many eyes which have been lost where a little cleanliness and a drop or two of atropine would have worked wonders for the patient, had they been used at once when the injury took place. Where there is an injury perforating the cornea with prolapsed iris, it should always be snipped off early and with the diligent use of atropine, or eserin. to try and pull the iris back into the anterior chamber to prevent adhesions in the wound which is so detrimental to vision and causing a long drawn out siege of treatment with possible complete loss of the eye in the end.

These adhesions take place very quickly and no time can afford to be lost if we do not expect bad results. Foreign bodies which become imbedded in the cornea always need prompt removal under the most thorough aseptic conditions, as they are so often the predisposing cause for corneal ulcer and their thorough removal followed by a boric acid wash for a few days until all signs of irritation have subsided.

If the foreign body has been deeply imbedded or has been in the cornea sometime, it is well to instill a drop or two of a one per cent. atropine solution and order colored lens for a few days—especially in people under forty years of age—

---

*Chairman's Address, Section on Eye, Ear, Nose and Throat, Twenty-sixth Annual Meeting, Tulsa, May 15, 1918.

but caution should be used in using atropine in people over forty years of age. The deeper a foreign body is imbedded in the cornea the less pain it is likely to cause the patient, as the lids pass over it without producing friction and irritation, therefore we sometimes find them that have been in there for days without the patients' knowledge of it until they consult you for dread of light and a red, irritated eye and beginning ulceration of the cornea around the foreign body.

Under these circumstances the foreign body and the ulcerated necrotic tissue should all be thoroughly removed under strict asepsis, being careful not to carry any other kind of infection into an already weakened tissue, and a drop or two of atropine solution instilled to quiet down the ciliary muscles and colored lens or many times better a bandage be applied for two or three days to keep the eye at rest. Rough handling of an eye spud when removing foreign bodies may scrape off much healthy epithelium, giving more room and chance for infection to take place. The instillation of a few drops of four 'per cent. cocaine solution and waiting five to ten minutes will produce sufficient anesthesia to remove them without pain to the patient and we should never attempt to remove a foreign body from the cornea without complete anesthesia and control of our patient and good light to see that all foreign substance is thoroughly cleaned out.

There are two all important things in both disease and injury of the eye—viz: *Cleanliness and rest.* Cleanliness by keeping the eye free from secretion with a good boric acid solution used as often as necessary to keep out the secretions and rest and protection by either a bandage—colored lens and instillation of atropine under proper circumstances. Atropine properly used will save many eyes both in disease and injury. Of course it is contra-indicated in glaucoma and injuries that have either perforated or threatened to perforate the cornea near the limbus, it is contra-indicated in deep-seated corneal ulcer in the same region, which might perforate and cause the iris to prolapse and become incarcerated in the cornea. It is one of our most useful drugs in simple corneal ulcer, iritis, and practically all cases of injury, dilating the pupil and pulling it away from the crystaline lens, thereby preventing adhesions to the lens which complicates matters always, and is further beneficial in quieting down the ciliary muscle and putting the eye at rest.

The rules or indications and contra-indications for the use of atropine and eserin are rather simple and should be remembered by every physician. Always dilate the pupil in injury or inflammatory conditions where the cornea, iris or ciliary body are involved, unless there is a deep ulcer or injury near the limbus which might perforate and cause a prolapsed iris. This holds good in people under forty years of age, but atropine should be used very guardedly in people after forty years of age, as it might possibly cause glaucoma.

It is a common practice among many physicians to prescribe a solution containing cocaine in both eye diseases and injuries where the eye is at all painful; this is very bad practice and especiallly so where there is an abrasion of the cornea or corneal ulcer, as cocaine has a drying and destructive action upon the epithelium of the cornea and has no curative or antiseptic action at all upon the disease and the relief from pain is of only very short duration, therefore, it should never be used in the eye except during some operative procedure or removal of foreign body and then the cornea carefully watched and kept flushed with boric acid solution to prevent cracking and peeling off of the epithelium; remembering this delicate membrane is our guard against infection, the same as the skin upon the hand or other parts of the body.

Among the acute infectious diseases there is one of which I wish to speak, and that is "Trachoma". There are today in Oklahoma hundreds of cases of trachoma running at large, which is a constant menace to the public, as this disease is infectious and is very prone to produce at least permanent damage to the vision if not blindness to the unfortunate victims who contract it. If we were able to get hold of and control these people it could soon be stamped out. But unfortunately it is a disease of the poorer classes who are usually ignorant and live under poor hygienic surroundings and haven't the means with which to get medical assiatance long enough to effect a cure, as it always runs over a considerable period of time before we can pronounce them cured, and these patients either drift from one doctor to another or quit treatment entirely; thus by using no sanitary precautions, they readily spread the disease.

There are many errors made regarding the diagnosis of trachoma. Many patients come to us stating they have granulated lids or have had them and recovered, when they neither have them then nor ever did have, for a patient who has had genuine trachoma has always the tell-tale scars on the upper lids. Many of these patients who think they have trachoma, or have been told so by a physician, are suffering generally from some error of refraction or milder eye disease— all of this is misleading to the laity and then when one does get real trachoma he cannot understand why the treatment is long and drawn out. A little more care should be exercised in making the diagnosis and those with trachoma should be strongly impressed with the seriousness of the disease and the damage they may do the public at large by not being careful to prevent infecting some one else.

Glaucoma is one of the most rapid diseases in the destruction of vision, especially the acute form. The intra-ocular pressure becomes so great that unless the tension is soon relieved blindness from optic atrophy will ensue. This disease has been known to completely destroy the vision of an eye in a few hours. Therefore, it should always be promptly recognized in order to save the vision. Unfortunately many of these patients think they have a so-called neuralgia in their head and do not realize the seriousness of their real condition until it is too late. The intense pain in the eye and the increased tension should never be mistaken by a physician for any other disease, especially in the acute type, but many cases of chronic glaucoma, which is not so actively destructive to vision, and has periodic attacks of pain, have been passed along with headache powders to relieve the pain, for sometimes years before it is recognized and permanent damage has been done to the vision.

It would be an excellent rule if physicians would always take the tension of the eyes when treating severe pain in the head, especially those in the frontal region. A little practice would soon enable one to tell if the tension was very high at least.

BLADDER DRAINAGE.

A new technic for bladder drainage is described by H. P. Jack, Hornell, N. Y. (*Journal A. M. A.*, April 27, 1918). It is an adaptation of the use of the Murphy' button, one half of which is inserted into the end of a large rubber tube, the rubber end surrounding the button closely about its shank. The other half of the button, surrounded down to its shank by a soft rubber ring, if desired, so that it will not cut through too quickly, is placed inside the bladder through a small slit, The bladder tissues are brought firmly about the shank of this half of the button, and the two halves are pushed closely together. This gives a perfect joint and enables one to use his drain as much or as little as he pleases. If not satisfied as to the perfect drainage, another and smaller tube may be introduced inside of the larger one, clear to the bottom of the bladder. Forty eight hours after this operation which is usually performed under local anesthesia, quinin and urea hydrochlorid, four-hour washings of the bladder are begun. · He has used this technic in ten cases of prostatectomy with utmost satisfactoin, and it has saved much suffering to the patient. He has never used the rubber ring suggested. The button has always remained in the tissues without cutting, for two weeks. Should it be desired to keep the button in place for a much longer period, the use of the ring is obvious. The incision into the bladder may be of sufficient length, to allow search for, and removal of stones, which is imperative.

CHAIRMAN'S ADDRESS—SECTION ON GENERAL MEDICINE; NERVOUS AND MENTAL DISEASES*

By A. B. LEEDS, M. D., Chickasha, Oklahoma

It is certainly a great pleasure, as well as a great honor, to preside as the Chairman of the Medical Section of the Oklahoma State Medical Association, at this meeting at Tulsa.

During these strenuous war times, it has been with some difficulty that your Chairman has been able to present the few authors and their papers, as he has had three different programs arranged and almost ready to submit to the Secretary of this association, only to have the call of patriotism and other duties shatter the program to pieces.

Finally, in desperation both to the Chairman of your section and the Secretary of this association, he made a personal appeal to some of his friends and they have more than answered this personal appeal, and I am sure that most of them did so at a sacrifice of time and business.

In considering what would, perhaps, be of the most interest at this time, outside of the needs of the Surgeon General for physicians applying to the Medical Reserve Corps, your chairman feels that a few words, relative to the great importance of what has been done in the investigation of Focal Infections, would be the most timely subject, just now, for him to discuss very briefly.

It is needless for me to tell you that during the last three or four years, since Billings and Rosenow promulgated the idea of the importance of foci of infection in the causation of many of the ills of mankind, this subject has received the earnest and careful consideration of many of the brightest minds in our profession and what conclusions and definite results have been obtained, in this investigation, will be the purpose of these remarks.

The suggested conclusions, which your chairman will make today, are not only based on a series of 1643 cases which has come under the personal observation of your chairman, but upon all the results mentioned in all the medical literature possible for him to secure and study.

It seems to be the consensus of opinion of all who have thoroughly and carefully investigated this subject that a great advance in the etiology of many pathological conditions was certainly made when the importance of focal infections was brought, so exhaustively, to the attention of our profession some few years ago.

To all of the investigators, this work has been exceedingly interesting, gratifying, and so often so startling that the results have been hard to believe.

The results obtained have, as a whole, been uniform and where all that was hoped for was not accomplished, further investigation demonstrated that there was either overlooked foci which had not been eliminated, or resistance that was very much lowered or practically nil, or the permanently damaged tissues or organs could not be brought to perform their normal functions.

While all of the investigators are not removing all of the foci, whether it be diseased tonsils, teeth, roots, draining sinuses, antrums, etc., at the same time that chronic pelvi are corrected, fibro-cystic ovaries are drained or removed, chronic or acute appendices are removed, the resection and drainage for emphysema is accomplished or in any pathological condition where surgical interference is indicated, there is no question but the results which are obtained by those who are removing all the foci, at the one operation, are more successful and a greater chance for a cure is given the patient.

---

*Twenty-sixth Annual Meeting, Tulsa, May 14, 1918.

Since there has been more rational co-operation between the wide-awake dentist, the surgeon and the internist, many of the previously so-called failures were found to be the result of leaving many foci, and these foci remaining were much more virulent and a more serious menace than those which had been removed.

The prerequisite for the treatment of these cases and what is absolutely necessary to effect a cure is the successful elimination of all the possible foci and to accomplish this result there must be a systematic, thorough, exhaustive and comprehensive examination as well as a very careful discrimination and differentiation used.

Personally, we do not consider any examination complete, much less satisfactory, until we have made an accurate deduction of the clinical picture presented and not only do we consider carefully the tonsils, teeth, peridental membranes, sinuses and antrums, particularly from the evidence of X-ray pictures, but so often we have to consider the relative effect of apparently normal looking tonsils and teeth upon the focal infection patient.

We wish to emphasize that no accurate diagnosis is possible nor can any rational treatment be instituted upon the usual casual or superficial examination of these focal infection patients, for so often and frequently virulent pus has been demonstrated at the enucleation of apparently normal looking tonsils, also the X-ray has shown apical granuloma, abesess and caries in teeth pronounced normal and viable by dentists.

The results obtained by the detection and removal of partially removed or buried tabs of tonsils and even whole so-called velar lobes, as well as unsuspected and overlooked impacted roots and impacted infected unerupted teeth, has demonstrated that greater care and thoroughness is imperative in the treatment of these cases.

Radical discouragement, both to the patient and the physician, has resulted from removing diseased tonsils and teeth without correcting diseased sinuses, antrums, gall-bladders, appendices, chronic fibro-cystic ovaries, infected prostates and other foci, for we have learned that the temporary improvement which may result from the removal of part of the foci will be followed by a gradual return of some or all of the previous symptoms, for a focal infection patient, who has been once sensitized is always more easily overcome and unless all the foci are removed you do not get, or need you expect, any permanent results.

We have been surprised to find, frequently, that the first evidence of any foci, in a focal infection patient, is some severe constitutional or other secondary disorder which imperils the health and life of this patient, yet on the other hand, an impacted infected root or tooth as well as an infected sinus or antrum often gives more evidence of a systemic disturbance than a chronic gall-bladder, appendix or a similar foci.

You need not anticipate a disappearance of all the clinical symptoms or the effecting of a cure, in a case of long standing, even after all the foci have been removed, until a period of, at least, from three to six months has elapsed and during the first twelve months, after the removal of all the foci, if for any reason the resistance of this patient should be lowered, you can expect a temporary return of some of the previous symptoms.

Also, in cases of long standing, particularly in adults, where there are diseased tonsils, one or more infected teeth are usually present and if there are any impacted roots or impacted unerupted teeth, they are quite often infected and a cure certainly means their removal.

Many cases that formerly would not have been benefited or cured have cleared up promptly after not only the removal of all the infected teeth but all roots and particles of roots as well as the curettage and treatment of the tooth sockets or even the bone itself, and if there is a return of any symptoms, in a case where diseased teeth have been removed, even within a period of three to six months, look for and remove a later infected tooth or teeth which previously showed normal.

Specifically, we say that the clinical picture of the patient, more than the apparent condition of the tonsils, determines the question of enucleation and the radical removal of all diseased teeth or area around these teeth is the only rational treatment.

In closing, your chairman would say to you, do not be satisfied with anything but a thorough and comprehensive examination and study of all your cases, and if you do not get the results anticipated, rest assured you have overlooked some foci and particularly, at this time, when your brother physician has answered the call of his country and left his work for you and others to do, do your duty by doing thorough and conscientious work, especially with these focal infection patients.

CHAIRMAN'S ADDRESS—SECTION ON PEDIATRICS AND OBSTETRICS*

By T. C. SANDERS, M. D., Shawnee, Oklahoma

I wish to thank you for the honor conferred one year ago at our annual meeting by selecting me your chairman, and especially do I wish to thank those of you who have cooperated with me in building my program.

I wish first to dwell upon the program phase of this section, offering a few suggestions and incidentally a few remarks, namely: I believe there should be a heartier and more generous response on the part of members toward the chairman in helping him to formulate and build his program each year.

Personally, I have found it quite a task to get up a program this year, having written numerous letters trying to enlist new members as well as the old and faithful, for papers and discussions. To some of my letters there was no response, and to many others, replies were much delayed, neccessitating delay on the part of the chairman in completing program. I fully realize in a sense this has been an unusual year in many respects, particularly the upset conditions in all lines incident to our terrible conflict in Europe, and that many of our brother physicians are nobly serving under Old Glory, and that most of us left at home are very busy men; still, if you will note, the most successful medical societies are made so by the busier men in their respective communities, who in spite of business stress, etc., can and usually do find time to prepare and read papers at their different meetings, and in many other ways promote the cause of medicine. Hence, I think it is up to us of this section (if we are to make it bigger and better each succeeding year) to cooperate with our chairman in every way, offering him advice and suggestions, and above all in being prompt in our response to any communication from him.

We have in this section combined two very, very important branches of the practice of medicine, fields in which there is always room for study and development, and fields which make up a large per cent. of the general practitioners' practice, as well as all of those who specialize in one or both branches, therefore, I believe for above reasons, this should and eventually will be one of the largest attended and most active sections of our state organization.

I also think it advisable, and would suggest same to this section, that in our election each year we also elect a vice-chairman, in order that the work would proceed just the same, in the event of the chairman going to war or for other cause of absence.

I would also urge that this section, as in some other sections, be furnished with a stenographer, in order that our proceedings and discussions may be properly cared for.

It now gives me great pleasure to take up the program for this year, which I feel sure from the character of the subjects of the different papers, and the men presenting them, will prove both very interesting and instructive to all of us.

*Twenty-sixth Annual Meeting, Tulsa, May 15, 1918.

CHAIRMAN'S ADDRESS—SECTION ON SURGERY*

By LeROY LONG, M. D., Oklahoma City

Gentlemen:

In speaking to you today I desire to call attention to a few things that I conceive to be of importance in connection with the work of the general surgeon.

At this moment I have in the hospital five patients with drainage tubes in their abdomens after operations for either a spreading peritonitis or an abscess resulting from a perforation in the course of an attack of appendicitis. Every one of these patients had been given cathartics, before being brought to hospital. Every one of them gave a history of acute abdominal pain as the initial symptom. Notwithstanding this, an effort was made in each case to purge the patient—in some of the cases there were repeated efforts.

One of these patients lives in Oklahoma City; the others are from various parts of the state. All of them had been under the care of physicians regarded as possessing at least average ability.

With one exception, a diagnosis of appendicitis had been made before the cathartic was ordered. In about half of the cases the family had given cathartics before the physician was called, but when he saw the patient the dose was repeated.

I do not wish to take up time here by going into an argument against the administration of cathartics in appendicitis. Surely it may be assumed that every surgeon worthy of confidence has long since taken a clear and decisive position against such a hazardous and death producing procedure. It would seem, however, that there are still many men in the profession who take this foolish—this dangerous—this criminal course, and it is plainly the duty of the surgeon who so often sees the disastrous consequences of such a course to improve every opportunity to call the attention of his brother physicians to its evils and the importance of avoiding them.

Some years ago I made the statement at a meeting at McAlester that it should be a surgical law that in the presence of an acute abdominal pain followed by nausea, a cathartic must not be given. The additional experience of the years since that time, with the picture of suffering and death as the result of this ill-advised procedure before me, constrains me to go a step further, and I now say to you that it should be a surgical law that cathartics must not be given in the presence of acute abdominal pain, no matter whether it is followed by nausea or not.

I have called attention to the dangerous use of cathartics in appendicitis because that is a common—almost a daily sin that is being committed. Appendicitis being by far the most frequent acute abdominal condition beginning with pain, the greater number of disasters following the giving of cathartics occur in connection with that disease, but I have seen the same thing in conneation with a perforation of a gastric or duodenal ulcer: in connection with an empyema of the gall bladder; in connection with intestinal obstruction; in connection, even, with a ruptured extra-uterine pregnancy.

There is another traditional and time-honored procedure to which even some surgeons continue to bow down as if it were a mystic god to be worshiped—and that is the routine administration of cathartics after operation in the abdomen. They are especially anxious that this be done if there is prolonged post-operative nausea, tympany or abdominal distress, and as a result we too often see cases of overlooked acute dilatition of the stomach, post-operative ileus, and only too frequently—death.

This fetich of giving a cathartic after operation is one before which all of us have, at one time or another, bowed down, and I must confess that it took me a

*Twenty-sixth Annual Meeting, Tulsa, May 15, 1918.

long time to get away from it. It took a long time because it seemed that a departure from it would be an iconoclastic procedure fraught with some risk since many of our great clinicians carried it out as a routine procedure. I recall that on one occasion while attending the clinic of one of the widely known gynecological surgeons in an eastern city, I asked him about his practice in connection with cathartics after operation. He replied that patients operated in the morning were started on half grain doses of calomel hourly at midnight.

Just before that time I had the misfortune of having a case of post-operative ilues. I operated for the ileus and, to my great joy, the patient recovered; that is, she recovered so far as saving her life was concerned, but she recovered with a crippled abdomen that will be an ever present menace the remainder of her days. However, I felt so elated over my success that I reported the case at a medical meeting, calling attention especially to the technique employed. Sometime afterwards, in a moment of mature and honest reflection, I wondered how much the routine post-operative cathartic might have had to do with the production of the ileus. Thereafter—tentatively, at first—I began to drift away from this false fetich at whose shrine I had been trying to find a place to worship with the numerous 'throng always found before it. As I gradually learned the value of gastric lavage, of the colon tube for gas, of the hypodermatic use of small doses of morphine as necessary to keep the patient comfortable, of forgetting about the bowels moving for several days, and then if necessary, a low enema of a few ounces of glycerine with enough warm water to make a pint—never over a pint—as I learned these things I renounced my allegiance to the foolish tradition of post-operative catharsis. Years have come and gone since that time, but, notwithstanding the considerable increase in the volume of my work, I have not had to record a single case of post-operative ileus, nor have I had any reason to feel otherwise than sincerely thankful that I have totally abandoned a procedure which I am convinced is fallacious and dangerous.

I must at this time call attention to the question of fee-splitting. It seems that there are still those who engage in this nefarious practice. In my judgment, there is just one thing for this section to do in this matter, and that is to drive the money changers from the temple. The man who secures his surgery in this way is a grafter and his presence among respectable people who are trying to render honest service should not be tolerated. The buying and selling of helpless patients must stop, and one way we can stop it is to put a black mark against the man who engages in it, and to ostracize him completely. Of course a hypocritical cry will go up that we are a coterie, of surgeons trying to dictate in personal matters, but we are a coterie, thank God, that is trying to place our specialty out of reach of the panderer and the highwayman.

But let us go even further in our service to the people than to try to protect them from those who would capitalize their misfortunes and buy and sell them. Let us realize in our souls the necessity of making the profession of medicine a truly altruistic profession. This does not mean that we should not charge liberal fees in the cases of those able to pay, but it does mean that we should see to it that the vast multitude who are so situated that they have practically no margin of financial safety are properly cared for when they need our services. I hope that no surgeon here would be guilty of making it necessary for the poor man to mortgage his home, or to pay usurious interest, or to take his children out of school in order to make money to pay for a necessary professional service. The surgeon who measures his success by the size of his bank account is no longer striving to reach what should be the ideals of our profession.

Since the beginning of the war in Europe, much important matter has been written about the proper treatment of wounds. Among the more prominent new procedures brought forward are the hypertonic salt solution of Wright, the hypochlorite solution of Dakin used after the method of Carrel and Dauchesne, the bismuth-iodoform-paraffin mixture of Rutherford Morrison and the powder of Vincent. Remarkably satisfactory results are reported by the partisans of these various procedures.

While there seems to be much difference of opinion with reference to the use and efficacy of these additions to the surgeons' armamentarium, it seems that there are certain important fundamental things concerning which all are agreed. One of the most important is the careful *debridement* in the case of lacerated wounds. This seems to me to be based upon sound surgical principles, for we must not forget the elementary fact that the healing of wounds depends in the last analysis upon the integrity of the cells of the body.

Another remarkable advancement has been in connection with the treatment of burns by the use of an impermeable covering consisting of a paraffin mixture. For many years some of us have tried to carry out the principle of this treatment by the use of vaseline and various petroleum preparations. This procedure appeals strongly, therefore, to those of us who have consistently opposed the painful and depressing so-called antiseptic treatment of extensive burns, as well as the treatment of deep and extensive burns by the no less painful and depressing open air or hot air methods.

Finally, our country is engaged in war against barbarism. It is engaged in war against a foe that has for four years systematically practiced every conceivable and beastly cruelty—yes, cruelties not even conceivable in the minds of a truly civilized people. Our boys are going and our doctors are going with them. As American citizens we are going to stand shoulder to shoulder with heroic France and her allies until the bestialism of the Hun is forever wiped from the face of earth.

In the very nature of things, all of us can not go to the front, but no matter where we are we must serve. Now is no time to think of laying up wealth. What we do must be done with one single end in view—the eventual victory of right over might.

Those of us who remain at home must serve, but let us remember that, no matter how hard we may try to do our duty at home, we can not make a sacrifice equal to that made by those who go away from home to serve in the Army or Navy. Realizing this, let those who serve at home see to it that the interests of the absent ones are protected in every possible way.

I thank you, gentlemen, for honoring me with the Chairmanship of your section. I thank those who will take part in this meeting. As we go away I shall anxiously look forward to another meeting when, I pray God, we may mingle together with the sweet realization that Prussian militarism has been destroyed and that peace reigns upon the earth.

PERINEAL LACERATIONS.

H. A. Bernstein, New York (*Journal A. M. A.*, April 27, 1918), criticizes the insufficiency of the majority of perineal operations, and advocates the detailed suturing of the muscle terminations of the two sides together. Each should be sutured separately. The application of tenacula, to draw the different parts of the tear into correct position, has been the first principle in all operations for secondary repair of the perineum, since the time of Hegar, and why it is always neglected in the primary operation is not apparent. After the muscles have been replaced, if the wound is deep, slack may be taken up in the connective tissue by one or two buried catgut sutures. With the guide sutures held in place for repair he unites the edges of the torn vaginal mucosa. The edges of the vaginal mucosa are joined with a continuous chromic gut suture, and the outer side of the perineum is repaired with the three or four silkworm-gut sutures deeply and widely inserted. In complete tears, it is necessary to insert a rectal tube about four inches into the rectum, and keep it there for about four days. The bowels should not be moved during this time. The operation requires no special experience, and he calls attention to the use of guide sutures to control the success of the operation.

SYMPTOMS AND DIAGNOSIS OF SYPHILIS OF THE BLADDER —CASE REPORTS*

By W. J. WALLACE, M. D., Oklahoma City

I think it is usually the custom for the chairman to give an address of some kind, but at this time the principal subject is one of patriotism and that will be given and has been given by men who can do justice to the cause so much better than I can, so I have decided I would just read you a paper on "Syphilis of the Bladder". That is, as I have been able to see it and study it. The data has been very limited, as far as I can find, so I will just read you what I have found and mine is merely the symptoms and diagnosis. I have not gone into the treatment at all; have not gone into the pathology; because I thought once I would mention pathology but I didn't know enough about it, at this present time, so I just left that off. I will just merely give you some symptoms and treatment, symptoms and diagnosis.

In my work, I am finding quite a few cases of syphilis of the bladder, that we have been treating for other things. The reason why I mentioned this paper at this time.

Syphilis of the bladder is a rather uncommon disease, or at least thought so by the average physician, and because of this idea many physicians are inclined to discount its existence entirely. Among the old European syphilologists there has been a wide difference of opinion; of the older school, Nogues, Desnos, and Minet deny the existence of the disease, while Casper, Legueu, Fournier, Guyon and Nitze have never reported a case. The majority of the American text books of today do not mention the disease at all, or if they do, merely in a casual way.

Up to 1902 only sixteen cases had been reported in European literature, while since that time only about twenty-two cases in all have been reported with about six cases in America. I believe this apparent increase is due to the fact that physicians in every branch of medicne have become more painstaking in their examination, and syphilologists are looking for more bladder lesions, whose presence a few years ago would not have been suspected.

We all remember when appendicitis masqueraded under the guise of various ailments, and when gall-bladder diseases were a rare occurrence. It is also in very recent times that certain diseases of the kidney and bladder have been recognized and specifically named, although I am not inclined to believe that syphilis of the bladder is as common as these maladies, though it is deserving of more investigation than it has received.

It does not seem unreasonable to presume that some of the large number of patients whom we see every day suffering with intractable or relapsing cystitis, may have an unrecognized syphilitic infection.

Symptoms.

The bladder is most frequently affected in the tertiary stage and cystitis is usually associated, as well as hematuria.

Pain: A majority of past authors have noted as an outstanding symptom the extreme sensitiveness of the bladder, especially so when the cystoscope and various solutions are introduced. This, I think, is wrong. The bladder is not as sensitive as it should be for such an inflamed thickened appearing mucosa. The pain we have is of a heavy, aching, not of the acute, cutting, as we find in some forms of bladder trouble. If ulcers or lesions are located on the side of the bladder, the pain is referred to the supra-pubic region, if on the base of the bladder, to the perineum; if on the

---

*Chairman's Address, Section on Genito-Urinary Diseases, Skin and Radiology, Twenty-sixth Annual Meeting, Tulsa, May 15, 1918.

trigone, referred to the cord and testicles; if at the internal sphincter, referred to the end of the penis. So the pain is in the proportion to the number of lesions and the location. If around the vesical orifice the pain, of course, is greater. But the pain is nearly always intensified by the accompaning cystitis, which sooner or later we have. I just want to lay a little stress on that point, the pain, I think is a very important feature to bear in mind. It is not in proportion in syphilitic bladder as in other things.

Urinary: Urgency and frequency of urine are always pronounced. The appearance of the urine is not unlike that found in other forms of bladder disturbances; it is dark, murky, cloudy in color, due to epithelial cells and mucous. The urine frequently contains more than the usual amount of blood for an ordinary cystitis. There is a small number of pus cells in proportion to the general symptoms; while we have the freqeuncy of urination, it is not as great, nor as painful as we would find in the tubercular bladder and not in proportion to the appearing pathology.

Hematuria: Hematuria always accompanies this condition, especially so by the time a patient presents himself to the physician. That is the first thing that frightens him and causes him to consult the doctor, as the previous attacks have been mild and he has taken some mild antispasmitic which has given him temporary relief, but the appearance of blood frightens him and he calls for special treatment.

So our three classical symptoms are, (2) pain, (3) frequency of urination, and (1) hematuria.

There are classical symptoms in this as, of course, in many other things, that would bring the patient to you, so of course, would the hematuria, a little bleeding, and of course you have our pain and frequency of urination.

Diagnosis: Diagnosis of syphilis of the bladder is usually neglected because the physician is not looking for it. It is probable now, with the many advances of recent years, that the profession will be more on the lookout for this condition. The diagnosis is difficult because there are other symptoms present besides those indicating syphilis, which are more distressing and disfiguring to the patient. So a chronic cystitis is usually taken for granted without a special or painstaking examination. The diagnosis is based upon the symptoms and history of the case, but must be confirmed by subjective, objective, cystoscopic, urinary and Wassermann examinations. After eliciting the subjective symptoms, we should, as a routine, cystoscope all patients presenting themselves with the above described symptoms. I have frequently diagnosed syphilis of the bladder by the cystoscopic examination alone. Baker emphasizes the fact that functional disturbances of the bladder which accompany syphilis of the nervous system, can be readily diagnosed by cystoscopic examination. I think that is very true in certain cases.

The character of the pain is a very important diagnostic point at this time, as we frequently find almost a complete anesthesia of the urethra and internal sphincter. This in itself is suggestive of an involvement of the central nervous system and would lead one to suspect a syphilitic condition. In other diseases of the bladder with symptoms of this character it is almost impossible to make a cystoscopic examination on account of the intense pain. Usually we can fairly well inflate the bladder with water enough to make our examinatiom. It is necessary to wash the bladder three to four times to clear it of the usual deposit, and I wish to say at this point that the bleeding is not in proportion to the intensely reddened, ulcerated bladder, as would be the case in other bladder lesions. Through our cystoscope we will usually see numerous tubercular-appearing nodes, with an occasional low grade ulcerated base, rather shiny in its appearance and not very deep. This is usually rather extensive, covering the trigonum and the base of the bladder. The ulcerations would most likely be mistaken for a T. B. but they are a little different in appearance. The next form is more typical of the gunma, usually a circumscribed deep-appearing sore, or there may be several scattered on the base or near the ureteral orifices or near the sphincter with a diffused, thickened tissue intervening. If closely observed, it will be found to be almost typical of a gumma in general.

Sometimes, though rarely, we will find a polypoid vegetation near the vesical orifice or base of the bladder with all the appearance of a beginning malignancy. Sometimes we can get a piece of this growth or the scrapings of the ulcers for our laboratory examination, which should always be hone, if possible.

Next, to complete our diagnosis, we should have urinary and Wassermann tests made as a routine on all extreme bladder cases.

Differential Diagnosis.

Differential diagnosis of syphilis of the bladder is necessarily difficult because of the small amount of literature on the subject. It is probable that a true diagnosis will seldom be made, unless one is familiar with the objective and subjective symptoms. Tuberculosis is the most frequent lesions for mistake. In tuberculosis we have ulcerating tubercles and painful condition, the ulcer bleeding easily and profusely and the bladder non-distensible, only containing from one to four ounces of water and examination being almost impossible, unless under general anesthesia. Tuberculosis of the bladder is secondary to other parts of the body. The next condition to consider is tumors of the bladder. These will be found to be either the benign or malignant, and in this it is very difficult to make our diagnosis at first. But in tumors of the bladder we have the spontaneous hemorrhage with no bearing on exercise or rest, with fragments in the urine which the laboratory test would show us. In the syphilitic bladder the ulcers do not bleed so freely nor are they so painful and the bladder can be distended to a fair size. You can wash the bladder and make a fair diagnosis and the patient's general condition is usually fairly good. So our next step now, after our cystoscopic examination, bearing in mind the things so similar to the syphilitic bladder, is to call on our laboratory and therapeutic tests for further assistance. Wassermann should be taken in every case and the urine and bladder scrapings sent to the laboratory to see if we can locate the spirochete or other causes just mentioned.

I wish now to submit a few case reports:

1. September 21, 1917. J. H. R., farmer, Centrahoma, age 27. Family history negative. Married four years. Has two children in good health. Three years ago had an attack of intense pain over region of kidney and in bladder. These attacks lasted off and on for six months, patient in bed toward latter part of attacks for a period of four weeks, lost considerable weight. Placed on treatment, kind not known, which helped but did not entirely cure him.

Present trouble: Attack began three weeks ago, over region of kidney and bladder with intense straining and tenesmus with frequent, painful and bloody urination. Passed considerable lumps with mucus but no calculi. Pulse 95, temperature 100. Patient seemed sallow and septic. Under general anesthesia, cystoscopic examination was made and the following condition found: prostate moderately enlarged, no stricture, considerable amount of blood resulting from examination, but after washing bladder several times was able to see a villous growth on right side near the internal sphincter and one near the right urethral orifice.

Anti-syphilitic treatment was instituted and the growth completely cleared and patient is now making his crop and apparently well.

2. July 24, 1917. Mrs. E. N. S., age 43. Husband died fourteen years ago, pneumonia. Has one child 16 years of age, good health. One miscarriage and one child dead at birth, the one living being her third pregnancy. History

of venereal diseases negative. December, 1916, was operated on, and both ovaries, tubes and uterus were removed.

Present trouble: Painful, frequent, and occasionally bloody urination. Urinary analysis as follows: reaction alkaline, S. P. G. 1030, small amount of albumen, sugar negative and a number of granular casts present. Cystoscopic examination revealed both urethral orifices thickened, a number of papules alternating with ulcers on the internal sphincter, as well as several in the urethra, trigonum thickened showing small nodes and three distinct ulcers, irregular in outline. The whole condition being very much like T. B. bladder. Wassermann positive. Diagnosed as tubercular syphilodermata of the bladder, which was cleared up under specific treatment.

3. May 5, 1917. M. G., age 24. Family history negative, within patient's knowledge. Past history negative as to venereal diseases.

Present trouble: May 15th, came to my office suffering with terminal hematuria, with some pain and sediment in the urine, claimed that while not sick, was not feeling well, and was frightened at sight of blood in urine.

Examination: Physical condition not quite up to normal, very nervous and apprehensive. Cystoscopic examination showed ulcerated and nodular tragonitis, with also a thickened and reddened condition in the bladder, also one distinct ulcer and a few small nodes at internal sphincter. Prostatic urethra showed several distinct erosions. While bladder was badly inflamed, there was not a great amount of pain in making cystoscopic examination. Urinary examination: albumen, small amount, sugar negative, acid reaction, S. P. G. 1028. Epithelial cells, but no casts. Wassermann was made, positive. Trouble has completely cleared under specific treatment.

Wish to add that after talking with patient's father, found that the latter contracted syphilis some 28 or 30 years ago, so I regard this as a case of inherited syphilitic condition of the bladder.

4. July 20, 1917. Mrs. L., age 30. Family history negative. All diseases of childhood, remained in good health until age of nineteen, at which time she began to have some pain over region of left kidney. Five years ago she had appendectomy, fixation of uterus, salpingectomy on left side. Ten days following this began to have trouble with bladder. Three weeks after operation, abdominal wound broke open. Two years later she had nephrectomy of left kidney which she claimed was a pus kidney. Bladder also was very badly inflamed at that time. Patient lost a good deal in weight and wounds healed very closely.

June, 1917, was operated on for intestinal obstruction with good recovery, but patient still suffered with bladder complication and the diagnosis was made for T. B.

On June 20, 1917, patient was referred to me for treatment of the bladder condition. Tenderness over region of bladder. Cystoscope revealed highly inflamed mucosa, two distinct ulcers at right urethral orifice, four ulcers on the trigone, left orifice thickened with several small ulcers. Internal sphincter contained several papules and four or five ulcers, all of which bled rather freely. Urethra congested but no ulcers. Urinary analysis: S. P. G. 1016, alkaline, no albumen, no sugar, casts present, bacteria present but no T. B. Sqaumous epithelium present, with pus and blood, looking very much like a T. B. bladder. Blood for Wassermann positive.

Anti-syphilitic treatment instituted. Patient apparently well and healthy.

5. E. L. J., age 28. Married and one child five years old. Family and past history negative. Referred to me for cystitis.

Cystoscopic examination showed papules and ulcers on the trigone, a group of small ulcers above the right urethral orifice, neck of bladder was inflamed with a few ulcers and small papules.

Attempted fulguration without success, also bladder washes and deep injections without relief. During this time I took blood for Wassermann and much to patient's surprise it was positive. Discontinued all local treatment, gave antisyphilitic treatment and the trouble healed.

6. May 5, 1917. Miner, age 40. No history of venereal diseases. Three years ago had a supra-pubic cystotomy for growth in the bladder. Apparently cured until three months ago when he began suffering with frequent and painful urination.

Examination showed an intensely reddened bladder, marked ulcerations over the base and trigonal regions with a white deposit covering same. At first appearance thought it malignant, and while he came for an opeartion, delayed same for further investigation. Blood for Wassermann positive. Patient was given two doses of salvarsan with other anti-syphilitic treatment and was very much improved, so much so that he left saying that he had to go back to his work. Heard from him a few months later and was still at work.

His original trouble evidently was a syphilitic polypoid growth.

7. January 1, 1918. J. P. P., blacksmith, age 29. Married two years but no children. Contracted gonorrhea 12 years ago, otherwise history negative.

November, 1916, was operated on for stone in bladder. No stone found, but a tumor was located and removed (papilloma). Returned home and remained well until two months ago, at which time he was referred to me for a similar operation.

Examination showed ulcerations and a villous growth on the neck of the bladder and extending down on the trigone. Several distinct nodules were near the growth. The growth was most too extensive for fulguration, and too, I suspected malignancy. Blood for Wassermann positive. Growth and bladder have cleared up under intensive treatmnet.

8. October 5, 1916. H. P., age 29. Family history negative. Gonorrhea 14 years ago, another attack February, 1916. No history of syphilis.

Present trouble: Difficult and frequent urination with much straining and small stream. Some pain over region of bladder when full.

Examination: Large, soft and tender prostate, stricture at the membranous urethra size 18. Gave treatment for stricture for two weeks at which time I was able under local anesthesia to introduce cystoscope and found the following condition: Reddened and thickened bladder walls, a distinct gumma the size of a dime near the left urethral orifice above and to the outside, with all the typical characteristics of a gumma in other regions of the body. Blood for Wassermann positive.

This is briefly the history of eight cases. On account of lack of space I shall not describe any further ones, but my records show that eighteen cases (these described included) have been sent to me for other bladder troubles with no history of ever having contracted syphilis.

So, in conclusion, syphilis of the bladder is more common than we have heretofore realized and no operation should be performed nor tumors fulgurated, without first taking blood for a Wassermann.

JOURNAL OF THE OKLAHOMA STATE MEDICAL ASSOCIATION

VOLUME XI   MUSKOGEE, OKLA., JUNE, 1918   NUMBER 6

PUBLISHED MONTHLY AT MUSKOGEE. OKLA., UNDER DIRECTION OF THE COUNCIL

DR. CLAUDE A. THOMPSON, EDITOR-IN-CHIEF

ENTERED AT THE POST OFFICE AT MUSKOGEE, OKLAHOMA, AS SECOND CLASS MAIL MATTER, JULY 28, 1912

THIS IS THE OFFICIAL JOURNAL OF THE OKLAHOMA STATE MEDICAL ASSOCIATION. ALL COMMUNICATIONS SHOULD BE ADDRESSED TO THE JOURNAL OF THE OKLAHOMA STATE MEDICAL ASSOCIATION, 308 SURETY BUILDING, MUSKOGEE, OKLAHOMA.

The editorial department is not responsible for the opinions expressed in the original articles of contributors.

Reprints of original articles will be supplied at actual cost, provided request for them s attached to manuscript or made in sufficient time before publication.

Articles sent this Journal for publication and all those read at the annual meetings of the State Association are the sole property of this Journal. The Journal relies on each individual contributor's strict adherence to this well-known rule of medical journalism. In the event an article sent this Journal for publication is published before appearance in the Journal, the manuscript will be returned to the writer.

Failure to receive the Journal should call for immediate notification of the editor, 307-8 Surety Building, Muskogee, Okla.

Local news of possible interest to the medical profession, notes on removals, changes in address, deaths and weddings will be gratefully received.

Advertising of articles, drugs or compounds unapproved by the Council on Pharmacy of the A. M. A. will not be accepted.

Advertising rates will be supplied on application. It is suggested that wherever possible members of the State Association should patronize our advertisers in preference to others as a matter of fair reciprocity.

EDITORIAL

THE TWENTY-SIXTH ANNUAL MEETING.

HOUSE OF DELEGATES AND COUNCIL.

The Council met May 14th at 1:30 P. M., Dr. W. Albert Cook presiding. The Secretary read his report for the year, which was accepted. An Auditing Committee composed of Drs. J. Hutchings White, J. L. Austin and J. T. Slover was appointed.

A report from O. J. Logan, Attorney in the Chiropractic Matter, was read. A committee consisting of Drs. Ed. James, R. L. Mitchell and F. Y. Cronk was appointed to make recommendations as to that matter.

HOUSE OF DELEGATES, May 14th. Dr. W. Albert Cook in the chair. Reading of minutes was dispensed with as they had been previously published.

Notice was given that the following Constitutional Ammendment was on call for vote at the next meeting of the House.

CONSTITUTION: AMENDMENT. Article 9, Section 4. "When a member of any component society moves into another county of this State he shall be amenable to and automatically become a member of the county society of the county where he resides".

To this there was offered the following amendment: "Provided that this shall apply only to matters of jurisdiction or inquiry as to alleged violations of the Constitution and By-laws and Code of Ethics, of any member who may be without the jurisdiction of his county society. That the State Secretary, after inquiry of the county societies interested, being advised that there is no objection thereto, shall carry such member as a member of the society to which he has moved. - That in the event a member moving into a new location is denied admission as a member of the society into whose jurisdiction he has moved, the following order shall be followed: (1) He shall be carried as a member of his original society, and shall forfeit no privilege of membership during the pendency and final settlement of his case. (2) On appeal from (a) either the member involved, (b) his original society or (c) the society denying him membership, the record from every person and society involved shall be transmitted to the Council and its verdict and order shall be final and binding on all concerned."

PROPOSED AMENDMENT TO THE BY-LAWS: To lie over twenty-four hours:

To amend Chapter five; ELECTION OF OFFICERS. After section three (3) add the following section:

Section 4. All officers except the President-elect, who shall take office at the first meeting after his predecessor has served a term of one year, shall assume office on the first day of January following their election, and shall, unless otherwise specified, hold office until December 31st following. All officers of this Association are required to promptly turn over to their successors all papers and records of their office on the day or immediately after they relinquish office.

Section 5. In the event any officer of this Association removes from the State, the vacancy thus created may be filled by appointment by the President, or if an officer has previously been elected to hold such office, such officer shall automatically assume the duties of the office to which he has been elected.

A PROPOSITION to reduce the councillor districts from thirteen to eight was offered as follows:

District 1. Texas, Beaver, Cimarron, Harper, Ellis, Woods, Woodward, Alfalfa, Major, Grant, Garfield, Noble and Kay.

District 2. Dewey, Roger Mills, Custer, Beckham, Washita, Greer, Kiowa, Harmon, Jackson and Tillman.

District 3. Blaine, Kingfisher, Canadian, Logan, Payne, Lincoln, Oklahoma, Cleveland, Pottawatomie, Seminole, and McClain.

District 4. Caddo, Grady, Comanche, Cotton, Stephens, Jefferson, Garvin, Murray, Carter and Love.

District 5. Pontotoc, Coal, Johnston, Atoka, Marshall, Bryan, Choctaw, Pushtamaha and McCurtain.

District 6. Okfuskee, Hughes, Pittsburg, Latimer, LeFlore, Haskell and Sequoyah.

District 7. Pawnee, Osage, Washington, Tulsa, Creek, Nowata and Rogers.

District 8. Craig, Ottawa, Delaware, Mayes, Wagoner, Cherokee, Adair, Okmulgee, Muskogee and McIntosh.

HOUSE OF DELEGATES, May 16th, 1918, 9:00 A. M. A roll of the House was called by the credentials committee. The Council committee to investigate and report suggestions as to changing the councilor districts reported favorably and the changes were adopted as heretofore offered. The House ordered that where there was only one councilor in a newly created district he should hold over and where there were two or more lots should be drawn to determine who should hold until the next election.

The House voted to accept the suggestions and adopted the changes.

The proposed change in the Constitution adding Section 4 to Chapter 9 was adopted.

The proposed change in the By-Laws adding Section 4 to Chapter 5 was adopted.

The Secretary was authorized to continue activity in the Chiropractic matter, and if necessary to report to the membership on any emergency arising which might require the cooperation of the individual members.

A War Historian was discussed and on motion such office was created. Dr. L. Haynes Buxton, Oklahoma City, was appointed to the position and instructed to make up a careful record of all physicians entering the service and arrange for permanent preservation of such roster.

The Auditing Committee reported that the books of the Secretary-Treasurer had been checked and found correct.

A resolution offered by Dr. M. A. Kelso was adopted as follows: Inasmuch as the United States is at war and thousands of our noble profession are in service in the army and thousands more are and will be called to duty at home and abroad, therefore be it resolved that the Oklahoma State Medical Association in convention assembled endorse the proposed law known as the Owen-Dyer Bill and that for the general welfare of the profession be it further resolved that we urge its early passage by Comgress.

Election of officers resulted as follows: President, L. J. Moorman, Oklahoma City; 1st vice-president, Ed. D. James, Miami; 2nd vice-president, H. M. Williams, Wellston; 3rd vice-president, Walter Hardy, Ardmore; Delegate to the A. M. A., LeRoy Long, Oklahoma City. Meeting place 1918, Muskogee.

Dr. Franklin Martin, Chairman of the Medical Section Council of National Defense, addressed the House in the afternoon. Adjourned.

GENERAL MEETING.
May 14, 1918, 8:30 P. M.

Invocation, Rev. J. W. Abel, Tulsa.

President Cook: We now have the pleasure of listening to **Honorable A. F. Ross,** representative of the Mayor.

Mr. Ross: Mr. Chairman, Members of the Society, Ladies and Gentlemen. Just before the convention convened this evening the chairman asked me, what on earth I was doing among this honorable, respectable set of people. He was not acquainted with the fact that my given name was Austin Flint. It has led me into many strange and curious places; it has involved me in a great many difficulties; it has been a great handicap for me to bear, but upon behalf of the Mayor of the City, and the people of the city, I bid you all welcome in our midst, welcome because you are members of your profession, and some of them who stand for the very high ideals of your profession. I am a porfessional man, and even into that high and dignified profession, it being the law, occasionally, accidentally there creeps and crawls those who are not a credit to it. It becomes our business in our organization to sweep them from our profession, to the end that we may be held in the high esteem to which all men know we are entitled. But seriously, my friends, humanity loves those benefactors, loves them out of gratitude, loves them naturally and irrestibly, and I imagine if there is a class of men uniformly loved for the benefactions conferred upon those among whom they live, surely it is those who in the dark hours of disease minister to those afflcited. It is a great profession and offers magnificient opportunities. My little knowledge of what had been achieved in the last quarter of a century gives me a right to make the statement that no profession in America has advanced so rapidly, or accomplished so much as the medical men of America. Those who belong to my profession find its secrets and know its ways by reading dusty volumes, by putting in so many hours of solid reading and hard work, but the secrets of the medical profession are as numerous as the leaves on the tree, and as different as the members of the human family, and surely it requires daring and spirit, as well as fundamental knowledge, to become a successful physician or surgeon. There is another reason, too, why at this particular time civilization is so far ahead, and it is due greatly to members of this profession. Never before has such a crisis come upon the world as at this particular time. Never has there been before this such a time, that by one fell blow our liberty, our civilization, all good that has arisen since men came out of the dark ages, was about to be destroyed overnight, and in that terrific contest, with those tremendous stakes, the men of your profession, and men of your caliber, are those who are going to make it possible to win, and when it is over and ended, then, believe me, my friends, no little credit of the victory will be due to him and him and him, and thousands who have gone before him, and thousands who will go after him.   We are glad always to have men of your kind, your character, your caliber, your patriotism, in our midst.   We want to be so kind, so generous, and so indulgent to you while you are here that it will be so pleasant you will want to come back again.

We tender you every member of your profession living in our city as a committee for your entertainment.   They have never failed, and I know they will not in the entertainment of you.   I want to say that you—each of you—are as welcome in our midst, as you are across the threshold of our home when disease lies therein.   I thank you.

The President: The gentleman who is to reply to the address of welcome needs no introduction to you—**Dr. John W. Duke,** State Commissioner of Health.

Dr. Duke: Mr. President, and Gentlemen of the Oklahoma State Medical Association, and Mr. Flint.   I sincerely congratulate you upon the name of Flint. The United States of America owes a debt to Austin Flint that it will never be able to pay.   I was taught by his son and grandson.   You must be a great man. Then, too, your most cordial welcome bids us cheer in your city.   We know you must be a great people to select a man like you to give us this flattering reception, even if you did not mean it.   We shall expect to cross the thresholds of your homes; we expect to eat at your tables, and I assure you we will leave all instruments, etc., in our own homes.

Gentlemen, this is a serious time.   I remember that last year in our association we wondered if we would see these men next year.   We see, some of them, and there are a great many of the old ones that are not here, and a great number of them in khaki, who are ready to give their lives for our protection, the protection of our homes, and our women and our children.

Oklahoma has responded generously in her call for medical men.   I wonder how many great and loyal men are in this room tonight who will respond to that call.   If this war continues, and I am afraid it will, perhaps in the next twelve months every man in the state of Oklahoma under fifty years of age will be compelled to join the colors.   The need is very urgent and the call should be heeded. We represent a great profession, it is needless for me to call your attention to that for each of you know in your own greatness that you must belong to a great profession.   To be a good doctor means a great deal of careful study.   A good lawyer 300 years ago would be a good lawyer today but a good doctor 300 years ago would be a very poor doctor today.   This profession is a progressive one.   It cannot be fastened down to any fixed rules.   There is always new information. So a good lawyer 300 years ago, if he was brought back to life and put on this earth, would be a good lawyer still, but science progresses so rapidly that this would not be the case with the doctor.   Science has made our profession a profession of which we are all very proud.

Now I wish to call your attention to a very important matter that has given me a great deal of concern.   I am going to take advantage of your presence to speak about it.   That is surgical hygiene.   The Surgeon General and the surgeons of the Public Health Service are very much concerned about this matter, and they get out circulars, and send many letters urging them to let no opportunity pass to call this matter to the attention of the medical profession and civilians.   It has been estimated from statistics gotten from cantonments in this country since the declaration of war by this country, that about 450,000 men who are in the camps in this country are suffering from syphilis.   Could the Kaiser do worse? He has not.   Your quota from Oklahoma in that number would be about 7,800. I need not call your attention to the very great danger that confronts our army from this appalling disease, but let me remind you that when you find one suffering from this dread disease you find five suffering from the other social disease. Multiply 7,500 by five and you will have the number suffering from social diseases.

Carry your imagination a step further and estimate how many women in this land are suffering from these two diseases, and how many men in civil life are suffering, and if this continues to spread what in the name of God is going to happen to us? You must teach your people that this is a disease transmitted from one to another by germs and should be quarantined and controlled the same as other diseases are; that it should be treated scientifically, and that all cases suspected should be treated with a prophylatic.

I hope all men present will take this matter up and lecture and do all you can to protect these soldier boys from this disease. I will leave it to you as how to proceed to do this in the community where you live, but there should be public meetings and you should address the people of the community, and there should be nothing left undone that would protect them and our soldier boys from this dread disease.

I shall not detain you longer and I thank you very cordially for your kind attention.

Major Homer T. Wilson, Camp Bowie, Texas: May I first express the appreciation I feel at the privilege of addressing this Association. I assure you it is an honor which I value highly, coming as it is my privilege to do, from your neighboring state, which is pleased to feel herself your big sister of the southwest. I cannot feel like I was a stranger, although up until today I have met very few of you. Again, having been for the last year and a half in Camp Bowie, associated with the Oklahoma and Texas Boys, it makes me feel very close to Oklahoma, and let me pause just long enough to say that in this whole country of ours there may be as good soldiers as these Oklahomans are going to make but there will not be any better.

(Reads paper which is to be submitted to Surgeon General before publication).

President: We will now have a discourse by one of our old crowd, who has been active in the service nearly ever since our last meeting. We will now listen to Captain L. S. Willour, President-elect.

Dr. Willour: Members of the Profession, I find myself in a very embarrassing position. Dr. Thompson told me to pick my subject and I chose orthopaedics.

(Reads paper which is to be submitted to Surgeon General before publication).

Dr. Willour: Ladies and Gentlemen, I am sure you are all acquainted with the next speaker, and I take great pleasure in introducing Captain Cook, our President (The President here delivered his address).

President: This concludes the program for the evening. All the sections will meet promptly at 9:00 o'clock in the morning and they want to get through by four o'clock so they can take a car ride over the city and to the Cosden Company. Tomorrow night there will be a dance at the Elks' club.

REPORT OF COMMITTEE ON TUBERCULOSIS.

At the last annual meeting of the State Medical Association, your Committee on tuberculosis called attention to the re-organization of the State Anti-Tuberculosis Association, under the new name, The Oklahoma Association for the Prevention of Tuberculosis, and recommended that the medical profession co-operate in the work of this association.

Since that time the Oklahoma Association for the Prevention of Tuberculosis has secured a full time, general secretary and its policies have been definitely determined. Inasmuch as two members of this committee are officially connected with the State Association for the Prevention of Tuberculosis, and since the declared policies are in keeping with the instructions received by this committee at the time of its inception, it has been deemed wise to unite our efforts in aiding the work of this Association.

The Red Cross Seal Campaign.

Through the Oklahoma Association for the Prevention of Tuberculosis, your committee has had a part in the Red Cross Seal Campaign which resulted in the accumulation of a fund amounting to $40,000.00. During this campaign 145,000 pieces of literature were distributed. About 1200 press notices were sent to various papers over the state. There were 127 agencies for the sale of seals covering 400 towns.

Education.

The money raised by the sale of Red Seals is to be employed chiefly for educational purposes. The association has planned an extensive educational program which is to penetrate every corner of the state. Special literature adapted to local needs, including literature for Indians and a pamphlet on open air schools. Lantern slides have been prepared for exhibition at the theaters. Moving pictures are also included in the educational program. The committee has attached the association's official announcement of this Educational Service to this report.

Legislation.

One of the ultimate results of education should be legislation. The Oklahoma Association has already succeeded in doing valuable work in preparing the way for legislation which will provide care for at least some of the tuberculous of the state, who are at present, not only without help, but a source of danger to others. Your committee recommends that the State Medical Association should co-operate with the Oklahoma Association for the Prevention of Tuberculosis in legislative matters.

The Public Health Nurse.

The association has planned to place six or seven public health nurses in the state under the direction of a supervisor. The scarcity of nurses, aggravated by war conditions, has made it very difficult to secure nurses trained in public health work.

Health Surveys.

The Oklahoma Association has secured the services of M. P. Horrowitz, of Cambridge, and Dr. Gayfree Ellison, of the State University, for the purpose of conducting health surveys in several of the larger towns in the state. These surveys in the hands of experts, receiving the co-operation of the State Board of Health, should have a wide educational value and do much toward elevating the standard of public health administration.

Dispensaries.

It is the purpose of the association to aid in establishing dispensaries in many of the towns and cities of the state. While the public health nurse and the dispensary render material service in the communities in which they operate, their chief value is educational.

Local Anti-Tuberculosis Societies and Committees have been organized in many of the towns and counties throughout the state. The Oklahoma City Anti-Tuberculosis Society has employed an experienced public health nurse and has a free tuberculosis dispensary already in operation. The dispensary is open three days in each week and has had an average daily attendance of ten patients. The records of this dispensary are very complete, both from the medical and sociological standpoints. Each patient receives a physical examination with an X-ray of the chest, and a complete blood examination, including a Wassermann and a complement fixation for tuberculosis.

In connection with this dispensary and with the co-operation of Dr. Cloudman, examining physician for the Oklahoma City Schools, and the X-ray laboratory of St. Anthony Hospital, certain members of your committee have undertaken to secure a physical examination and an X-ray of the chest in one hundred apparently healthy school children. Findings in the healthy school children to be compared with the records of the children examined in the dispensary. The purpose of this study is to help determine the true value of the X-ray in diagnosis of thoracic conditions and particularly tuberculosis.

L. J. Moorman.

Lelia E. Andrews.

REPORT OF COMMITTEE ON NECROLOGY.

To the President and Members of the Oklahoma State Medical Association.

Gentlemen:—

Some one has said, "When we attempt to penetrate the mystery of death we stand helplessly before a closed door, no ray of light reaches us from this portal, our physical eyes are not adjusted to see beyond the realm of time into the vast region of eternity, only with the eyes of faith can we pierce the veil and see the Great Beyond."

At this time it is our custom to pause, and pay tribute and honor to those of our members who have passed away; who have finished their work; who have passed through the Valley of the Shadow; who have entered the gate through which we all must go, but whose influence remains with us, and all those with whom they have been associated will remember them for what they have done.

Today our attention is called to those who have recently died for Humanity and Liberty, and as we read the list of Heroes who have died in khaki we feel they have not died in vain, that the offering of our brave young manhood of this country on the Altar of Liberty is a fitting expression of the supreme sacrifices they are capable of making.

Medical Heroes are common, yet in the most instances, they go unnoticed, unhonored, and their virtues unsung. The physician needs not War to set the stage for their display of heroism or acts of gallant courage. His profession calls for courage from start to finish, and unselfish devotion to those who need him. Never a night too dark or stormy, never a hill too steep, never a road too dangerous, when duty calls.

Yes, those of our colleagues whose names appear in the list below, braved the storms and those who knew them as their family Physician, their Friend, their Helper, will remember them and love and honor them, and commemorate their virtues to the rising generation. We would go and in spirit visit their last resting places and meditate, knowing that in only a little while, we too, will be in the land of the true, where we live anew, in the Beautiful Isle of Somewhere.

Those of us who have died since our last meeting, are as follows:

Dr. T. J. Lee, Rocky.
Dr. G. E. Miller, White Oak.
Dr. Bruce Younger, Marietta.
Dr. Bruce Watson, Perry.
Dr. J. M. Brown, Muskogee.
Dr. T. C. Barnes, Marlow.
Dr. D. U. Wadsworth, Tulsa.

Dr. D. D. Weiser, Apache
Dr. Porter Norton, Mangum.
Dr. J. C. Johnstone, Blackwell.
Dr. Commodore Farrington, Shawnee.
Dr. J. H. Rinehart, Meridian.
Dr. B. F. Fortner, Vinita.
Dr. Walter Penquite, Chickasha.

Respectfully submitted,

Martha Bledsoe,

J. W. Pollard.

REPORT OF SECRETARY-TREASURER-EDITOR

To the House of Delegates, Council and Members of the Oklahoma State Medical Association:

I herewith sumbit my report of the transactions of my office from May 1, 1917, to April 30, 1918:

Membership: Our association has held its membership numerically speaking very well considering that approximately three hundred physicians, nearly all of them members, have joined the Medical Reserve Corps and are now either in France, England or the various Army cantonments throughout the country. Our membership April 30, 1917, was 1363; April 30, 1918, it was 1386. Many county societies paid, by authority of the Council, the sum of two dollars for members in active service, which sum is deemed sufficient to carry the expense generated. A not inconsiderable number paid their dues directly before this rule was made.

The Journal: Closes the most prosperous year we have ever had. Comparison shows that we received in 1917 for advertising $2,756.07; the year ending April 30, 1918, shows that source of revenue alone has increased to $3,157.83. I call your attention now to the fact that this may be made much greater if you will patronize your advertisers and show them the cooperative spirit their patronage deserves. None but the best class of business is accepted and when all things are equal the man paying you money for advertising space deserves your business over one who pays your Journal nothing.

The Chiropractic Case: At our last meeting authority for the expenditure of such sums as might be necessary was granted the Council. The estimates made by the attorneys at that time were far exceeded, as the checking of the petitions proved to be a very laborious task, requiring the services of a highly competent clerical force and many weeks were devoted to the work.

This case is now in the Supreme Court with every reasonable prospect that it will be decided in our favor, as it is very similar to the Muskogee State Fair Bill case, which was recently decided against the petitioners for submission to the people. If, however, the case should be decided adversely, it will be necessary to meet the issue at the next general election when in the course of operation of the law it would be submitted to the people.

It is pertinent to state here that many county societies took no interest whatever in this case, refusing or failing to carry their small share of an assessment or appeal which the Council decided should be made for additional sums in order not to too severely cripple our cash reserve. In one or two instances this attitude was assumed by county societies from whose counties a large number of signers to the Chiropractic petition were obtained.

The Medical Reserve: Through the good offices and cooperation of the American Medical Association, a great deal of work incident to securing suitable material for the Medical Reserve Corps was accomplished. This required so much unusual effort and correspondence, that when added to the usual routine of the office the year ends as the most laborious in our history.

Finances: The condensed table attached below is a true statement of the receipts and disbursements since our last meeting to April 30, 1918.

The cash books, duplicate deposit slips, cancelled vouchers and all matters pertaining to the office in detail have been submitted to the Council committee for auditing:

RECEIPTS:

Balance April 30, 1917	$ 2,283.52	
Advertising	3,157.83	
Account Chiropractic	276.00	
Time Deposits Surrendered	1,500.00	
Interest on Time Deposits	51.34	
County Secretaries	4,505.58	$ 11,774.27

EXPENDITURES:

Telephone, telegraph, express	$ 13.72	
Office Supplies	116.30	
Postage	198.00	
Printing Journal, extras, etc.	3,296.82	
Stenographic and Clerical Work	412.70	
Reporting Meetinge	140.13	
Chiropractic Expense	1,737.54	
Refund County Secretaries	4.50	
Councilors, Delegates and Committee Expense	466.17	
Secretary's Salary	900.00	
Press Clippings	27.00	
Treasurer's Bond	10.00	
Auditing Books	10.00	
Transfer, Medical Defense Fund	1,375.00	
Certificate of Deposit, Com. Natl. Bank	500.00	
Liberty Bond	500.00	
		$ 9,697.88

May 1, 1918, Balance Cash on Hand	$ 2,076.39	
Certificate of Deposit	1,000.00	
Liberty Bond	500.00	

TOTAL CASH RESOURCES, Medical Assn $ 3,576.39

MEDICAL DEFENSE FUND
Receipts.

May 1, 1917, Balance on hand in Bank	$ 503.00	
April 30, 1918, Oklahoma State Medical Assn	1,375.00	
April 30, 1918, Interest, Time Deposit	100.00	
		$ 1,978.00

Expenditures

July 17, 1917, Attorneys' Fees	$ 300.00	
September 22, 1917, Attorneys' Fees	50.45	
April 17, 1918, Attorneys' Fees	50.00	
April 30, 1918, Time Deposit, Com. Nat'l Bank	1,000.00	$ 1,400.45

May 1, 1918, Balance Cash in Bank		577.55
Time Deposit, Commercial National Bank		3,000.00

TOTAL CASH RESOURCES, May 1, 1918 $ 3,577.55
TOTAL CASH RESOURCES ALL FUNDS $ 7,153.94

Respectfully submitted,

C. A. Thompson, Secy-Treas.

ADDRESS OF DR. FRANKLIN MARTIN, CHAIRMAN MEDICAL SECTION, COUNCIL OF NATIONAL DEFENSE.

I really do not see why you need anyone from Washington when you have a man like the one who has just addressed you. I feel sure that we will have him at Washington within the next few weeks. Anybody who can make an appeal like Dr. Buxton is entitled to addresses not once a month, but every day.

It is worth a great deal to me even though the time is short, and I had to get in at the last hour, to meet these physicians of Oklahoma. When we get right down to bed rock, Oklahoma is really the heart of America; Oklahoma is the place where the real Americans made their last stand. You have among you the only real Americans that are left, the old Aborigines, and when I come into a city like this, one like no other city in the country except the Capitol of the Nation, I cannot help feeling like taking off my hat and congratulating you from the bottom of my heart. But the more American we are the more is our responsibility at this time. I wonder if you realize the task that we have before us. I wonder if you realize what the emergency is; I wonder if you realize in every respect what we are up against in this fight. The reason I ask that is because it does seem to me that some of us are not stirred to the depth you should be stirred to in this crisis. Some of you may be very good actors; you may be able to drown your facial expressions; you might be very successful in obscuring your thoughts, in a good poker game for instance, because if you are not I fear some of you are too complacent; you do not understand how serious this is. I come from Washington, I associate every day in Washington with the men who are trying to do this thing right, the men who are struggling sixteen hours a day, struggling until they are practically frazzled from work, in the endeavor to organize our great Nation for the great struggle before them, and there I think some of us have gotten some idea of the size of this job. Do you realize that possibly there has been a propoganda that has excited in our souls an idea of self confidence? What in God's name are you confident about? What have we done? What have the Allies done, except on that little line on the western front, compared with the wonderful feats of the Germans?. Germany has us almost thrashed, and some of us have not discovered it. Just one little break at the front now and we have not two or three years of war, but we have a war that must go on for ten years, until we, in our complacancy, get ready to fight. Germany, with her wonderful efficiency—and you have to take off your hat to German efficiency—thirty years ago had Belgium mapped, every town, every community, everything in that particular community or township or hamlet. They had that map prepared. She has just finished rolling that map out; the same of Servia, and Servia is organized and Germanized. Then Poland is broken and Germanized; then the Balkan states, organized and Germanized; finally Rumania organized and Germanized. What happens? She lays down the maps; takes the obstreperous ones back in her territory, putting her trusted ones there, and it becomes Germanized. She gets her sustenance from there; she takes everything she wants, and she pays for that in paper. She takes it back to the interior organization, and then sells it back to these people for gold. The Imperial Bank of Germany has almost double the amount of gold she had in August, 1914.

That is exactly what Germany is up to; that is what she has done to France; the territory she has covered; it is exactly what she will do to England if she gets there; it is what she will do to the rest of France if she gets there. She has her maps for every place, and My God you cannot beat it, unless we beat it like we have beaten everything in this conutry, by being a little smarter.

Have you had any word recently that would indicate that Germany is going to do anything else? We feel down deep in our hearts, all of us who are working know, that if we can hold on a little longer until we get good and ready that we can help to stop this thing, and when we get it stopped we can proceed to unroll our maps. Unfortunately we have not had a map. Unfortunately we do not know how to organize like Germany. Fortunately we have enough men in this country to organize and give them something of their own game when the time comes. Now think of this; this is worth while, it may be of some comfort. As I said, we have been trying to play the game in Washington, I say "we" but I have had a very little of it, but the President and those with him in his council have been trying to play it in a disinterested big way. Who ever asks or questions the politics of a man who is sent to do some big job? The President does not. The President in appointing his first advisory committee appointed seven. In that the old fashioned politics were supposed to be in vogue. They figured out three Democrats, three Republicans, and the other they did not figure out. Now they do not figure out the question of politics. Does any one ever ask the politics of the men who are to fill the positions of trust in these times? Don't you see it is a big game? We are getting every big man we can. That is what we are trying to do in a smaller way in this medical game. The first thing is that we cannot in any way be interested in what the service is going to pay us. We have got to place this claim in a big non-politic way. Every man enrolled in the service becomes in a day, not a Republican, not an Oklahoma citizen, but a soldier of the United States. Everyone who is placed on the committee of the Council of Defense—you are not representing the American Medical Association, or your county medical society, but you are serving the Government. Your President appoints. You are permitted in this state to serve the United States Government, and your appointment is just as much a government position as mine is, and you serve with just as much expense paid as I have, namely one dollar a year.

.Now who has been doing the work in your state, and why have they been doing the work? The chairman of your committee of National Defense is Dr. L. H. Buxton; Horace Reed, Secretary; LeRoy Long, Assistant Secretary; W. E. Dicken, Treasurer; W. D. Berry, Muskogee; John W. Duke, Guthrie; C. R. Hume, Anadarko; Claude A. Thompson, Muskogee; Chas. L. Reeder, Tulsa; T. H. McCarley, McAlester; J. M. Workman, Woodward; Ellis Lamb, Clinton; A. S. Risser, Blackwell; J. H. Barnes, Enid; B. L. Mitchell, Vinita; C. H. Webber, Bartlesville; J. S. Fulton, Atoka; Ney Neel, Mangum; R. H. Henry, Ardmore; A. K. West, Oklahoma City; E. O. Barker, Guthrie.

Members in active Camp and Hospital service: Major A. L. Blesh, Major Fred H. Clark, Major Floyd J. Bolend, Captain R. V. Smith, Captain L. S. Willour, Captain H. C. Wooley, Captain Rex J. Bolend, Captain W. A. Cook, Lieutenant A. L. Guthrie, Lieutenant L. M. Sackett.

This list has been revised and a number added to it. Now that committee was appointed by me at the suggestion of the Council of National Defense, and that committee is a part of the Government. This is a letter to me from the President of the United States when your committee, and 350 men, met last week in Washington, representing the Council of National Defense, with every state in the Union but one represented, and this is what the President says:

"My Dear Dr. Martin:
"Thank you for telling me of the approaching meeting of the State Committees of the medical section of the Council of National Defense. Will you be kind enough to convey to them when that convention convenes, a message of sincere appreciation from me, of their services as authorized governmental agencies of the army, navy, public health service, and the American Red Cross, and of the part they have played in the preparation for war.
"Will you not, at the same time, convey to them my warm personal greetings.
"Cordially and sincerely yours,
"Woodrow Wilson".

Woodrow Wilson, the Secretary of War, the Council of War, the Surgeon General, and the head of the Red Cross definitely understand that these committees are authorized directly from the President, therefore each of you on the committee of National Defense is a Government official. Furthermore, your county committees that were organized nearly two years ago, one year before we were at war even, were also taken over by the Council of National Defense, and each member of the county committee is really serving the Government, and as fast as your members are taken away, one by one, as they will be, and must be taken, they must be accepted as honorable soldiers. We have in the Council of Defense an addressograph with every one of your names; we have over 4000 counties, and the name of every man in these committees, and in 48 hours, with our addressograph, and our governmental printing office, we can get a message to every one of you. The proof of that is in this pamphlet I hold in my hand. We had our meeting in Washington a week ago and here, with the government printing office, we have the complete transactions, including the speeches. Every thing said is outlined in that meeting. This shows the definiteness of our organization. Do not for God's sake get the idea that we have no organization. We have a very definite one, and it is backed by the President of the United States.

Now what do we want from Oklahoma? The Surgeon General of the Army, and let me stop right here and try to say what I feel in my heart for the Surgeon General of the Army. Can you imagine a time in history when the man who had been honored more than any other scientist in this country, should be the Surgeon General of the United States, and when you realize that, could anything be more just than to have the very man we have? A man with a judicial mind. A man with the largest kind of a mind. Do you realize the Surgeon General's job is the biggest job in the army except the job held by the Secretary of War? Do you realize he will have first 18,000 men, then he will ask for 25,000, then for 30,000 medical officers. Then he will have over 200,000 enlisted men; then he will have 20 per cent. of all the men in the armies when the big fight comes. That is the big thing he has to do. Do you expect any little narrow fellow to do this work? No. There never would be a bigger tragedy in the world. Two weeks of failure in the Surgeon General's office would be worse than any German victory. He had thirty men in his office a few years ago, and that number has now increased until five large buildings in Washington are now used for the office staff. With his big personality and his strength of character he went before the Committee of the Senate and he said—"Things are not as we would like to have them; we have made mistakes; we began last year with 400 and we now have 14,000. We have had some difficulties with our hospitals, some of them have not the refinements we wish, but gentlemen if you will just have a little patience we will get all these things done. If it had not been for that great big, honest, lovable man we would have had a scandal in our administration that would have gone to the high heavens. He stopped it. They had it framed to have a scandal that would out stench the one of '98, but he stopped it. The old fashioned rumors are about but we do not pay much attention to them. The President of the United States knows the worth of General Gorgas and every member of the National Defense knows the value of General Gorgas. Every big man who has been to Washington realizes the importance and strength of General Gorgas, and we are for General Gorgas first and last for the next Surgeon General of the Army. Any man that would dare for one minute to suggest that anyone else could possibly fill his place would be so filled with conceit I am sure he would be unsafe for the community.

Now what do we want of the doctors? First the doctors who have gone, God bless them, the men between twenty-two and thirty-five, a great many of these men have gone. Some of them have not. They must go. There is no reason in the world why such a man should not go. He is a marked man unless he does go, unless physically afflicted, and will be mighty unpopular. The next will be the man between thirty-five and forty-five. The men who have since last year been writing the Surgeon General numerous letters. He receives many every morning. Doctor I am so and so, in such a town; forty-one years of age; I want to serve my country and am writing you a letter, but there is something the matter. I have three children in college; my mortgage is due and it is so it cannot be adjusted; my interest is now being paid; I have a private hospital that will go to pieces and the community will suffer if I go; I am Dean of _ _ _ _ _ _ _ _ _ _ medical school. It would go to pieces if I went to the front. Now I want your advice.

I say get your things in shape just as rapidly as possible and tell us when you can go in, and many of them have said "we will go in six months, or a year". Many of them say—"Let me know when you really want me." Now gentlemen I am here to answer your letters. The time is up; the call is here; we want you now, and if the mortgage is not adjusted it would be better to go and not have it adjusted than to have your country organized by the Huns. Now how many can go at this call? If you all went in Oklahoma we would be embarrassed. Oklahoma has 2,634 doctors. You have sent 342. We want you to send 100 now from Oklahoma, and we want this 100 out of this group of men who have been waiting; the men who were really up against it, and who have been waiting to get straightened out.

Now I will say to you that if you take your examination, make your application and file your papers and say you want six weeks or two months you are very likely to get this consideration.

Then here comes the rub in many cases. You do not want to spend the time in training camps at home. Now tell me what in the devil would you do over there if you had not spent time in a training camp at home? Let me say to you wives who are sending your doctors to this three months training, after they have been taught to stand up and breathe and put on their clothes and eat, and to take care of themselves you will be mighty proud of them. Then you must know the paper work that goes with military business or you are lost. There is something to learn besides the salute. While it is difficult it is not as difficult as the work in those three months, and do not ask to go to France until you have had training.

Now besides having recorded in your examination papers what you preferred to do, it would be a very good thing to write to me, at the National Council of Defense, and say you are about to receive your Commission; that you are an eye specialist; that you are 42 years of age, and you will be placed in the position where you can do the best work.   That is almost of as much value to the Surgeon General's office as anything we can get. So when you make your application it is perfectly right that you should ask that you are assigned to the thing you are best qualified to do. If your letter is not replied to in a week remember this pile of correspondence. We try to answer every letter every day but it is impossible when your letters involve going into file. It is a big job because you are not the only one. There are 22,000 others.

Now as you are all going into the war you are more or less interested in the man who cannot get in. The unfortunate man who, from a physical standpoint, or because of some actual demand upon his time at home that is real; that brings us to the other corps, the Volunteer Medical Reserve Corps. That takes in every man between 22 and 55, who cannot for any reason get into the army, and it also accepts the woman, and it also accepts all individuals over 55 years of age who wish to volunteer. How do you get into that corps? Write a letter to me and I will send the papers immediately. They explain themselves; you fill them out and return to us immediately. We look over your reasons; if you have applied for a commission in the army we look up your application. We then make a list of those who are eligible and we then send them to the state committee, a committee of five. They go over these names and state whether they are what they claim to be. For instance, we eliminate those who are necessary for work at home, college work, industrial work, etc. This committee looks up your credentials and says whether you are necessary or not. It will be decided largely on your own statement of the case. Now that gives everybody an opportunity. Take the army examination and go into the army. If you cannot and are of age, go into the volunteer service. We will send you an insignia. Your right to stay at home will not be questioned. It cannot be.

Now one thing more, you have in this state probably a statesman who is more a friend of the medical profession than any other in the United States, and that is Senator Owen. Now we soon discovered 18,000 of us who were in the reserve corps, that the highest we could get was the Majority. We sent abroad Mayo and men of his class to serve in Europe. We found that we were serving side by side with men who were Colonels and Major Generals. We found that England gave her medical officers rank up as high as Lieutenant-Generals. We found that England had many Major Generals; that France had the same, that Japan had the same; that Italy had the same; that Germany had the same; but we were limited to the Major. Our regular officer cannot be above the Colonel except one and that is the Brigadier General, so it was up to us to do something to put those men in a place where they would not be humilitated, always sitting at the foot of the table. So we decided to have a bill. We know that Senator Owen got through the Chamberlin Bill for the medical men and was their true friend. I sent for him and we got Dwyer of St. Louis, two surgeon generals, Dr. Vaughan, Dr. Mayo and Dr. Simpson and we wrote what is now the Owen-Dwyer bill. For every 200 men we get two officers with a Major. For one thousand we get five, for 14,000 we would have 70 officers, and a corresponding number of Colonels and so on. That is less than in any other branch of the army so we are not asking for anything we should not have. We wrote this bill and Dwyer and Owhn accepted it and introduced them, one in the House and one in the Senate, on February 5th, and they are just about ready to be reported out of the committee. They have been criticised from every standpoint but the Surgeon General of the Navy and the Surgeon General of the Army are definitely for the bill. I took the matter up with the President of the United States, with all the papers, and all the data, leaving all the matter with him and asked him very earnestly to look over the papers and see if it was the thing to do. I will read the letter I received from him in regard to same:

"My Dear Dr. Martin—

"I read very carefully your memorandum of Feb. 27th about the rank accorded members of the Medical Corps of the Army and have written letters to the chairman of the Military Committee, of the House and Senate, expressing the hope that the bill and resolutions may be passed.

"Sincerely,
"Woodrow Wilson."

Now that is what the President of the United States has done after careful consideration of the bill. Now I do not know that you can possibly do anything better than doing exactly what the President would himself. I do not believe one can complain if you do what he did. Write to Senator Chamberlin, chairman of the Senate committee, and Representative Dent, chairman of the Military committee of the House. If I were you I would send a night telegram to that wonderful man, your own Senator, and tell him how glad you are he is back of you. I asked him one day if this sort of thing could be overdone. He said never—we are always glad to hear from our constituents—they would not ask if they did did not want it. Now if we could get thirty or forty messages out tonight, they would cost us about $2.25 each, which is not much in this state, it would have a very decided influence over the committee of the House and Senate and would warm the heart of the man who has done this work so well for you.

I have only one more thing to ask and that is an appeal to you to get ready to go. We have all made up our minds that we have got to go, but I want to impress upon you the necessity of getting ready right away. Let us get this 100 men for Oklahoma and help your committee in this state. You know your committee, help your committee to get a line on these men, your county committee, and your state committee, and whenever you find a man who waits, who wants to go and needs a little encouragement write me a letter. Those of you who have made up your minds please do not leave this city until you have had an examination by a real expert and receive papers and instructions in a way that will not go awry. I thank you.

PERSONAL AND GENERAL NEWS

Dr. J. W. Scarborough, Mangum, has moved to Lawton.

Drs. M. M. DeArman and General Pinnell announce the opening of a general hospital at Mimi.

Dr. Fowler Border, Mangum, has established a convalescent hospital in addition to the Border Hospital.

Drs. W. E. Dixon and S. C. Davis announce the formation of a partnership at Oklahoma City. Dr. Davis was formerly from Clinton, but has just returned from an extended stay for study in the east.

Dr. F. W. Jones, Verden, and Miss Blanche Armstrong, Oklahoma City, were married May 8th. Mrs. Jones was formerly head nurse at the University Hospital. They will make their home in Verden.

Pushmataha County physicians organized a medical society at Antlers April 20th, electing H. C. Johnson president and Ed.W. Guinn, secretary, Antlers; J. A. Burnett, vice-president, Crum Creek; E. S. Patterson, Antlers, Geo Robinett, Nolia, and J. L. Lawson, Clayton, Censors; P. E. Wright, Albion, and B. A. Huckabay, Tuskahoma, delegates.

Dr. H. B. McKenzie, one of the oldest physicians of Enid and father of Dr. Walton McKenzie of that city, died April 25th from pneumonia. Dr. McKenzie had lived in Enid since its opening, coming to the city in 1893 and had been identified with many important civic advancements of Enid. He was an active member and one of the organizers of the Baptist Church of Enid and stood high in the esteem of his fellow citizens.

The Chicago Medical Society wishes to invite the Physicians of the Army and Navy and the examining boards of the various states as their guests during the meeting of the A. M. A. Headquarters will be "Parlor A," La Salle Hotel. You are assured it will afford the Medical Society much pleasure to have the physicians engaged in the service visit Chicago during this meeting and will spare no means to make their visit pleasant.

MISCELLANEOUS

PHYSICIANS INVITED TO CHICAGO.
War Department.
Office of the Provost Marshal General,
Washington.

May 27, 1918

1. On June 13th and 14th, 1918, in Chicago, during the annual meeting of the American Medical Association, two half-day sessions have been arranged for those charged with the selection of registrants, including physicians, lawyers, board members and clerks of boards.

2. This meeting will be convened at the Studebaker Theatre, June 13th, at 2:00 P. M., and will be addressed by representative men from the legal and medical professions who have had valuable experience with the Questionnaire and Local, District and Medical Advisory Board work.

3. On Friday, June 14th, at 9:00 A. M., there will be a session for the Medical Aides to Governors, for informal discussions. Medical Aides will be officially ordered to attend.

4. At 10:00 A. M., medical members of Local, District and Medical Advisory Boards will meet for the discussion of questions pertinent to the execution of the Selective Service Regulations; and special consideration will be given to the forthcoming new "Standards of Physical Examinations". At each of these meetings representatives of this office will be present to participate and give such instructions and advice as may be necessary.

5. If you will kindly cause this information to be disseminated through the usual channels, it is believed that in addition to the thousands of physicians who attend the annual convention of this Association, many others, whether medical men or not, interested in the Selective Service, who are within reasonable distance, will appreciate the opportunity to be present.

By Hubert Work,   E. H. CROWDER,
   Major, M. R. C.   .   Provost Marshal General.

205   JOURNAL OF THE OKLAHOMA STATE MEDICAL ASSOCIATION

TRIAL TUBES OF CHLORAZENE.

It is interesting to learn that The Abbott Laboratories of Chicago are sending to physicians, on request, convenient trial tubes of ten Chlorazene tablets. In view of the growing importance of the Dakin discoveries, we suggest to our readers that they avail themselves of this generous offer.

'COUNCIL ON PHARMACY AND CHEMISTRY—ATRICLES ACCEPTED.

Merck and Company: Creosol-Merck, Guaiacol Carbonate-Merck. Quinine Dihydrochloride-Merck, Thymol Iodide-Merck.

PROPAGANDA FOR REFORM.

Some Nostrums. Continuing its policy of giving the public the facts in regard to worthless, injurious or misleading advertised nostrums, the Louisiana State Board of Health has analyzed the following "patent medicines". Dermillo, a skin and complexion nostrum composed of zinc oxid, calcium carbonate, starch and salicylic acid in water, colored and perfumed. Wendell's Ambition Pills, a "great nerve tonic," containing strychnin, ferrio oxid, pepper, cinnamon and ginger, and probably a little aloes. Orchard White, a toilet preparation to be mixed with lemon juice, reported to be a mucilage containing bismuth citrate, boric acid, alcohol and gum tragacanth. Exelento Quinine Pomade, a hair preparation found to consist chiefly of petrolatum, some liquid petrolatum, a trace of oil of gaultheria, sulphur, amd among other things, a trace of quinin. Sloans' Liniment, which appeared to be composed essentially of oil of turpentine, oil of camphor, oil of sassafras and capsicum. Vick's Vap-O-Rub, which appeared to be a mixture of petrolatum with camphor, menthol and oil of thyme, eucalyptus and turpentine. La Creole Hair Dressing, a perfumed solution containing lead acetate, sulphur and glycerin, alcohol and water. Prescription A-2851 for Rheumatism, formerly said to have been known as Eimer and Amend's Rheumatic Remedy, which appeared to be a sherry wine containing 7.5 per cent. potassium iodid (Journal A. M. A., April 6, 1918, p. 1024).

Gauiodine. Examination of Guaiodine, a preparation of the Intravenous Products Co., Denver, in the A. M. A. Chemical Laboratory shows that, instead of containing free "colloidal" iodine as claimed, the preparation is essentially an iodated fatty oil, containing iodin. The referee of the Committee on Pharmacology reported to the Council on Pharmacy and Chemistry that equally misleading, in view of the Laboratory's findings, are the implied claims that the antiseptic action of Guaiodine corresponds to that of free iodine. Guaiodine is advertised chiefly for the treatment of gonorrhea by means of obviously false claims. The Council declared Guaiodine inadmissible to New and Nonofficial Remedies because of false statements as to composition and action (Journal A. M. A., April 6, 1918, p. 1026).

Neoarsphenamine. The Federal Trade Commission has granted an importing license to the Diarsenol, Company, Inc., 475 Ellicott Square, Buffalo, for neodiarsenol, the Canadian brand of neo-arsphenamine. License to manufacture neoarsphenamine has also been issued to The Takamine Laboratories, New York, to the Farbwerke-Hoechst Co., New York, and to the Dermatological Research Laboratories, Philadelphia. The safest and most effective products, provided one has mastered the technique, are the arsphenamines—not the neoarsphenamines (Journal A. M. A., April 6, 1918,p. 1027).

American-Made Acetylsalicylic Acid. At the request of the Council on Prarmacy and Chemistry an examination of the market supply of American-made acetylsalicylic acid has been made in the A. M. A. Chemical Laboratory by P. N. Leech. The investigation shows that there are on the American market, made by American firms, several brands of acetylsalicylic acid that are just as good as, if not better than, the widely advertised Aspirin-Bayer. About a year ago the Council on Pharmacy and Chemistry deleted Aspirin-Bayer from New and Nonofficial Remedies. Since the Bayer aspirin patent expired in February, 1917, thereby making it possible for manufacturers legally to produce and sell acetylsalicylic acid in the United States, the Council established standards for the quality of this unofficial drug. As a result, the following products have been found to meet these requirements and are included in New and Nonofficial Remedies: Aspirin-L. and F., Acetylsalicylic Acid-Squibb, Acetylsalicylic Acid-Merck, Acetylsalicylic Acid-Milliken, Acetylsalicylic Acid-M. C. W., Acetylsalicylic Acid-Monsanto and Acetylsalicylic Acid-P. W. R. (Journal A. M. A., April 13, 1918, p. 1097).

Unduly Toxic Arsphenamin. In view of the reports in current medical literature of untoward results from the use of arsphenamin and neoarsphenamin, Dr. G. W. McCoy, Director of the U. S. Hygienic Laboratory, Washington, D. C., requests that samples of any lot of these arsenicals which have shown undue toxicity be forwarded to the Hygienic Laboratory for examination (Journal A. M. A., April 13, 1918, p. 1110).

Hall's Catarrh Cure. Another victim fails to get the hundred dollars offered in cases in which this preparation failed to effect a cure. The promoters informed its victim that before paying the guarantee, he would have to prove that his case was one of simple catarrh not complicated by any other disease and that he had taken sufficient of the cure (Journal A. M. A., April 13, 1918, p. 113).

Antipneumococcus Vaccine. The work by Lister in the diamond mines of Kimberley, South Africa, gives promise of a successful method of inoculation against lobar pneumonia. Lister finds that the pneumonia prevalent among the workers in the diamond mines is due mainly to three groups of pneumococci, and that inoculation with a vaccine made from the three groups prevents the occurrence of pneumonia as caused by members of these groups (Journal A. M. A., April 20, 1918, p. 1163).

ROSTER OF MEMBERS OF COUNTY SOCIETIES, 1918.

ADAIR COUNTY

D. A. Beard_____Westville
D. P. Chambers_____Stilwell
B. F. Collins_____Nowata
B. H. Hines_____Evansville, Ark
J. M. Lane_____Sand Springs
P. H. Medearis_____Procter
J. A. Patton_____Stilwell
Jas. A. Robinson_____Centralia
A. J. Sands_____Watts
R. L. Sellars_____Westville
T. S. Williams_____Stilwell

ALFALFA COUNTY

H. B. Ames_____Burlington
Z. J. Clark_____Cherokee
W. H. Dersch_____Carmen
Milton T. Evans_____Aline
J. S. Hibbard_____Cherokee
H. E. Huston_____Aline
L. T. Lancaster_____Cherokee
H. A. Lile_____Aline
E. J. Reichley_____Helena
T. A. Rhodes_____Cherokee
J. M. Tucker_____Carmen

BEAVER COUNTY

M. H. Levi_____Liberal, Kansas

BECKHAM COUNTY

T. T. Clohesy_____Berlin
J. M. Denby_____Carter
A. A. Huntley_____Sweetwater
J. A. Jester_____Elk City
I. A. Lee_____Erick
J. M. McComas_____Elk City
Thomas. D. Palmer_____Elk City
K. R. Rone_____Elk City
M. Shadid_____Carter
H. K. Speed_____Sayre
J. E. Standifer_____Elk City
De Witt Stone_____Sayre
V. C. Tisdal_____Elk City
J. D. Wardord_____Erick
O. W. Wendell_____Sayre
J. E. Yarbrough_____Erick

BLAINE COUNTY

J. S. Barnett_____Hitchcock
Henry Blender_____Okeene
J. W. Browning_____Geary
M. W. Buchanan_____Watonga
F. R. Buchanan_____Canton
H. W. Doty_____Watonga
G. T. Green_____Drumright
W. F. Griffin_____Greenfield
V. R. Hamble_____Homestead
J. B. Leisure_____Watonga
E. F. Milligan_____Geary
L. H. Murdock_____Okenee
J. A. Norris_____Okeene
A. F. Padberg_____Canton
D. F. Stough_____Geary

BRYAN COUNTY

J. R. Allen_____Caddo
D. Armstrong_____Durant
J. L. Austin_____Durant
J. A. Bates_____Kemp
W. C. Bates_____Achille
J. E. Dorsett_____Hendrix
H. B. Fuston_____Bokchito
C. J. Greene_____Durant
J. K. Griffith_____Kemp
John A. Haynie_____Durant
J. H. Kay_____Kenefick
J. R. Keller_____Calera
D. C. McCalib_____Utica
H. McKinney_____Durant
W. H. McCarley_____Colbert
C. S. Mullenix_____Roberta
S. W. Rains_____Platter
H. E. Rappolee_____Caddo
J. L. Reynolds_____Durant
E. W. Richardson_____Colbert
J. L. Shuler_____Durant
J. B. Smith_____Durant
O. E. Stringer_____Achille
A. J. Wells_____Calera
H. W. Yeats_____Durant
C. C. Yeiser_____Colbert

CADDO COUNTY

P. H. Anderson_____Anadarko
J. H. Beucler_____Apache
Jesse Bird_____Cement
S. Blair_____Apache
W. E. Booth_____Sickles
B. D. Brown_____Apache
Joseph R. Bryan_____Cogar
Lieut. T. Sam'l Campbell_____
R. S. Cannon_____Hydro
J. H. Cantrell_____Carnegie
Claude S. Chambers_____Anadarko
W. T. Dardis_____Ft. Cobb
    157 E. 31st St., New York, N. Y.
F. Dinkler_____Ft. Cobb
Ed. W Downs_____Hinton
M. H. Edens_____Anadarko
W. A. Ewing_____Ft. Cobb
Gus R. Griggs_____Lookeba
W. T. Hawn_____Binger
J. J. Henke_____Hydro
Chas. R. Hume_____Anadarko
R. E. Johnson_____Bridgeport
W. W. Kerley_____Anadarko
C. W. Lane_____Okanogan, Wash.
    U. S. Indian Service
Chas. B. McMillan_____Gracemont
P. L. McClure_____Ft. Cobb
P. B. Myers_____Apache
J. W. Padberg_____Carnegie
W. B. Putman_____Alfalfa
R. D. Rector_____Anadarko
F. W. Rogers_____Carnegie
P. L. Sanders_____Carnegie
Lieut. R. Earl Smith, M. R. C._____Ft. Sill
    Post Hospital
A. H. Taylor_____Anadarko
Wade H. Vann_____Cement
Lieut. J. W. Wheeler, M. R. C.,_____Ft. Sill
A. J. Willard_____Cyril
S. E. Williams_____Hydro
R. W. Williams_____Anadarko

CANADIAN COUNTY

T. M. Aderhold_____ElReno
C. D. Arnold_____ElReno
W. B. Catto_____ElReno
F. H. Clark_____ElReno
H. C. Brown_____Okarche
J. A. Hatchett_____ElReno
P. F. Herod_____ElReno
Thos. Lane_____ElReno
H. C. Masters_____ElReno

W. R. Miller_____Calumet
W. J. Muzzy_____ElReno
D. P. Richardson_____Union City
Jas. T. Riley_____ElReno
N. E. Ruhl_____Peidmont
R. E. Runkle_____ElReno
S. S. Sanger_____Yukon
G. W. Taylor_____ElReno
L. G. Wolff_____Okarche

CARTER COUNTY

G. W. Amerson_____Milo
E. R. Barker_____Healdton
J. T. Barnwell_____Graham
Jesse C. Best_____Ardmore
F. W. Boadway_____Ardmore
T. S. Booth_____Ardmore
J. H. Cameron_____Healdton
J. L. Cox_____Ardmore
T. W. Denham_____Ardmore
Thos. W. Dowdy_____New Wilson
R. O. Early_____Ardmore
L. D. Gillispie_____Springer
G. E. Goodwin_____Ardmore
David A. Gregory, M. R. C., Washington. D. C.
Walter Hardy_____Ardmore
W. G. Hathaway_____Pooleville
Robert H. Henry_____Ardmore
H. A. Higgins_____Springer
D. G. Johnson_____Ardmore
J. A. Martin_____Healdton
J. C. McNees_____Ardmore
J. W. Shelton_____Ardmore
J. H. Smith_____Healdton
Dow Taylor_____Woodford
F. P. Von Keller_____Ardmore
T. H. Ware_____New Wilson
J. W. Webb_____Berwyn
R. S. Willard_____Ardmore

CHEROKEE COUNTY

T. P. Allison_____Tahlequah
J. S. Allison_____Tahlequah
A. A. Baird_____Park Hill
W. G. Blake_____Tahlequah
B. Duckett_____Hulbert
J. T. Duckworth_____Tahlequah
H. B. Fite_____Tahlequah
   U. S. Naval Station, New Orleans, La.
Israel Hill_____Gideon
L. E. McCurry_____Tahlequah
B. L. Morrow_____Salina
C. A. Peterson_____Tahlequah
J. M. Thompson_____Tahlequah

CHOCTAW COUNTY

E. R. Askew_____Hugo
T. L. Chambliss_____Soper
R. L. Gee_____Hugo
C. H. Hale_____Boswell
K. P. Hampton_____Soper
G. E. Harris_____Hugo
T. A. Heartgrave_____Soper
W. N. John_____Hugo
George I. Marsh_____Ft. Towson
V. L. McPherson_____Boswell
J. S. Miller_____Hugo
J. D. Moore_____Sawyer
W. M. Oliver_____Boswell
J. W. Phillips_____Miami
C. H. Swearingin_____Hugo
H. H. White_____Hugo

Reed Wolfe_____Hugo
W. M. Yeargan_____Soper

CLEVELAND COUNTY

C. S. Bobo_____Norman
T. M. Boyd, Embarkation Camp, Hoboken, N. J.
G. M. Clifton_____Norman
J. L. Day_____Ft. Clark, Texas
Gayfree Ellison_____Norman
J. J. Gable_____Camp Pike. Ark.
   1st. Lieut. M. R. C., Base Hospital.
S. H. Graham_____Camp Bowie, Texas
D. W. Griffin_____Norman
Ruben M. Hargrove_____Norman
J. B. Lambert_____Lexington
R. D. Lowther_____Norman
J. R. McLaughlin_____Norman
W. J. Melton_____Shamrock
E. A. Morgan_____R. F. D. No. 6. Norman
C. E. Northcutt_____Lexington
R. E. Thacker_____Lexington
A. A. Thurlow_____Norman
J. P. Torrey_____Norman
J. M. Williams_____Norman

COAL COUNTY

Frank Bates_____Coalgate
T. H. Briggs_____Atoka
W. E. Brown_____Lehigh
W. T. Blount_____Tupelo
Albert Cates_____Tupelo
J. B. Clark_____Coalgate
L. A. Connor_____Coalgate
R. D. Cody_____Centrahoma
J. S. Fulton_____Atoka
H. G. Goben_____Lehigh
J. J. Hipes_____Philips
W. A. Logan_____Lehigh
J. A. Nelson_____Centrahoma
F. E. Rushing_____Coalgate
F. E. Sadler_____Coalgate
W. B. Wallace_____Coalgate

COMANCHE COUNTY

C. W. Baird_____Lawton
Jackson Broshears_____Lawton
E. B. Dunlap_____Lawton
L. T. Gooch_____Lawton
E. S. Gooch_____Lawton
Fred Hammond_____Lawton
J. R. Hood_____Indihaoma
C. P. Hues_____Lawton
J. G. Janney_____Lawton
Chas. W. Joyce_____Fletcher
L. C. Knee_____Lawton
C. M. Martin_____Elgin
L. A. Milne_____Lawton
E. B. Mitchell_____Lawton
D. A. Myers_____Lawton
J. A. Perisho_____Cache
G. Pinnell_____Miami
F. Shoemaker_____Washington, D. C.
   U. S. Indian Service

COTTON COUNTY

N. O. Benson_____Randlatt
M. T. Clark_____Walters
L. B. Foster_____Walters
A. B. Halsted_____Temple
C. F. House_____Hastings
R. J. Rice_____Randlett
G. O. Webb_____Temple

CRAIG COUNTY

F. M. Adams_____Vinita
Louis Bagby, M. R. C.,_____Ft. Riley, Kansas
C. P. Bell_____Welch
J. O. Bradshaw_____Welch
N. L. Cornwall_____Bluejacket
J. W. Craig_____Vinita
P. W. Hays_____Vinita
A. W. Herron_____Vinita
F. L. Hughson_____Vinita
W. W. Jackson_____Vinita
W. R. Marks_____Vinita
R. L. Mitchell_____Vinita
C. S. Neer_____Vinita
D. W. O'Leary_____Welch
E. A. Pickens_____Grove
J. H. L. Staples_____Bluejacket
D. B. Stough_____Vinita
Chas. F. Walker_____Grove
C. J. Wells_____Jonesville, Mich.

CREEK COUNTY

Amos Avery_____Sapulpa
J. W. Bone_____Sapulpa
D. W. Conger_____Mounds
O. S. Coppedge_____Depew
O. C. Coppedge_____Bristow
G. C. Croston_____Sapulpa
Melvin Fry_____Drumright
H. S. Garland_____Sapulpa
I. E. Gladden_____Kiefer
Harry Haas_____Sapulpa
Ben C. Harris_____Sapulpa
J. W. Hoover_____Sapulpa
Ellis Jones _____Keifer
H. B. Justice_____Sapulpa
E. W. King_____Bristow
D. T. F Laidig_____Drumright
W. P. Longmire_____Sapulpa
J. M. Mattenlee_____Sapulpa
C. L. McCallum_____Sapulpa
Levi P. Murray_____Milfay
Wm J. Neal_____Drumright
M. H. Newman_____Oklahoma City
C. B. Reese_____Sapulpa
S. W. Reynolds_____Drumright
Chas. T. Schrader_____Bristow
B. C. Schwab_____Sapulpa
W. F. Snograss _____Bristow
G. A. Stafford_____Kiefer
R. M. Sweeney_____Sapulpa
Z. G. Taylor_____Mounds
John M. Wells_____Bristow
Geo. H. Wetzel_____Sapulpa
F. R. Wheeler_____Mannford

CUSTER COUNTY

T. A. Boyd_____Weatherford
S. C. Davis_____Clinton
J. Matt Gordon_____Weatherford
K. D. Gossom_____Custer
Ellis Lamb_____Clinton
C. H. McBurney_____Clinton
Robert McCullough_____Arapaho
P. G. Murray_____Thomas
W. W. Parker_____Thomas
O. H. Parker_____Custer
McLain Roger s_____Clinton
N. P. H. White_____Clinton
J. J. Williams_____Weatherford

DEWEY COUNTY

E. J. Hughes_____Vici
W. E. Seba_____Leedey

GARFIELD COUNTY

W. A. Aitken_____Enid
A. Anderson_____Kremlin
J. H. Barnes_____Enid
J. W. Baker_____Enid
H. P. Bishop_____Carrier
G. A. Boyle_____Enid
Amin Boutros_____Enid
L. L. Bunker_____M. R. C.
Lee W. Cotton_____Enid
F. P. Davis_____Enid
J. W. Francisco_____Enid
W. W. Gill_____Ringwood
G. O. Hall_____Enid
D. S. Harris_____Drummond
J. H. Hays_____Enid
W. E. Haygood_____Bison
T. B. Hinson_____Enid
J. W. Huddleson_____Enid
F. A. Hudson_____Enid
W. L. Kendall_____Enid
M. A. Kelso_____Enid
W. E. Lamerton_____Enid
S. A. Looper_____Oklahoma City
J. E. Mahoney_____Enid
S. N. Mayberry_____Enid
A. L. McInnis_____Enid
E. N. McKee_____Enid
H. B. McKenzie_____Enid
W. H. McKenzie_____Enid
Waldo P. Newell _____Hunter
A. S. Piper_____Enid
P. A. Smithe_____Enid
R. J. Swank_____Enid
C. E. Thompson_____Enid
A. E. Wilkins_____Covington
E. J. Woolff_____Waukomis

GARVIN COUNTY

T. C. Branum_____Pauls Valley
J. R. Calloway_____Pauls Valley
Lieut. John R. Calloway_____Pauls Valley
    8th Cavalry, Sierra Blanca, Texas.
John Darst_____Wynnewood
J. O. Erwin_____Pauls Valley
Lewis Gaddy_____Stratford
W. C. High_____Maysville
G. L. Johnson_____Pauls Valley
A. P. Kever_____Lindsay
E. H. Lain_____Paola
N. H. Lindsey_____Pauls Valley
J. K. Lindsey_____Elmore City
H. P. Markham_____Pauls Valley
J. C. Matheney_____Lindsay
J. B. McClure_____Lindsay
C. P. Mitchel_____Lindsay
J. B. Morgan_____Foster
E. E. Norvell_____Wynnewood
C. M. Pratt_____Maysville
B. W. Ralston_____Lindsay
M. E. Robertson_____Brady
A. J. Robinson_____Pauls Valley
W. E. Settles_____Wynnewood
J. B. Shannon_____Pauls Valley
A. H. Shi_____Stratford
E. Sullivan_____Pauls Valley
J. W. Tucker_____Purdy
M. M. Webster_____Stratford

H. P. Wilson_____Wynnewood
J. A. Young_____Maysville

GRADY COUNTY

J. C. Ambrister_____Chickasha
H. C. Antle_____M. R. C.
Wm. R. Barry_____Camp Pike, Ark.
R. J. Baze_____Chickasha
Walter J. Baze_____Chickasha
Martha Jane Bledsoe_____Chickasha
N. C. Boon_____Chickasha
Wm. Le Roy Bonnell_____Chickasha
W. R. Bowman_____Quapaw
W. H. Cook_____Chickasha
C. P. Cox_____Ninnekah
E. L. Dawson_____Chickasha
D. S. Downey_____Chickasha
L. E. Emanual_____Chickasha
T. Fuller_____Amber
G. R. Gerard_____Ninnekah
R. J. Gordan_____Ninnekah
P. J. Hampton_____Rush Springs
R. R. Hume_____Minco
F. W. Jones_____Verden
A. B. Leeds_____Chickasha
J. S. Little _____Minco
W. H. Livermore_____Chickasha
S. O. Marrs_____Chickasha
W. J. Mason_____Pocasset
C. E. Smith_____Chickasha
G. H. Thrailkill_____Miami
A. C. White_____Chickasha
L. H. Winborn_____Tuttle

GRANT COUNTY

I. V. Hardy_____Medford
C. H. Lockwood_____Medford
J. F. Martin_____Deer Creek
D. D. Roberts_____Nash
B. W. Saffold___ _____Gibbon

GREER COUNTY

C. W. Austin_____Brinkman
G. F. Border_____Mangum
G. F. Bray_____Reed
G. P. Cherry_____Mangum
W. D. Dawson_____Granada, Colo.
M. M. De Arman_____Miami
W. O. Dodson_____Willow
H. W. Finley_____Reed
R. L. Holt_____American Expeditionary Forces
                    France.
Thos. J. Horsley_____Mangum
O. R. Jeter_____Brinkman
E. S. Kilpatrick_____Vinson
J. B. Lansden_____Granite
Frank H. McGregor_____London, Eng.
Ney Neal_____Mangum
T. J. Nunnery_____Granite
L. E. Pearson_____Reed
E. M. Poer_____Jester
T. L. Willis_____Mangum
G. W. Wiley_____Granite

HARMON COUNTY

C. E. Collins_____Gould
S. W. Hopkins_____Hollis
J. E. Jones_____Hollis
J. S. McFaddin_____Hollis
J. B. Patrick_____Vinson
W. C. Pendergraft_____Hollis
R. L. Pendergraft_____Hollis
W. T. Ray_____Gould
Jas. W. Scarborough_____Gould
O. J. Street_____M. R. C.

HASKELL COUNTY.

J. E. Billington_____Brooken
A. B. Callaway_____Stigler
A. M. Chambers_____Quinton
W. C. Gilliam_____Keota
Emmett Johnson_____Kinta
T. B. McClure_____McCurtain
S. E. Mitchell_____San Antonia, Texas
    Camp Hospital, Flying Dept., Kelly Field
W. G. Ramsey_____McCurtain
R. F. Terral_____Stigler
E. Thomas_____Quinton
T. B. Turner _____Stigler
M. Van Matre_____Keota
J. R. Waltrip_____Kinta

HUGHES COUNTY

Fred B. Hicks_____Wetumka
C. A. Hicks_____Wetumka
John W. Lowe_____Holdenville
P. E. Mitchell_____Wetumka

JACKSON COUNTY

E. A. Abernathy_____Altus
R. F. Brown_____Headrick
D. C. Buck_____Eldorado
J. J. Caviness_____Altus
W. H. Clarkson_____Blair
E. S. Crow_____Olustee
T. H. Harbin_____Olustee
J. B. Hix_____Altus
R. H. Hyde_____Eldorado
J. T. Lowe_____Humphreys
R. H. Mayes_____Duke
J. W. McCrary_____Martha
L. H. McConnell_____Elmer
E. P. Miles_____Hobart
S. P. Rawls_____Altus
W. H. Rutland_____Altus
W. P. Rudell_____Altus
W. E. Sanderson_____Altus
C. G. Spears_____Altus
S. P. Strother_____Holdenville
J. S. Stults_____Olustee
H. R. Taylor_____Eldorado
R. Z. Taylor_____Blair
D. E. Wilson_____Elmer

JEFFERSON COUNTY

T. E. Ashinghurst_____Waurika
W. M. Browning_____Waurika
A. G. Cranfill_____Grady
J. T. Derr_____Waurika
W. J. Dossey_____Ringling
F. M. Edwards_____Ringling

A. R. Lewis _____Ryan
C. W. Maupin _____Waurika
J. W. Moore _____Waurika
J. M. Stephens _____Hastings
L. B. Sutherland _____Ringling
S. O. Taylor _____Ringling
G. C. Wilton _____Ryan

JOHNSTON COUNTY
Guy Clark _____Milburn
J. J. Clark _____Milburn
W. P. Cottrell _____Milburn
S. A. Croker _____Tishomingo
S. E. Cummings _____Ravia
J. M. Ellis _____Wapanucka
H. B. Kniseley _____Tishomingo
J. T. Looney _____Tishomingo
T. W. Stallings _____Tishomingo
F. B. Stobaugh _____Mannsville
F. A. White _____Madill

KAY COUNTY
W. K. Bell _____Blackwell
A. P. Gearhart _____Blackwell
H. O. Gowey _____Newkirk
A. R. Havens _____Blackwell
A. L. Hazen _____Newkirk
J. C. Hawkins _____Blackwell
W. M. Johnson _____Peckham
Allen Lawrey _____Blackwell
J. A. Jones _____Tonkowa
S. S. McCullough _____Braman
D. W. Miller _____Blackwell
Geo. H. Niemann _____Ponca City
E. J. Orvis _____Blackwell
A. S. Risser _____Blackwell
E. E. Wagoner _____Tonkowa

KIOWA COUNTY
A. Barkley _____Hobart
J. M. Bonham _____Hobart
J. R. Bryce _____Snyder
J. R. Dale _____Hobart
M. Gray _____Durant
J. T. Hamilton _____Snyder
A. H. Hathaway _____Mt. View
H. E. Hollis _____Snyder
J. A. Land _____Lonewolf
W. R. Leverton _____Hobart
F. F. Martin _____Roosevelt
Wm. McIlwain _____Lonewolf
W. W. Miller _____Gotebo
J. A. Muller _____Snyder
W. A. Nunnery _____Roosevelt
J. R. Preston _____Mt. Park
G. W. Stewart _____Hobart
A. L. Wagoner _____Hobart
B. H. Watkins _____Gotebo
A. J. Weeden _____Mt. View

KINGFISHER COUNTY
E. R. Cavett _____Kiel
C. W. Fisk _____Kingfisher
C. O. Gose _____Hennessey
J. A. Overstreet _____Kingfisher
J. W. Pendleton _____Kingfisher
Newton Rector _____Hennessey
A. L. Share _____Kingfisher
C. E. Wagner _____Hennessey

LATIMER COUNTY
E. L. Evins _____Wilburton
E. B. Hamilton _____Wilburton
G. A. Kilpatrick _____Wilburton
S. C. Talley _____Red Oak
J. A. Munn _____Wilburton
R. L. Rich _____Red Oak
H. L. Dalby _____Wilburton
J. F. McArthur _____Wilburton
T. L. Henry _____Wilburton

LE FLORE COUNTY
C. B. Billingsley _____Cowlington
G. R. Booth _____Le Flore
N. W. Campbell _____Poteau
E. A. Campbell _____Heavener
E. L. Collins _____Panama
S. C. Dean _____Howe
Calhoun Doler _____Bokoshe
W. M. Duff _____Braden
J. J. Hardy _____Poteau
Harrell Hardy _____Bokoshe
George Hartshorne _____Spiro
A. J. Hunt _____Howe
W. Z. McLaine _____Heavener
H. C. Mahar _____Spiro
R. W. Minor _____Williams
A. M. Mixon _____Spiro
G. A. Morrison _____Poteau
C. R. Morrison _____Cameron
John Plumlee _____Junction City, Kans.
R. M. Shepard _____Talihina
E. E. Shippey _____Wister
J. B. Wear _____Poteau
B. D. Woodson _____Poteau

LINCOLN COUNTY
J. W. Adams _____Chandler
W. H. Davis _____Chandler
F. B. Erwin _____Wellston
P. F. Erwin _____Wellston
R. H. Hannan _____Prague
S. E. Gayman _____Tyron
C. L. Kerfoot _____Prague
A. M. Marshall _____Chandler
C. M. Morgan _____Chandler
F. H. Norwood _____Prague
W. A. Pendergraft _____Carney
H. M. Williams _____Wellston
F. W. Wyman _____Stroud

LOGAN COUNTY
C. B. Barker _____Guthrie
Pauline Barker _____Guthrie
E. O. Barker _____Guthrie
C. F. Cotteral _____Guthrie
J. L. Dorough _____Coyle
J. W. Duke _____Guthrie
L. A. Hahn _____Guthrie
J. L. Houseworth _____Guthrie
Benton Lovelady _____Guthrie
J. L. Melvin _____Guthrie
C. S. Petty _____Guthrie
H. T. C. Richmond _____Marshall
W. W. Rucks _____Guthrie
David Stevens _____Guthrie
A. A. West _____Guthrie

LOVE COUNTY
D. Autry _____Marietta
W. V. Batson _____Marietta
T. J. Jackson _____Marsden
A. E. Martin _____Marietta

MAJOR COUNTY

Victor Anderson_____Fairview
B. F. Johnson_____Fairview
Elsie L. Specht_____Fairview

MARSHALL COUNTY

A. E. Ballard_____Madill
C. B. Ballard_____Kingston
M. D. Belt_____Woodville
T. A. Blaylock_____Madill
J. A. Collins_____Willis
F. M. Crume_____Lark
W. Lee Davis_____Kingston
W. H. Ford_____Kingston
J. I. Gaston_____Madill
T. M. Gordon _____Kingston
W. D. Haynie_____Powell
J. L. Holland_____Madill
E. F. Lewis_____Kingston
J. E. Reid_____Madill
J. A. Rutledge_____Woodville
W. H. Ussery_____Lebanon
O. E. Welborn_____Kingston
S. P. Winston_____McMillan

MAYES COUNTY

J. L. Adams_____Pryor
W. C. Bryant_____Choteau
J. E. Hollingsworth_____Strang
J. D. Leonard_____Strang
J. L. Mitchell_____Pryor
E. L. Pierce_____Locust Grove
Carl Puckett_____Pryor
F. W. Smith_____Pryor
W. J. Whitaker_____Pryor
L. C. White_____Adair

MURRAY COUNTY

J. A. Adams_____Sulphur
H. C. Bailey_____Sulphur
I. N. Brown_____Davis
A. P. Brown_____Davis
R. Dunn_____Davis
J. C. Luster_____Davis
A. V. Ponder_____Sulphur
W. H. Powell_____Sulphur
J. M. Salter_____Sulphur
J. H. Simmons_____Sulphur
J. T. Slover_____Sulphur
G. W. Slover_____Sulphur
W. M. Tucker_____Sulphur

MUSKOGEE COUNTY

S. W. Aiken_____Muskogee
H. T. Ballantine_____Muskogee
W. D. Berry_____Muskogee
T. L. Blakemore_____Muskogee
A. J. Brewer_____Coweta
Benj. H. Brown_____M. R. C.
Edwin Davis_____Haskell
J. M. Dwight_____Muskogee
C. E. DeGroot_____Muskogee
J. J. Dial_____Muskogee
E. Dill_____Boynton
R. N. Donnell_____Muskogee
A. N. Earnest_____Muskogee
A. W. Everly_____Muskogee
F. W. Ewing_____Muskogee
R. C. Farris_____Porum
O. W. Fischer_____M. R. C.
W. P. Fite_____M. R. C.
F. B. Fite_____Muskogee

W. E. Floyd_____Muskogee
S. J. Fryer_____Muskogee
C. M. Fullenwider_____Muskogee
J. B. Graves_____Council Hill
J. G. Harris_____M. R. C.
A. W. Harris_____Muskogee
Chas. W. Heitzman_____Muskogee
C. L. Hill_____Miami
J. J. Hollingsworth_____Muskogee
Sessler Hoss_____Muskogee
O. E. Howell_____Oktaha
W. R. Joblins_____Porter
R. E. Jones_____Braggs
Emma S. Keith_____Muskogee
Forrest S. King_____Muskogee
O. C. Klass_____Muskogee
John E. Lee_____Haskell
J. B. Lightfoot_____Miami
A. J. Lovell_____Dalhart, Texas
P. S. Mitchell_____Yale
Milton Morrow_____Muskogee
P. P. Nesbitt_____Muskogee
Wm. B. Newton_____Muskogee
J. T. Nichols_____Muskogee
J. G. Noble_____Muskogee
I. B. Oldham_____Muskogee
J. H. Plunkett_____Porum
Jas. Grant Rafter_____Muskogee
B. W. Randel_____Okmulgee
D. M. Randel_____Muskogee
John Reynolds_____Muskogee
C. V. Rice_____Muskogee
C. T. Rogers_____Muskogee
H. C. Rogers_____Muskogee
J. Hoy Sanford _____M. R. C.
H. A. Scott_____Muskogee
J. F. Smith_____Haskell
J. W. Sosbee_____Webbers Falls
A. L. Stocks_____Muskogee
Joseph H. Stolper_____M. R. C.
C. A. Thompson_____Muskogee
M. K. Thompson_____Muskogee
W. T. Tilly_____Muskogee
J. S. Vittum_____Muskogee
G. C. Wallis_____Ft. Gibson
F. L. Walton_____Muskogee
J. C. Warmack_____Muskogee
F. E. Warterfield _____M. R. C.
J. Hutchings White_____Muskogee
Fred J. Wilkiemeyer_____Muskogee
J. H. Woodcock_____Miami

McINTOSH COUNTY

Dyton Bennet_____Texanna
G. W. Graves_____Hichita
L. I. Jacobs_____Vivian
N. P. Lee_____Checotah
Lieut. D. E. Little_____Eufaula
J. R. McCollock_____Checotah
W. S. Minor_____Pierce
Lieut. A. B. Montgomery_____Charlotte, N. C.
    Camp Green.
B. F. Rushing_____Hanna
J. N. Shaunty_____Eufaula
F. L. Smith_____Fame
A. J. Snelson_____Checotah
W. A. Tolleson_____Eufaula
B. J. Vance_____Checotah
J. C. Watkins_____Checotah
G. W. West_____Eufaula
W. F. Womack_____Chetocah

McCLAIN COUNTY

O. O. Dawson_____Wayne
I. N. Kolb_____Dibble
T. C. McCurdy_____Purcell
W. C. McCurdy_____Purcell
C. B. Smith_____Washington
J. W. West_____Purcell

McCURTAIN COUNTY

J. B. Chastain_____Davis
A. W. Clarkson_____Valliant
O. O. Hammond_____Broken Bow
W. F. Hill_____Idabel
C. R. Huckabay_____Valliant
W. Burns McCaskill_____Idabel
C. T. McDonald_____Broken Bow
W. A. Miller_____Liberty, Mo.
J. T. Moreland_____Idabel
W. A. Moreland_____Idabel
R. H. Sherrill_____Broken Bow
C. F. Shuford_____Broken Bow
R. D. Williams_____Idabel
N. D. Woods, Jr._____Millerton

NOBLE COUNTY

S. F. Brafford_____Billings
Robt. A. Cavitt_____Morrison
F. L. Keeler_____Perry
L. Kuntz_____Perry
B. A. Owen_____Perry
L. D. Stewart_____Perry
J. T. Williams_____Billings

NOWATA COUNTY

R. I. Allen_____Nowata
J. E. Brookshire_____Nowata
J. R. Collins_____Nowata
E. F. Collins_____Nowata
D. D. Howell_____Nowata
D. M. Lawson_____Nowata
W. M. Nairn_____Nowata
M. B. Scott_____Delaware
L. T. Strother_____Nowata
J. P. Sudderth_____Nowata
J. G. Thomas_____Alluwe
C. A. Walters_____Nowata
Geo. A. Waters_____Lenapah

OKFUSKEE COUNTY

C. M. Bloss_____Okemah
C. C. Bombarger_____Paden
W. H. Davis_____Castle
W. C. Griffith_____Weleetka
R. Keys_____Castle
J. A. Kennedy_____Okemah
H. A. May_____Okemah
A. O. Meredith_____Bearden
L. A. Nye_____Okemah
J. M. Pemberton_____Okemah
J. R. Preston_____Weleetka
J. S. Rollins_____Paden
A. J. Stephenson_____Okemah

OKLAHOMA COUNTY

J. M. Alford_____Oklahoma City
Leila E. Andrews_____Oklahoma City
F. M. Bailey_____Oklahoma City
C. E. Barker_____Oklahoma City
A. Bee_____Oklahoma City
A. L. Blesh_____Oklahoma City
Rex Boland_____Oklahoma City

T. A. Buchanan_____Oklahoma City
T. C. Burns_____Oklahoma City
L. H. Buxton_____Oklahoma City
F. K. Camp_____Oklahoma City
A. B. Chase_____Oklahoma City
C. P. Chumbley_____Oklahoma City
W. R. Clement_____Tulsa
H. H. Cloudman_____Oklahoma City
C. E. Clymer_____Oklahoma City
A. J. Coley_____Oklahoma Ciyt
Paul H. Crawford_____Oklahoma City
W. C. Cummings_____Oklahoma City
L. R. Cunningha_m_____Oklahoma City
A. E. Davenport_____Oklahoma City
E. F. Davis_____Oklahoma City
C. R. Day_____Oklahoma City
F. R. DeMand_____Oklahoma City
W. E. Dicken_____Oklahoma City
W. E. Dixon_____Oklahoma City
E. G. Earnhart_____Oklahoma City
J. T. Edwards_____Oklahoma City
R. T. Edwards_____Oklahoma City
C. D. Ferguson_____Oklahoma City
E. S. Ferguson_____Oklahoma City
C. J. Fishman_____Oklahoma City
T. H. Flesher_____Oklahoma City
W. A. Fowler_____Oklahoma City
Fred F. Fulton_____Oklahoma City
Geo. Fulton_____Oklahoma City
Ruth Gay_____Oklahoma City
R. B. Gibson_____Oklahoma City
H. H. Gipson_____Oklahoma City
A. L. Guthrie_____Oklahoma City
Karl Haas_____Harrah
J. E. Harbison_____Oklahoma City
J. S. Hartford_____Oklahoma City
A. C. Hirshfield_____Oklahoma City
G. W. Hinchee_____Oklahoma City
J. R. Holliday_____Oklahoma City
R. M. Howard_____Oklahoma City
R. L. Hull_____Oklahoma City
George Hunter_____Oklahoma City
S. M. Hunter_____Oklahoma City
L. E. Inman_____Oklahoma City
A. D. Johns_____Oklahoma City
W. J. Jolly_____Oklahoma City
J. F. Kelly_____Oklahoma City
J. F. Kuhn_____Oklahoma City
E. S. Lain_____Oklahoma City
Geo. A. La Motte_____Oklahoma City
W. M. Langsford_____Oklahoma City
Wm. Langston_____Oklahoma City
T. L. Lauderdale_____Oklahoma City
N. E. Lawson_____Oklahoma City
C. E. Lee_____Oklahoma City
W. P. Lipscomb_____Oklahoma City
R. E. Looney_____Oklahoma City
Ross D. Long_____M. R. C.
LeRoy Long_____Oklahoma City
T. R. Longmire_____Oklahoma City
J. T. Martin_____Oklahoma City
J. C. Mahr_____Oklahoma City
J. H. Maxwell_____Oklahoma City
J. F. Messenbaugh_____Oklahoma City
D. D. McHenry_____Oklahoma City
O. Perry McNair_____Oklahoma City
G. D. McLean_____Oklahoma City
S. L. Morgan_____Oklahoma City
L. J. Moorman_____Oklahoma City
J. Z. Mraz_____Oklahoma City
L. A. Newton_____Oklahoma City

N. R. Nowling_____Oklahoma City
D. D. Paulus_____Oklahoma City
J. R. Phelan_____Oklahoma City
C. R. Phelps_____Oklahoma City
J. S. Pine_____Oklahoma City
J. M. Postelle_____Oklahoma City
Horace Reed_____Oklahoma City
J. A. Reck_____Oklahoma City
J. W. Riley_____Oklahoma City
Lea A. Riely_____Oklahoma City
M. M. Roland _____Oklahoma City
J. B. Roloter_____Oklahoma City
W. L. Russell_____Oklahoma City
L. M. Sackett_____Oklahoma City
W. T. Salmon_____Oklahoma City
H. V. L. Sapper_____Oklahoma City
F. M. Sanger_____Oklahoma City
W. M. Sanger_____Oklahoma City
S. N. Stone_____Oklahoma City
M. Smith_____Oklahoma City
M. E. Stout_____Oklahoma City
F. B. Sorgatz_____Oklahoma City
E. S. Sullivan_____Oklahoma City
W. M. Taylor_____Oklahoma City
C. B. Taylor_____Oklahoma City
H. Coulter Todd_____Oklahoma City
Cary Townsend_____Oklahoma City
E. L. Underwood_____Oklahoma City
Curt von Wedel_____Oklahoma City
O. J. Walker_____Oklahoma City
W. J. Wallace_____Oklahoma City
M. W. Weir_____Oklahoma City
Eva Wells_____Oklahoma City
W. W. Wells_____Oklahoma City
Willis K. West_____Oklahoma City
L. M. Westfall_____Oklahoma City
A. W. White_____Oklahoma City
K. J. Wilson_____Spencer
A. A. Will_____Oklahoma City
Henry J. Worrell_____Oklahoma City
Geo. J. Wood_____Jones
A. D. Young_____Oklahoma City
A. M. Young_____Oklahoma City

OKMULGEE COUNTY

I. W. Bollinger_____Henryetta
J. E. Bercaw _____Okmulgee
Virgil Berry_____Okmulgee
H. D. Boswell_____Henryetta
Harry E. Breese_____Henryetta
W. G. Brymer_____Dewar
Oscar Burrow_____Wetumka
E. C. Bryan_____Okmulgee
A. W. Coleman_____Dewar
W. M. Cott_____Okmulgee
T. O. Crawford_____Beggs
A. H. Culp_____Beggs
J. G. Edward_____Henryetta
A. H. Herr_____Okmulgee
F. H. Hollingsworth_____Beggs
A. R. Holmes_____Henryetta
W. S. Larrabee_____Henryetta
G. Y. McKinney_____Kusa
C. M. Ming._____Okmulgee
W. C. Mitchener_____Okmulgee
R. Mooney_____Henryetta
W. N. Nagle_____Henryetta
J. P. Nelson_____Coalton
W. B. Pigg_____Henryetta
J. Lee Riley_____Henryetta

Ira W. Robertson_____Henryetta
N. N. Simpson _____Henryetta
W. L. Stephenson_____Henryetta
Wm. A. Thompson_____Kusa
G. W. Tilly, M. O. T. C., Ft. Oglethrop, Ga.
L. B. Torrance_____Okmulgee
J. O. Wailes_____Morris
Virgil W. Wallace_____Morris

OSAGE COUNTY

W. H. Aaron_____Pawhuska
T. M. Berry_____Hominy
J. F. Clark_____Avant
K. L. Colley_____Big Heart
T. J. Colley_____Hominy
J. M. Ennis_____Pawhusha
G. W. Goss_____Pawhuska
W. F. Herron_____Hominy
F. F. Jones_____Pawhuska
Ira Mullins_____Hominy
Q. B. Neal_____Pawhuska
J. G. Shoun_____Fairfax
D. A. Shoun_____Fairfax
Benj. Skinner_____Pawhuska
A. J. Smith_____Pawhuska
H. L. Summers_____Osage
Harry Walker_____Pawhuska
Roscoe Walker_____Pawhuska
Divonis Worten_____Pawhuska
David A. Yates_____Avant

OTTAWA COUNTY

J. D. Bewley_____Miami
T. W. Brewer_____Miami
W. J. Clark_____Douthitt
D. L. Connell_____Picher
A. M. Cooter_____Miami
Jas. R. Dawson_____Afton
Fred E. Deal_____Miami
Geo. A. DeTar_____Miami
T. J. Dodson_____Picher
John C. Dovell_____Miami
J. S. French_____Afton
E. F. Garlington_____Olustee
Geo. I. Garrison_____Quapaw
J. B. Hampton_____Commerce
R. H. Harper_____Afton
J. C. Jacobs_____Miami
Ed. D. James_____Miami
E. A. Leasure_____Fairland
Earl Lightfoot_____Mineral, Kansas
C. O. Lively_____Tar River
G. P. McNaughton_____Miami
W. L. McWilliams_____Miami
B. B. Mason_____Picher
Blair Points_____Miami
W. M. Rivers_____St. Louis
G. H. Rutledge_____Afton
W. A. Sibley_____Tar River
Ira Smith_____Commerce
W. B. Smith_____Fairland
G. E. Smith_____Miami
Luther W. Trout_____Afton
R. F. Von Cannon_____Miami
J. T. Wharton_____Picher
J. Clay Williams_____Picher
M. P. Willis_____Commerce
F. L. Wormington_____Miami

PAWNEE COUNTY

W. E. Arnold_____Jennings
C. W. Ballaine_____Cleveland
L. C. Barber_____Ralston
C. E. Beitman_____Skedee
J. R. Fleming_____Sinnett
N. W. Gaymond_____Ralston
D. J. Herrington_____Terlton
H. B. McFarland_____Cleveland
G. H. Philips_____Pawnee
J. A. Roberts_____Cleveland
E. T. Robinson_____Cleveland
R. E. Weller_____Pawnee

PAYNE COUNTY

C. W. Bacon_____Yale
C. H. Beach_____Glencoe
J. H. Cash_____Glencoe
L. A. Cleverdon_____Stillwater
Benj. Davis_____Cushing
E. M. Harris_____Cushing
R. W. Holbroke_____Perkins
W. B. Hudson_____Yale
Eli Hughes_____Stillwater
D. F. Janeway_____Stillwater
H. C. Manning_____Cushing
H. McQuown_____Stillwater
J. C. Morris_____Cushing
J. B. Murphy_____Stillwater
C. E. Sexton_____Stillwater
C. D. Simmons_____Stillwater
W. E. Stewart_____Cushing

PITTSBURG COUNTY

E. N. Allen_____McAlester
F. J. Baum_____Savanna
R. L. Browning_____Haileyville
C. J. Brunson_____Adamson
J. A. Burnett_____Crum Creek
A. E. Carlock_____Hartshorne
T. S. Chapman_____McAlester
G. R. Connaly_____Blocker
J. E. Davis_____McAlester
J. W. Echols_____McAlester
M. H. Foster_____Alderson
J. Paul Gay_____McAlester
W. C. Graves_____McAlester
J. Worth Gray_____Quinton
A. Griffith_____McAlester
J. O. Grubbs_____N. McAlester
W.[P. Hailey_____Haileyville
Chas. T. Harris_____Kiowa
A. J. Harris_____McAlester
J. C. Johnston_____McAlester
L. C. Kuyrkendall_____McAlester
W. P. Lewallen_____Canadian
T. H. McCarley_____McAlester
J. N. McLendon_____McAlester
J. P. McRae_____McAlester
R. A. Munn_____Kiowa
T. T. Norris_____Crowder
Lieut. T. J. Palmer_____Ft. Riley, Kansas
R. K. Pemberton_____McAlester
O. W. Rice_____Alderson
W. W. Sarnes_____Hartshorne
C. C. Shaw_____McAlester
J. A. Smith_____McAlester
Graham Street_____McAlester
E. H. Troy_____McAlester
G. S. Turner_____Krebs
F. L. Watson_____McAlester

Capt. L. S. Willour_____Waco, Texas
        Camp McArthur
McClellan Wilson_____McAlester

PONTOTOC COUNTY

A. G. Akers_____Army
Wm. D. Akers_____Army
W. B. Berninger_____Atwood
N. B. Breckenridge_____New Mexico
J. G. Breco_____Ada
S. L. Burns_____Maxwell
R. T. Castleberry_____Ada
J. Sham. L. Cummings_____Ada
B. B. Dawson_____Ada
W. D. Faust_____Ada
Edith Harrison_____Stonewall
Fred Harrison_____Stonewall
T. A. Hill_____Roff
J. L. Jeffress_____Roff
R. F. King_____Ada
M. L. Lewis_____Ada
M. C. McNew_____Ada
H. D. Meredith_____Ada
C. L. Orr_____Ada
L. M. Overton_____Fitzhugh
S. M. Richey_____Francis
S. P. Ross_____Ada
T. S. Sturdivant_____Vanoss
B. F. Sullivan_____Ada
Catherine Threlkeld_____Ada
W. C. Threlkeld_____Army
H. J. Weeden_____Sasakaw
C. S, Wilkerson_____Roff

POTTAWATOMIE COUNTY

R. M. Anderson_____Shawnee
G. H. Applewhite_____Camp Cody, N. M.
W. A. Ball_____Wanette
M. A. Baker_____Shawnee
G. S. Baxter_____Shawnee
F. Bence_____Shawnee
C. B. Bradford_____Shawnee
W. C. Bradford_____Shawnee
R. A. Brown_____Prague
W. R. Butler_____Maud
J. M. Byrum_____Shawnee
Z. T. Calhoun_____McComb
H. G. Campbell_____Asher
F. L. Carson_____Shawnee
G. W. Colvert_____Tecumseh
U. S. Cordell_____Romulus
J. Culbertson_____Maud
R. R. Culbertson_____Maud
J. E. Cullom_____Earlsboro
J. L. Fortson_____Tecumseh
W. M. Gallaher_____Shawnee
L. J. George_____Stuart
E. E. Goodrich_____Tecumseh
E. J. Gray_____Tecumseh
G. E. Hartshorne_____Ft. Riley Kansas
J. E. Hughes_____Shawnee
R. C. Kaylor_____McLoud
A. C. McFarling_____Shawnee
W. N. McGee_____Shawnee
A. H. Owen_____Meeker
W. D. Phillips_____Maud
H. M. Reeder_____Shawnee
E. E. Rice, American Expeditionary Forces,
        France.
J. H. Royster_____Wanette

T. D. Rowland _____San Antonio, Texas
        Kelly Field No. 2
G. H. Sanborn_____Shawnee
T. C. Sanders_____Shawnee
J. H. Scott_____Shawnee
J. M. Stooksbury_____Shawnee
Jas. H. Turner_____Shawnee
H. A. Wagner, American Expeditionary Forces
      France.
J. A. Walker___Camp McArthur, Waco, Texas
J. E. Walker_____Earlsboro
H. H. Wilson_____Shawnee

PUSHTAMAHA COUNTY
Edw. Guinn_____Antlers
B. M. Huckabay_____Tuskahoma
H. C. Johnson_____Antlers
J. S. Lawson_____Clayton
E. S. Patterson_____Antlers
George Robinett_____Nolia
P. E. Wright_____Albion

ROGER MILLS COUNTY
B. M. Ballenger_____Hamburg
W. L. Cary_____Rankin
Lee Dorrah_____Hammon
J. P. Miller_____Cheyenne
G. H. Wallace_____Cheyenne
W. I. Wimberley_____Hammon

ROGERS COUNTY
F. A. Anderson_____Claremore
A. M. Arnold_____Claremore
Caroline Bassman_____Claremore
J. C. Bushyhead_____Claremore
H. L. Callahan_____Collinsville
J. E. Ewell_____Catoosa
C. V. Elliott_____Inola
J. H. Haley_____Catale
W. F. Hays_____Claremore
H. L. Hillis_____Collinsville
W. A. Howard_____Chelsea
Lawson Hughes_____Collinsville
Henry F. Knabb_____Foyil
J. F. Means_____Claremore
W. S. Michael_____Collinsville
E. Pleas_____Collinsville
L. C. Presson_____Collinsville
S. C. Rutherford_____Inola
J. C. Smith_____Catoosa
W. E. Smith_____Collinsville
J. M. Stemmons_____Oolagah
Geo. Strickland_____Claremore
J. C. Taylor_____Chelsea
J. G. Waldrop_____Claremore
John W. Wright_____Collinsville

SEMINOLE COUNTY
W. R. Black_____Seminole
T. F. Harrison_____Wewoka
S. N. Holliday_____Hazel
W. T. Huddleston_____Konowa
W. P. Jenkins_____Wewoka
H. A. Kiles_____Konowa
W. L. Knight_____Wewoka
E. R. McAlester_____Seminole
J. H. Perkins_____Wewoka
M. M. Turlington_____Seminole
M. A. Warhurst_____Seminole

SEQUOYAH COUNTY
J. C. Breedlove_____Muldrow
C. Bryant_____Vian
M. D. Carnell_____Okmulgee
J. A. Cheek_____Sallisaw
T. W. Collins_____Muldrow
A. A. Hicks_____Muldrow
V. W. Hudson_____Sallisaw
W. M. Hunter_____Vian
S. B. Jones_____Sallisaw
S. A. McKeel_____Sallisaw
J. A. Morrow_____Sallisaw
Chas. H. Morris_____Vian
J. T. Sandling_____Vian
T. F. Wood_____Sallisaw

STEPHENS COUNTY
J. P. Bartley_____Duncan
John G. Cowman_____Comanche
H. A. Conger_____Duncan
Edward DeMeglio_____Oklahoma City
M. F. Dicker_____Comanche
H. C. Frie_____Duncan
S. S. Garrett_____Dixie
P. M. Haraway_____Marlow
C. M. Harrison_____Comanche
W. S. Ivy_____Marlow
D. Long_____Duncan
A. R. Mavity_____Marlow
D. M. Montgomery_____Marlow
R. L. Montgomery_____Marlow
J. A. Mullins_____Marlow
J. W. Neiweg, 1st Lieut., M. R. C., Ft. Riley, Ks
S. A. Rice_____Alma
C. C. Richards_____Marlow
W. S. Spears_____Velma
J. I. Taylor_____Loco
E. B. Thomason_____Velma
J. O. Wharton_____Duncan
S. H. Williamson_____Duncan

TEXAS COUNTY
R. B. Hayes_____Guymon
Wm. H. Langston_____Guymon
Jas. M. McMillin_____Goodwell
Wm. J. Risen_____Hooker

TILLMAN COUNTY
J. E. Arrington_____Frederick
W. J. Brinks_____Manitou
G. A. Comp_____Manitou
W. A. Fugua_____Grandfield
A. J. Hays_____Frederick
C. A. Howell_____Manitou
L. A. Mitchell_____Frederick
F. E. Rosenberger_____Grandfield
T. F. Spurgeon_____Frederick
R. E. Wilson_____Davidson
Harper Wright_____Grandfield

TULSA COUNTY
C. M. Ament_____Sapulpa
P. N. Atkins_____Tulsa
C. H. Ball_____Tulsa
W. W. Beesley_____Tulsa
Walter Beyer_____Tulsa
J. C. Bland_____Tulsa
F. M. Boso_____Tulsa
W. W. Brodie_____Tulsa
H. S. Browne_____Tulsa
Paul R. Brown_____Tulsa
J. Raymond Burdick_____Tulsa

J. P. Butcher _____Tulsa
C. E. Calhoun_____Sand Springs
Geo. P. Campbell_____Sand Springs
L. H. Carlton_____Tulsa
H. C. Childs_____Tulsa
J. W. Childs_____Tulsa
E. L. Cohenour_____Tulsa
T. B. Coulter_____Tulsa
F. S. Clinton_____Tulsa
Geo. H. Clulow_____Tulsa
W. Albert Cook_____Tulsa
Fred.Y. Cronk_____Tulsa
Geo. M. Davis_____Bixby
B. J. Davis_____Sand Springs
Robert A. Douglas_____Tulsa
R. W. Dunlap_____Tulsa
W. F. Dutton_____Tulsa
Arthur V. Emerson_____Tulsa
O. A. Flanagan_____Tulsa
R. A. Felt_____Tulsa
H. W. Ford_____Tulsa
Onis Franklin_____Broken Arrow
Henry Gessler_____Tulsa
J. B. Gilbert_____Tulsa
Fred A. Glass_____Tulsa
J. F. Gorrell_____Tulsa
Ross Grosshart_____Tulsa
H. B. Gwin_____Tulsa
Thos W. Haskin_____Tulsa
S. De Zell Hawley _____Tulsa
E. F. Hayden_____Tulsa
J. S. Hooper_____Tulsa
M. A. Houser_____Tulsa
J. S. Hume_____Tulsa
Chas. D. Jackson_____Tulsa
L. D. Latham_____Tulsa
J. H. Laws_____Broken Arrow
C. P. Linn_____Tulsa
R. S. Linn_____Tulsa
N. W. Mayginnis_____Tulsa
P. H. Mayginnis_____Tulsa
B. Margolin_____Tulsa
P. A. Mangum_____Tulsa
W. D. McVicker_____Tulsa
S. S. Mohrman_____Tulsa
J. H. Morgan_____Tulsa
H. D. Murdock_____Tulsa
S. Murray_____Tulsa
Frank C. Myers_____Broken Arrow
B. N. Oden_____West Tulsa
C. D. O'Hern_____Tulsa
C. A. Pigford_____Tulsa
Horace P. Price_____Tulsa
C. L. Reeder_____Tulsa
R. E. L. Rhodes_____Tulsa
J. W. Rodgers_____Tulsa
W. H. Rogers_____Tulsa
A. W. Roth_____Tulsa
Emile Roy_____Tulsa
R. R. Smith_____Tulsa
R. V. Smith_____Tulsa
M. P. Springer_____Tulsa
J. C. Stevens_____Drumright
E. F. Stroud_____Tulsa
W. J. Trainor_____Tulsa
R. S. Wagner_____Tulsa
G. A. Wall_____Tulsa
J. E. Wallace_____Tulsa
H. P. Ward_____Leonard
B. F. Watterson_____Bixby

J. E. Webb_____Tulsa
P. C. White_____Tulsa
Daniel White_____Tulsa
A. Ray Wiley_____Tulsa
C. Z. Wiley_____Tulsa
W. W. Woody_____Tulsa
Walter E. Wright_____Tulsa
S. F. Yoho_____Tulsa

WAGONER COUNTY

S. R. Bates_____Wagoner
A. E. Carder_____Coweta
Isabelle Cobb_____Wagoner
G. R. Gorden_____Wagoner
C. E. Haywood_____Wagoner
G. W. Jobe_____Wagoner
C. E. Martin_____Wagoner
G. C. Moore_____Dallas, Tex.
J. E. Orcutt_____Coweta
T. J. Shiner_____Wagoner
W. W. Walton_____Coweta

WASHITA COUNTY

B. W. Baker_____Cloudchief
W. D. Bennett_____Sentinel
A. H. Bungardt _____Cordell
E. E. Darnell_____Colony
G. A. Dillon_____Dill
J. E. Farber_____Cordell
J. S. Freeman_____Rocky
J. H. Harms_____Cordell
A. J. Jetter_____Foss
J. W. Kerley_____Cordell
J. M. McQuaid_____Lookeba
A. S. Neal_____Cordell
A. M. Sherburne_____Cordell
E. F. Stevens_____Foss
Wm. Tidball_____Sentinel
E. S. Weaver_____Dill
A. Weber_____Bessie
T. C. White_____Canute
J. W. Witt_____Colony

WASHINGTON COUNTY

J. V. Athey_____Bartlesville
J. T. Bartley_____Bartlesville
S. J. Bradfield_____Bartlesville
Elizabeth Chamberlin_____Bartlesville
H. G. Crawford_____Bartlesville
T. B. Dickson_____Ramona
J. C. Dunn_____Bartlesville
O. I. Green_____Bartlesville
L. D. Hudson_____Dewey
W. H. Kingman_____Bartlesville
J. D. Kiser_____Bartlesville
W. E. Koppenbrink_____Bartlesville
Arthur North_____Bartlesville
S. M. Parks_____Bartlesville
W. E. Rammel_____Bartlesville
W. H. Shipman_____Bartlesville
O. S. Somerville_____Bartlesville
J. G. Smith_____Bartlesville
B. F. Staver_____Bartlesville
F. R. Sutton_____Bartlesville
H. C. Weber_____Bartlesville
G. F. Woodring_____Bartlesville
W. C. Wyatt_____Bartlesville
H. E. Yazel_____Bartlesville

WOODS COUNTY

J. A. Bowling------------------------Alva
A. J. Butts-------------------------Skiatook
E. P. Clapper----------------------Waynoka
D. B. Ensor-------------------------Hopeton
O. R. Gregg-------------------------Waynoka
A. E. Hale-----------------------------Alva
Isaac Hunt-------------------------Freedom
R. Z. Linney-------------Charlotte, N. C.
L. S. Munsell------------------------Beaver
S. H. Welch------------------------Dacoma
C. T. White----------------------------Alva

WOODWARD COUNTY

C. L. Amos-------------------------------May
W. J. Bamber------------------------Arnett
A. J. Brace--------------------------Sharon
H. S. Cockrell----------------------Mooreland
C. E. Davis------------------------Woodward
J. C. Duncan------------------------Forgan
R. L. Edmonds-----------------------Arnett
P. G. Eiler-------------------------Quinlan
C. J. Forney-----------------------Woodward
R. K. Goddard------------------------Supply
B. C. Hill---------------------------Supply

W. H. Jones---------------Ashland, Kansas
J. W. Messersmith--------------------Floris
E. M. Miller------------------------Buffalo
O. C. Newman-----------------------Shattuck
P. P. Oliver----------------------Boise City
J. L. Patterson------------------Naco, Ariz.
Fred Patterson---------------------M. R. C.
O. A. Pierson---------------------Woodward
J. P. Powell-----------------------M. R. C.
Floyd L. Racer---------------------M. R. C.
J. W. Rollo-----------------------Shattuck
W. L. Rose-----------------------Woodward
Wm. Slusher-------------------------Gage
J. M. Steele-------------------------Kenton
Albert A. Stoll-------------Longton, Kansas
H. E. Stecher------------------------Supply
C. W. Tedrowe---------------------M. R. C.
T. B. Triplett--------------------Mooreland
H. Walker--------------------------Rosston
D. Watts----------------------------Laverne
G. A. Westfall----------------------Supply
F. Z. Winchell-----------------------Buffalo
R. A. Workman--------------------Woodward
J. M. Workman--------------------Woodward

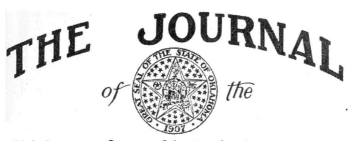

THE JOURNAL of the

Oklahoma State Medical Association

VOLUME XI   MUSKOGEE, OKLA., JULY, 1918   NUMBER 7

RADIUM AND ITS APPLICATION IN MEDICINE AND SURGERY.*

By EVERETT S. LAIN, M. D.

Associate Professor and Head of Department of Dermatology,
University of Oklahoma School of Medicine,
Oklahoma City

Most physicians of today are fairly versed upon some of the properties of radium or may have seen cases which have been treated successfully or otherwise with this agent. Therefore, they have already formed opinions as regards its present or future value in the field of medical and surgical therapeutics. It is not our desire to influence these opinions either for, or against, the therapeutic value of this agent, but only endeavor to present this subject in a briefly historical manner followed by some conclusions arrived at after a two years personal experience with this new agent. These conclusions are also based upon the many reports from various physicians who have been using radium for a much longer period. Also, I have had the pleasure of interviewing many of these physicians in their offices and in medical associations where the subject of radium and its field of usefulness was discussed.

Insofar as I am aware, this is the first attempt of any member of this society to present this subject before this, our State Association. Therefore, it shall not be out of place to refresh your memory briefly upon the history of the discovery of radium and some of its physical properties.

Several years prior to the discovery of radium, the radioactivity of several new elements in nature associated with their crude compounds had been demonstrated by a French physicist, Henri Becquerel. In the study of two of these elements, namely: Uranium and thorium, which were extracted from pitch blende and carnotite, he found that the residue remaining contained an even more radioactive and fluorescent substance than had yet been known. Soon after, extensive experiments were carried on in various French laboratories where the properties of these new and radiant metals were studied. One of the most active laboratories in which these experiments were being performed was that of the physical laboratory of the University of Paris. In this laboratory a man and wife labored side by side, known to Paris inhabitants only as Professor and Madame Curie. Possessing a well trained, scientific mind which was directed by an untiring zeal for knowing the wherefore of all things, they endeavored to make a reduction of uranium beyond that of any other laboratory, and brought forth another flourescent element which they named polonium. True to the curious nature of woman, Madame Curie was not yet satisfied with this another element derived

*Read before the Annual Meeting, Oklahoma State Medical Ass'n, Tulsa, May 15, 1918.

from pitch blende, and carried her reductions of the residue to a still further degree, which now brought forth a more potent radio-active and luminescent metal than had yet been discovered. This she reasoned is the prime element in all similar radio-activity, therefore it must be the root or radium. It is stated, a few years later this lady again exemplified the nature of her sex when she became so prominent socially and so widely known as a scientist that she found it expedient, and did obtain a divorce from her husband.

Radium is a metal of whitish-grey color, specific gravity 226.4, melts at a temperature of 700 centigrade and will decompose water innerjetically. It is said that a piece of radium will generate enough heat to raise its equal weight in ice water to a point of boiling in one hour of time.

The life of pure radium is estimated from one million to several hundred millions of years. Its original source of supply was the pitch blende mines of Northern Bohemia, though in recent years there have been located several mountainous elevations in Colorado which have yielded considerable amounts of carnotite which under a process of reduction also gives up radium in appreciable quantities. The reduction of these compounds requires large quantities of reagents, and is no small task of labor, extending over many days of time, even in the largest laboratories. It is estimated that to produce a gram of radium it requires 350 tons of crude ore and many tons of chemical reagents, such as sodium carbonate, hydrochloric and sulphuric acids. Therefore, the labor and expense in its process of reduction justifies in a manner the seemingly unreasonable price which it commands.

It has been learned that some of its unreduced compounds, such as radium bromide, chloride and sulphate, are for all practical purposes just as effective as the pure element. Therefore, the majority of placques, tubes and other forms of applicators which are upon the market and are used by physicians of today do not contain pure radium, but only these compounds, which are valued by their contents of so many milligrams of radium element.

The radio-activity of this new element is in many respects similar to that of the X-ray. However, with this essential difference, the three principal kinds of rays of radium can be separated or eliminated by metal screens, and its dosage can be far more accurately regulated than those of the X-ray. Its radio-active rays are divided into three kinds according to their properties and degree of penetration, or effects upon cellular life, namely: the alpha, the beta, and the gamma. The alpha rays represent the least penetrating, the most rapidly acting, and are easily screened. The beta rays are more penetrating and dissoluting, slowly acting and more difficult of screening. The gamma rays are the most deeply penetrating, taking several days for cellular reaction, slowly and deeply dissoluting, and are not easily screened even by the heaviest of metals such as silver, gold or lead. The convenience for application of radium around the eye or within the natural openings of the body such as the mouth, throat, vagina, rectum, etc., makes it of especial value in the treatment of early malignancy, which so frequently develops in these parts.

Since its discovery in the year of 1902, radium has been passing through the usual number of uses and abuses in the hands of the scientific as well as the unscientific, which accounts in a large measure for the many contradictory statements in the earliest reports as regards its success or failure in the various diseases in which it has been tried.

The study of radium and its medical and surgical application has now passed its fifteenth year. During this time much has been proven and demonstrated as regards its histology and histo-pathology when applied to animal tissue. It has been learned that it influences cellular life in varying degrees according to which of the rays have been used, controlled by the different screens, the distance of the applicator from the tissue affected, and the length of time in which it is applied. When applied to animal tissue its first effects are that of stimulation to both normal and pathological cells.

If the time of this application is extended or a more intense portion of the ray is used, its second effects are that of inflammation, followed by exudate, degeneration and absorption. In the latter or second degree of reaction, the pathological cells begin a process of degeneration while the normal yet remain intact. To this repeatedly demonstrated and histological fact we are partially indebted for the successful treatment of benign and malignant neoplasms.

The third degree is that of inflammation, exudation, degeneration, absorption, and maybe necrosis, of both normal and pathological cells, ofttimes accounting for the unhealed lesions or so-called burns.

To physicians who were previously experienced in the application and effects of X-ray, the taking up of this new therapeutic agent was but a transition from an active to a more active one, which agent is found to be far more convenient and successful in certain regions and for certain diseases in which the X-ray treatment was not all that could be desired.

In giving a few conclusions as regards the partial or specific value of this new addition to therapeutics, I do not presume you to believe that my experience during the past two years, covering a limited number of cases, should be taken as a final word upon what may or may not be done with radium.

During the past two years I have attempted no experiments upon new diseases, but have in a large measure followed the methods and suggestions of such men as Russell H. Boggs, Pittsburg; Isaac Levin of New York; Samuel E. Sweitzer of Minneapolis; Frank E. Simpson of Chicago; R. L. Sutton of Kansas City, and others who have had a wider experience and extending over a longer period of time.

Under the diseases which are favorably influenced for a short or long period of time, I shall classify: arthritis, goiter, exophthalmic, Hodgkin's disease, sarcomas, fibromas, psoriasis, leukemia, chronic eczemas, pruritis, etc. Under those which are influenced favorably in a more or less permanent manner and those in which this agent should be a first choice for certain stages, types or locations, I mention epitheliomas, carcinomas, sarcomas, lupus, leukoplakia, keloids, Naevi, keratomas, mucus-cysts and various other similar neoplasms, both benign and malignant.

Its convenience of application and ofttimes most marvelous results in the treatment of malignant neoplasms which so frequently develop around or upon the eyelids or in the various cavities of the body, such as the nares, mouth, ears, urethra, vagina and rectum, makes it the agent of first choice in many cases. It is also one of our most valuable post operative treatments in all forms of sarcoma and carcinomas as well as in tuberculosis of the superficial and accessible structures.

Summary.

1. Radium has the most powerful radio-active properties of any element yet discovered.

2. It has passed through the usual experience or attempts at curing the incurables or relieving the hopeless.

3. It has certain definite effects upon normal and pathological cellular life and when applied with careful observance of these laws, certain beneficial effects may be expected.

4. Radium is a most valuable addition to our therapeutics and is not excelled by any other agent, for the treatment of certain diseases, or stages of neoplasms when such are yet localized.

The following photographs with accompanying notes illustrate the ordinary and satisfactory effects in a few of the above mentioned diseases.

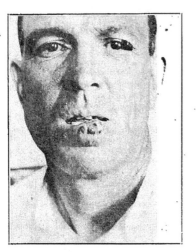

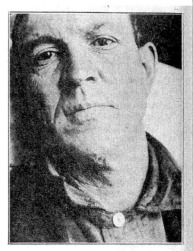

Case No. 1—Epithelioma of the lip, induration about one inch in diameter. Treated July, 1917.

Case No. 1—As patient appeared several weeks ago.

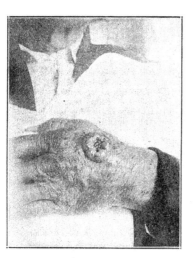

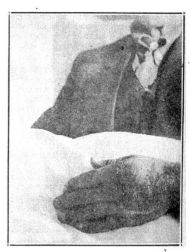

Case No. 2—Squamous celled Epithelioma on hand. Treated November, 1917.

Case No. 2—As hand appears to date.

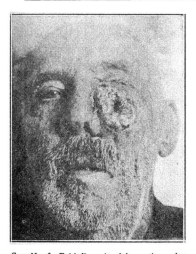

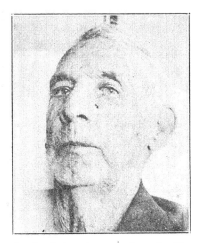

Case No. 3—Epithelioma involving entire malar
surface and portion of lower lid, alae of nose,
left side. Treated November, 1917.

Case No. 3—As patient appeared recently. No
remains of former lesion except small sinus
which has ceased to discharge.

DRIED VEGETABLES.

The usefulness of desiccation of vegetables for food in expeditions, etc., has
for its excuse the greater ease of transportation and conservation, and M. H.
Givens, New Haven, Conn. (*Journal A. M. A.*, June 8, 1918), discusses the subject from the physiologic point of view. In considering the value of food today,
its inorganic constituents should receive consideration as well as its protein, fat
carbohydrate and vitamin content. A brief review of the literature on this special
point is presented. The student of dietetics recognizes that were it not for the
use of milk, eggs and a few green vegetables our food intake would be very deficient in available lime. The author's study of the subject was planned to supplement our somewhat deficient knowledge regarding the composition of desiccated
vegetables. The method of drying and the analytic procedures are described.
A table is given of the percentage composition of vegetables, as purchased and
air-dried, arranged according to decreasing nitrogen content, which is at best,
Givens says, only a rough index of the protein contained. The variation in nitrogen,
according to the plant or parts of the plant, is striking. The starch plants, as
potatoes and carrots, have a low protein content; while others, like spinach, lettuce
and cabbage, contain a relatively high content in the dried state.   There is also
a noticeable difference in the amount of nitrogen in the different parts of the same
plant, the tops, roots, etc.   In the case of some vegetables, the nitrogen content of
the dried product is in striking contrast with that of the original material, owing to
the large loss of water, and the author calls attention to the possible loss of inorganic elements in cooking methods. The physiologic importance of calcium in
feeding growing organisms is universally recognized. The calcium statistics, reported by Givens, are in accord with the comparable figures for such of these materials as Sherman and Forbes have analyzed. The high calcium content of the
green vegetables is strikingly in contrast with that of the tubers and roots. There
may be a loss of inorganic constituents, particularly calcium, in the cooking of foods
and in the preparation of some of them for drying.

CARCINOMA OF THE MASTOID--CASE REPORT.*

By C. M. FULLENWIDER, M. D., Muskogee, Okla.

Fortunately, carcinoma of the middle ear or mastoid is an exceedingly rare occurrence. Newhart in a paper before the American Academy of Ophthalmology and Oto-Laryngology, last year quotes Zeroni's monograph (1899) in which he reports five cases of his own and one hundred twenty-one from the literature, of which however a considerable number were carcinoma of the external ear. Newhart was able to find thirty-four cases in the literature since Zeroni's paper and by inquiry fifty-one cases from the practice of American otologists. The growth in the majority of cases is of the squamous celled variety. A large number follow chronic suppuration. A few cures have been reported following operation. The close proximity of vital structures limits the scope of operative procedures so that an early diagnosis is essential for complete removal of the growth. The following case represents my only experience with the disease. It has been of such interest to me that I venture to report it to the society.

Mrs. J. A. E. Came to me in the fall of 1916 suffering from a chronic purulent discharge from the left ear which dated from an acute attack of otitis media seven years before. Hearing was reduced to loud voice at one foot. Granulations showed through a large perforation in the tympanic membrane and there was a mass of granulations covering a fistula on the floor of the canal and another on the posterior wall. The discharge was rather profuse and foul. I expressed the opinion that nothing short of the radical mastoid operation would cure the discharge but as the patient wished to avoid operation if possible, agreed to try conservative treatment for a time. I found extensive destruction of the bony walls of the canal and in repeated sittings was able to cut away practically all of the posterior wall of the external auditory canal and apparently nearly all of the mastoid contents. The bridge was left in place and the outer region of the mastoid near the cortex could not be reached. The exposure of the mastoid contents was so wide and the wound did so well for a time that I thought that a cure would result. The outer portion, under the cortex, continued to give trouble by the persistent recurrence of granulations and frequent slight hemorrhages. Finally the superior canal wall next to the tympanum began to sag and the patient began to complain of dizziness. On September the radical operation was performed. The mastoid was found to be extremely large and divided by a rather prominent ridge over the sinus. All of the portion anterior to the ridge, and the tympanic cavity itself, was filled with rather firm, tough granulation tissue which bled freely. The lining of the cells posterior to the sinus ridge was smooth and the cell filled only with a yellowish serous fluid. Everything was removed down to hard bone except over the inner part of the facial ridge, where the nerve was found exposed, and the inner wall of the tympanic cavity. On attempting to remove the ossicles, it was found that the slightest traction on them produced marked facial twitchings. They were removed by dissecting them out of the granulations with a small paracentesis knife. The tympanum was then cleared as thoroughly as possible. There was no facial paralysis and at no time could the fistula symptom be elicited, though the labyrinth was active.

For a time healing progressed satisfactory. About one-half of the wound had become covered with epidermis, when granulations began to trouble again. An area adjacent to the exposed facial nerve, one in the upper outer angle of the cavity and another in the tip of the mastoid, refused to become covered and granulations recurred as often as they were removed, and removal caused an increasing amount of hemorrhage. Finally an area in the roof of the antrum, which had seemed to be firmly healed, became thick and swollen and then broke down, the probe showing roughened bone.

---

*Prepared for 26th Annual Meeting, Oklahoma State Medical Ass'n, Tulsa, May 14-16, 1918.

On October 5th, 1917, the wound was reopened. The cavity was cleaned out with the curette. The granulations cut with a feeling of resistance. The cut surface showed small yellowish spots scattered through the tissue. The posterior portion of the mastoid which had been free at the first operation was now filled with the granulations, and in clearing them away, a large defect in the bone was found and the dura uncovered. Tissue removed was submitted to Dr. F. J. Hall, who reported it to be squamous cell carcinoma. Ten days later, the patient was seen by Dr. Geo. E. Shambaugh, who advised against further operative interference. At his suggestion, a specimen of the tissue was submitted to another pathologist, who confirmed the first diagnosis. It was decided to use radium. Seventy-five milligrams were placed in the cavity and left for twelve hours. This exposure was repeated on two subsequent occassions. The improvement was marked. Apparently the growth was stopped and while the tissue never became covered with epidermis, it took on the appearance of thin scar tissur. In February of this year, a small recurrence began to show deep in the roof of the tympanum. A small capsule of radium was inserted but this time without effect. Within the last few weeks, the growth has spread to the soft tissues both above and below the ear and facial paralysis has made its appearance. Pain which had been slight in the early stages, is now so severe as to require morphia, and the patient has rapidly lost strength.

Looking back over the case I realize that my suspicions should have been aroused much sooner than they were. The tissue removed at the first operation, should have been examined microscopically, as it should be at all radical mastoid operations. I do not think such an examination would have changed the result in this case, as it was already too late, but in another case it might give warning in time.

ANTIPNEUMOCOCCIC SERUM.

N. E. Wayson and G. W. McCoy, Washington, D. C. (*Journal A. M. A.*, June 8, 1918), say that antipneumococcic serum, as developed by Neufeld, has not been accepted as an entirely satisfactory therapeutic agent. Cole and his coworkers, however, have renewed the interest in the serum by the differentiation of types of pneumococci, and the use of the specific univalant serum. Clinical evidence has accumulated tending to encourage the use of Cole's Type I serum in cases in which the corresponding infecting organism has been determined. "The official control of this product by protection tests has thus far been confined to serum produced by the immunization of horses against type I pneumococci. Polyvalent serums are required to show the same protective against Type I organisms as is the specific serum. The evidence of the manufacturers' protection tests are accepted for the potency of serums made by immunizing animals against pneumococci of Types II and III." As it seemed desirable to have all serums claimed to be effective offered for sale officially examined in the government Hygienic Laboratory, an order of such testing was given by the Secretary of the Treasury and was carried out by the authors on 104 lots of serums made by the various laboratories, representing both commercial and noncommercial manufacturers, the details of which are given. These indicate that there is little preference between serum produced by institutions for interstate sale, and that made by noncommercial manufacturers. There is no inherent difficulty in producing the serum on a commercial basis, and while the summary of results shows that the method of testing adopted by the Hygenic Laboratory resulted in a greater number of failures in serums to pass satisfactorily, the irregularities are inherent in the test, and not due to slight modifications. While the mouse test seems irregular in its results, it is believed that it affords, in its present state, a valuable measure of potency of antipneumococcic serum, when properly controlled, and that that available in the market is as potent as that from other sources.

SOME SUGGESTIONS ON THE CAUSE OF CANCER.

By ARTHUR W. WHITE, A. M., M. D., Oklahoma City

Quite recently as a result of some of the continuous studies on the cause of malignancy, some new conclusions seem to have developed. In going over the literature on cancer for the past few months this phase of the question appealed to me a little more than any other at this time except, possibly, the question of metastasis, about which seemingly nothing has been written for some considerable time.

What is contained in this paper is drawn principally from conclusions reached by Leo Loeb, Doctor Spain, Fibiger and Bulkley—from observations on tissue and tumor growth.

Tissue growth is started by external factors, which bring about similar or identical results in the tissue, even though the causes themselves differ. These are considered primary causes and are referred to by most of these men as "formative stimuli" in order to distinguish them from functional stimuli. It may be that both the formative and functional stimuli are the same, acting in a similar manner; the difference in result depending on the difference in strength and time and in the systems on which they act.

The primary causes may be either physical or chemical. The physical are either mechanical or electrical, the rays of which are held by the tissues. The chemical causes are produced somewhere in the organism itself. Even in the case of parasitic organisms the change is partly through chemical agencies which they produce; there may also be a mechanical effect.

Loeb has shown that chemical stimulus brings about changes in the affected tissue. These changes are partly chemical as is shown by increased oxidation and partly physical as shown by increased water content in the cells.

Doctor Spain demonstrated that small quantities of various rays produce stimulation on various tissues, while large quantities cause destruction.

If a strong stimulus be applied to tissues, which are under an otherwise unfavorable condition, an abnormal response takes place with the formation of giant cells, and syncytia. If the conditions of nourishment to these tissues become still more unfavorable, necrosis results.

It seems that these conditions apply both to normal tissues under abnormal conditions and to tumors, but are much more evident in malignant tumor. Further, that these same physical factors when acting over a long period, on normal tissue produce tumors or cancers. Fibiger has found it possible to produce cancer experimentally by the application of physical and physico-chemical factors, as already referred to. Apparently from his report the transformation from normal tissue to cancer was a slow one passing through several intermediate steps.

The formative stimuli act the same upon tumors and cancers as upon the normal tissues, which may it seems to me in a measure, explain why the cancer mortality under surgical management increased from 63 per 100,000 in 1900 to 81.8 in 1916, or over 28 per cent.

Loeb was able by cuts, incomplete extirpation, transplation of tumors, etc., to excite new growths in tumors both benign and malignant; which teaches us that a tumor probably should not be sectioned for examination, unless that tumor be removed quite soon thereafter, also it may explain why following the disturbance, incident in an operation, of a small cyst or other tumor we have later developing a malignancy.

Chemical formative stimuli undoubtedly play a considerable part in the natural growth and development of normal tissue.

The difference in the growth of certain organs in the young and the old, and in different races of people, and in different climates seems to suggest the difference not only in the chemical substances circulating in the blood which affect the growth not only in normal tissues under normal conditions, but also the tissues under abnormal conditions, that is with reference to nourishment, oxidatio■, etc., but also that there is a varying resistance on the part of the tissues in certain systems against the effect of these chemical formative stimuli. Analagous substances seems to favor growth or delay of tumors in several typrs of animal life. The amphibia for example. We see from Loeb's reports some indications that during pregnancy tumors may assume large proportion in the rat, while in the mouse pregnancy seems to exert a very unfavorable influence on the growth or development of transplanted tumors so that it may be in the future that original and secondary, (or primary and metastatic tumors), will be considered as separate and distinct things.

The corpus luteum bears a specific relation to the uterine wall and the mammary gland in the normal course of metabolism, also artificially given it has a definite effect upon the ovary in its essential function, that of ovulation. So that this probably comes under the second class, that of metastatic conditions. A Japanese investigator recently in some experiments with corpus luteum on the hen demonstrated beyond question that it has a positive inhibitory action on ovulation. It has been proven experimentally in the case of cancer of the mammary gland in mice that there can be no doubt that these special substances play an important part in changing normal into cancerous tissues. By extirpation of the ovaries at maturity the spontaneous development of cancer of the breast, so common in certain strains of mice, can be almost altogether prevented.

There is another class of substances which prevent growth, as for example iodine, which according to Marine prevents compensatory hypertrophy of the thyroid, likewise according to Pearl calcium seems to counteract certain effects of the corpus luteum substances, as well as having a tendency to somewhat inhibit the growth of inoculated tumors. Again certain of these formative stimuli established in the etiology of tumor growth may bring about a converse condition, as for example assuming that heredity forms a part, along this line, the development of the stimulus may reach the point where it prevents the growth of tumor for one or two generations, when having lost its power or met new conditions in succeeding generations again acts as a productive factor.

In considering them a fully established cancer, it might be concluded that cancer is tissue growth in which a chemical stimulus probably not very different from that necessary to normal development is constantly at work producing changes which accompany all growths. So that internal secretions may be responsible for the production of cancer. It has been an accepted fact for some time that long continued stimulations may produce cancer; whether the chemical stimulus must be transmitted to the cells by an outside agency or whether long continued stimulation of tissue ultimately leads to such a change in the cell that the cell itself is unable to produce continuously the substance, which propagates the growth, is probably the thing yet to be decided.

Of the attempts to unite the various facts into consistent theory of tumor and tissue immunity and growths, only two recent ones seem to have attracted any particular attention, one by E. E. Tyzzer explains the immunity as due to a local anaphylactic reaction, that is some substance is given off by the tumor cells which combines with the body fluid. The other by Loeb has to do with the mutual chemical incompatibility of the body fluids of one individual with the tissues of the other, forming abnormal products which are induced to produce dense fibrous tissue.

Williams remarks "a mass of evidence could be adduced to show that cancer is a disease of hypernutrition;" this may mean when taken with the findings of others that normal nutrition can be overdone, or that the complex of modern civilization with all its temptations and errors in regard to eating and drinking, together with the nervous strain and the absence of physical exercise, does produce such a disturbance of the normal internal stimuli as to produce new growths.

At any rate the fact remains that while cancer is very infrequent among primitive people and among animals living in the state of nature, it is on the increase in morbidity and mortality with the increase of civilization. There can, therefore, be hardly any other conclusion than that this dire disease depends largely upon the conditions developed by or associated with our artificial existence, to which is given the name "modern civilization."

CANCER OF THE UTERUS.

By ROSS GROSSHART, M. D., Tulsa, Okla.

Cancer of female uterus and its appendages has been the destruction of women in great numbers, and it behooves the medical and surgical profession to relieve this condition by improving our methods as follows:

Until we know the true etiology of this malady we will not be able to prevent or cure all cases—but if we will use intelligently the known remedies we can prevent in a great measure the horrors and suffering of the female race.

First—let's be honest with our patients and strive to make an early diagnosis by careful history, by manual examination and observation. Don't try to prove or disprove your diagnosis by taking a microscopical specimen—safer to do complete hysterectomy as far as the patient is concerned on suspicious cases. Had better remove a few benign uteri at the age we find these disputed diagnoses than to allow one to go on and die with cancer.

These cases that are on the border line are as a rule around 40 years of age and have as a rule had their family, and you are not cheating the woman out of anything, and probably saving her a great amount of suffering, provided, the condition does not prove malignant. A uterus diseased sufficiently to simulate cancer will surely give trouble at menopause, which can be averted by removal.

Summing up what I have tried to say in short: A woman 35—irregular bleeding with leukorrhea—do not prescribe douches; make a diagnosis.

A suspicious diagnosis having been made, do not curette because a patient wants you to, and because you do not feel capable of doing major surgery. Be honest and do not jeopardize her life by allowing her to dictate to you; or your craving for money lead you astray, by doing a more simple operation (which always sounds good to a patient).

The female race would be better off if two out of three cases proved benign than to allow the third to die with cancer. An early operation is simple—mortality low. No damage to patient's future, and a happy menopause and complete relief of mind.

Operative Procedure.

Some of the readers of this article would probably like to have my idea of the operative procedure, which I will gladly give without hestitation. I would mention vaginal hysterectomy only to condemn it for cancer.

Surgery: If the malignancy is diagnosed early—sterlization of vagina—cauterize cervix, make incision through culdesac and around cervix. Push bladder away from uterus, do not cause undue manipulation of uterus. Control hemorrhage. Place iodoform gauze in vagina. Prevent contaminated air reaching peritoneal cavity. Open belly and complete hysterectomy by clamping and incising between same. Put ligature of soft catgut No. 2 on blood vessels; start at one side with continous ligature. Cover raw surfaces with peritoneum to opposite side after you have transplanted round ligaments into wall of vagina. Close belly without drain. If your cancer has been extensive, do a Wertheim after the description in text book. You will find it easier to leave the uterus intact by starting from vaginal side.

RELATIVE ETIOLOGY AND PATHOLOGY OF CANCER.

By W. FOREST DUTTON, M. D., Tulsa, Okla.

That cancer is deserving of continual study is made very clear when we understand the enormous number of lives lost anually by this cause. The special monograph, "Mortality from Cancer and other Malignant Tumors" (Bureau of the Census, 1914), shows that 52,420 deaths were assigned to these causes during the calender year 1914. This number of deaths occurred in that portion of the United States embraced in the registration area for deaths—this represents only 66.8 per cent. of the total population of continental United States. The 52,420 deaths is equivalent to a death rate of 79.4 per 100,000 people living. Assuming that this death rate is applicable to the entire country, it would mean that 78,730 deaths, if all deaths were registered, would have occurred in the United States during 1914 (F. L. Watkins).

W. Roger Williams (Natural History of Cancer, 1019) states that there has been an increase in the cancer death rate from 3 to 5 per cent. during the past thirty years.

In England the deaths, in males over 35 years of age in 1907, show that 1 man out of every 11, and 1 woman out of every 8 died of cancer.

The Aetna Insurance Company record shows that from 1870 to 1906, the death rate from cancer increased from 2.6 to 7.3 per cent. The general increase in the death rate per 100,000 population from cancer in the registration area of the United States between the years 1890 to 1900 was 12.1.

The increase of cancer in the males falls mainly on the alimentary tract, especially the stomach. The increase in the females affects the alimentary tract, breast, and uterus.

The etiological factors worthy of consideration should be considered under the following heads:

1. The occurrence of cancer in the animal and plant kingdoms.
2. Its distribution according to race and country.
3. The relation of certain localities in the same city and country.
4. Its relation to age and sex.
5. The frequency with which certain organs and tissues are affected.
6. The influence of heredity.
7. The influence of occupation and diet.

Cancer in animals bears some similarity to that found in human cancer. This has been fully demonstrated by a process of continued transplantation of its cultural cells.

Carcinoma has been frequently observed in the thyroid of trout, in the kidney of a frog, and in the glands of the skin of the *triton cristatus*.

Jensen (Second International Congress on Cancer at Paris, 1910) reports on tumors which appear to depend upon a persistent and abnormal proliferative power of certain cells on the growth of the beet. He also states that it may be transplanted. Smith has reported a like tumor growing in plants known as crown gall, which he believes to be true tumor due to the presence of bacteria.

L. Hecke (Wiener Klin Woch., 1912) discusses the relation of Smith's discovery to human cancer, and stated that it is questionable if it justifies a conclusion of an etiological factor in human cancer. Malignant tumors are frequently found in mammals. Those animals with which we are most familiar, the dog, horse, mouse, and rat, are frequently affected with cancer. The question of the identity of animal tumors with human cancer has not been successfully answered.

Van Houseman asserts that animal growths do not correspond to human cancer. Apolant (Berl. klin. Woch., 1912) maintains that the features of animal cancer answers our standards for the disease as it occurs in the human race. He includes their histological structure, their invading characteristics, their clinical course, and their ability to form metastases.

It has been found impossible to transplant animal tumors into human beings. All attempts have failed to inoculate human cancer into mice. Metchnikoff was unable to inoculate human cancer into apes. The attempt to inoculate animal tumors into animals of different sprcies has been unsuccessful.

Cancer occurs among all races. It does not show any special predilection for any one race, or locality. Actual statistics reveal that cancer is infrequent in Africa and the South Sea Islands. Rayburn reports that cancer is unknown in Buenos Ayers. A great many authorities believe that cancer occurs more frequently in the higher classes of society. According to statistics from civilized countries the upper strata of social endeavor suffers more than the lower.

Cancer is a disease of decadence. It belongs peculiarly to the later years of life, yet those prematurely aged, by disease, or heredity, are equally prone to to the disease.

The consideration of the distribution of cancer in the human body is of significant importance from an etiological standpoint. This phase of the subject is intimately connected with the relative frequency of cancer in the male and the female.

Cancer without doubt is far more frequent in the female. This fact is accounted for in the large number of cancers found among women in the uterus and breast. The stomach in the male appears to be the most frequently affected organ. Statistics show the stomach, uterus, breast, and abdomen, in order, in both sexes to be most often attacked.

The influence of age upon cancerous conditions is of much importance. The majority of cases of cancer occur in persons from 50 to 60 years of age. Cancer is rare among children. Cases have been reported in children of 5 years.

Hereditary influences in the development of cancer play an important part in the etiology. Paget maintains that heredity is a well known factor in the causation of cancer while Pierson of Middlesex Hospital in London asserts that heredity is a negligible factor. Le Doux Lebarde reported, in the famous case of Madam Z., 15 cases out of 26 offspring of this woman who had cancer, 1 of 7 males, and 14 out of 19 females. According to the "Fourth Scientific Report of the Imperial Cancer Research Fund," "Precise evidence is advanced of the existence of a hereditry predisposition to the development of spontaneous cancer." "It can be inferred with some probability that it is a local or circumscribed tissue predisposition, in virtue of which the mammary tissue is prone to pass from mere proliferative reaction to continuous or cancer proliferation." There is abundant evidence to show that predisposition is transmitted to one organ. This has been proven by observation of certain groups of animals. It is now generally accepted by many authorities (Leven, Bashford, Tyzzier, and others) that hereditary influence has an important bearing on the causation of cancer.

The question of the existence of an exciting cause as a factor in cancer has long engaged the minds of investigators. The relation of trauma to cancer has been recognized by many. Phelps (Annals of Surg,. 1910,) maintains that there is no connection between trauma and cancer. Coley (Annals of Surg., 1911) believes that there is an etiological connection between trauma and cancer. He has observed 970 cases in which a definite history of trauma existed 225 times, or 23 per cent. In 117 cases of the 225, or 52 per cent, the tumor developed within one month after the injury. There is without question the closest relation existing between injury and the development of certain melanotic sarcomas from pigmented moles. Coley personally observed 250 cases of carcinoma in which there was a history of antecedent trauma in 82, or 32.8 per cent; 120 of these were carcinoma of the breast.

The conclusions of Coley and others (McWilliams, Segoud, Ziegler, and Liebes) are that a local trauma of any kind, from chronic irritation to a single contusion, is very often the exciting cause of malignant tumors.

Haberfield (Zeitsch. f. Krebsforshung, 1908) discusses the question of the relation between chronic inflammation of the stomach, gall-bladder, and lungs to cancer. He bases his statements upon the microscopic findings in stomachs in autopsies of 662 cases of gastric cancer. In 106, or 16 per cent., of the cases were found conditions showing that the disease originated from ulcer. MacCarty of the Mayo Clinic (Surg., Gynecol. and Obstet., May, 1910) maintains there is evidence in the microscopic sections of 70 per cent. of gastric cancers, that the latter have originated in ulcer.

In reference to cancer of the biliary passages, Haberfield says that he found stones 119 times in 164 primary cancers. Seiger (Virchow's Archiv., 1893) found gall-stones in 94 out of 99 cases of primary cancer of the common duct. A study of statistics on the subject of cancer demonstrates a close connection between the development of cancer and the various forms of chronic inflammation. Cancer of the stomach is preceded by ulcer; cancer of the biliary passages by the history of chronic cholelithiasis; cancer of the breast by mastitis; and cancer of the cervix uteri by the history of cervical laceration, erosions, or irritative discharges.

The data given does not prove that any one definite etiological factor is the cause of cancer, yet, the one factor is constantly associated with the disease. The great variety of conditions that precede cancer would lead to the conclusion that it is a pathological disturbance associated with normal cell life. The statistics on the influence of occupation on carcinoma are few and unreliable. It appears from the statistics, that are available, that laborers, clergymen, smiths, nurses, and midwives, are the most frequently affected.

Diet has apparently no relationship to the cause of cancer. No diet has been found that appears to affect the progress of this disease. It is, therefore, unwise with our present knowledge to make deductions upon cancer metabolism.

A great many theories have been advanced concerning the *essential nature of cancer*. The *parasitic theory*, after years of painstaking labor and observation by the most competent investigators, has been practically abandoned. No single parasite has been found that will measure up to the standard necessary for the assumption of definite parasitic demonstration.

The clinical course of cancer is diametrical against the parasitic hypothesis. The multiplicity of the forms of chronic inflammatory processes which bear on etiological relation to cancer; its spontaneous development from normal tissue; the formation and growth of metastases, and the immunity of different characters existing among the lower animals indicate the nonspecifity of the cancer organism.

The *autogenic theory* is one based upon a conception which is far more complete. It presents a reasonable explanation of facts surrounding the development of malignant disease. This theory has been divided into two different forms, or phases of two conceptions.

Thiersch, 1865, evolved the idea of the difference in the longevity of the various tissues, and the effect upon one tissue of a disturbance in connection with another. He asserted that the "rarefaction" of the connective tissue stroma is accountable for the growth of cancer.

In 1877, Cohnheim described the existence within the tissues of isolated groups of embryonic cells, and it may be called the embryonic hypothesis. He believed that tumors and cancers arose from unused fragments of tissue, or residues, some of which may be due to faults or embryonic irregularities. Although this theory offers the solution of many difficult problems it does not present the least evidence of a concrete character on the etiology of cancer.

Ribbert combines in a finished theory the essential ideas of Cohnheim and Thiersch and is deserving of special attention. His hypothesis presents as the essential cause leading to the development of cancers an inflammatory process surrounding the proliferating areas. The epithelial cells are separated from each other by the products of such process, and from the single tissue of which they are a part. Then they begin their unlimited proliferation. In many cases it is an isolated complex of embryonal cells which is so acted upon by the chronic inflammatory process.

Janeway, after much detailed study, does not believe that the idea of either Ribbert or that of Bassman include all the factors demanded in the origin of cancer. He maintains that the laws controlling the life, growth, and metaplasia of the normal epithelial cells themselves include in the many cases all that may be needed for the transition into cancer. He concludes that the transition into cancer must be regarded in the nature of a degeneration. The excessive proliferative powers replace normal physiological functions and the degeneration is dependent at times upon the existence of previously isolated cell-complexes. At times it depends upon inflammatory processes of the surrounding connective tissue stroma, and, of more importance, upon no discoverable lesion external to the epithelial cells undergoing change into cancer. He concludes that the individuality of the cells of the organism is a determining factor.

The pathogensis of cancer has always been a fascinating subject of inquiry. Although the subject becomes chimerical when the investigator is imbued with the mirage of theory, yet, this speculation has led to much work of tangible value in special lines. Cancer may occur wherever epithelial tissue is present. The essential part is the invasion of neighboring tissues by groups of cells which present a greater or less deviation in their appearance from the normal cells. The various forms of these growths depend upon the different relation of these cells to each other and to the connective tissue stroma, and to the amount and character of the stroma. The cells of carcinoma generally simulate the epithelium of the tissue in which they arise. Thus it may be acinous, or adenomatous, or alveolar, and at times the epithelial elements may be so excessively developed that the tumor appears to be practically solid with cells. Growths such as these may occur in any glandular organ, but more particularly in the breast, intestines, gall-bladder, and lungs.

It is not the purpose of the author at this time to discuss the different forms of cancer, but briefly to give his views upon carcinoma in a general way.

The study of cancer proper is the study of the cell itself. Primarily cancer is a functional disturbance, and secondarily pathological.

Briefly a reiteration of the predisposing causes will be made. Heredity (according to Mendel's Law) plays an important role insofar as the parents transmit the features, physique, low vitality, and poor construction of any organ or tissue. The caucasians, as a race, are more prone to carcinoma because of the fact that they are more subject to trauma, and to the abuses of civilization. Carcinoma is more frequent in women on account of the frequent injuries to the breast and uterus, and in addition continuous evilation of these organs. As to the affection of other organs with cancer, they are attacked in about the same proportion as men.

Geographical distribution has little if any influence upon the occurrence of cancer, all things being equal.

Any occupation, in which individuals are constantly in contact with irritating substances, predisposes to cancer. Among those may be mentioned soot, tar, paraffin, arsenic, lead, and vanadium.

The exciting causes are, irritation; altered resistence of connective tissue due to trauma and affecting the epithelial cells; infections producing altered resisting function; and chronic irritation.

Irritation of the cell first stimulates its nutritive function affecting every part of the cytoplasm by its inherent conductive powers. As this condition progresses a defensive action of the cell takes place. This intensive defense produces, as it were, an endotoxin due to the hyperactivity of the nuclear dominance over the cytoplasm.. The barrier between the cell and the. irritating agent is broken. Then there is liberated, either by osmosis or the broken cell wall, the endotoxin which in turn becomes the irritant and the toxin. By this process the cells are stimulated to unusual proliferative activity. This progressive growth is manifest by the metastases in the lymph channels and glands in the part affected and the neighboring tissues.

Many forms of carcinoma occur and various subdivisions have been suggested, but, in general, notwithstanding the arrangement of cells, they all present the same essential charcteristics.

After the cell wall is broken, degeneration begins, hence the destruction of tissue. There is the possibility of cancer "plants" existing as the result of rapid degeneration. The affecting agent is the cancer serum or "juice," and its main objective is like tissue devitalized by low resistence. The affinity of the cancer toxin for devitalized epithelial cells of the same individual and not for those of another is convincing evidence that cancer is not inoculable or communicable.

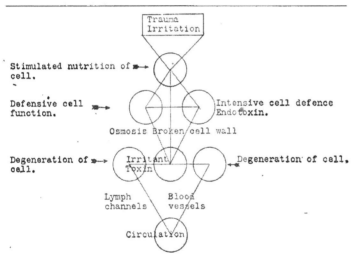

Graphic summary of the phenomena of the pathology of cancer.

Conclusions.

1. Heredity influences the development of cancer because of the predisposition of certain local or circumscribed tissue.

2. Cancer is a disease of decadence. It belongs peculiarly to the later years of life, yet those whose tissues are prematurely aged by disease or heredity are equally prone to the disease.

3. All races are susceptible to cancer.

4. Cancer occurs in organs most frequently subject to continuous irritation, or to trauma.

5. Diet has no relationship to cancer other than the ingestion of irritating substances.

6. Parasites have no etiological relation to cancer except that they may be the source of chronic irritation or inflammation.

7. Cancer is primarily a local disease.

8. The toxin of the cancer cell, or cells, may primarily affect the neighboring cells through cellular osmosis.

9. Cancer cell degeneration is often identical with its antecedent.

10. It has been proven practically impossible to transplant human cancer into animals or to other individuals.

11. Cancer tissue cannot be transplanted from one part of the body to another. Cancer tissue *per se* is not capable of transplantation unless it contain cancer toxin, hence the fallacy of transplantation of cancer from one individual to another.

12. A carcinomatous toxin may be disseminated by the natural metastatic channels.

13. The lymp-channels and glands act as a barrier to the rapid spread of cancer as they do in various other diseases; and when these are destroyed by disease, rapid dissemination takes place through the blood current.

14. Cancer serum or "juice" from one part of the body will, when injected into another part of the body, produce cancer.

15. Cancer in one part of the body renders all epithelial cells in other parts of the body inactive and susceptible to cancer toxin.

16. Cancer is non-inoculable and non-communicable.

AN ENGLISH APPRECIATION OF AMERICAN M. R. C. OFFICERS.

Colonel Furbush, of the Surgeon-General's Office, sends the following excerpts from a letter which he received from Lieut.-Gen. T. H. Goodwin, Director-General of the British Medical Service. The letter is dated May 8:

"This is only a short line as I am extremely busy. I would like to give ycu an extract from a letter which I have just had from G. H. Q. in France. It runs as follows:

'The casualties amongst Medical Officers during the week have been 23, of whom 3 were killed. 5 of the casualties were amongst Mediacl Officers of the U. S. A. attached to British battalions or field ambulances, 4 being "gas" casualties and one "missing" casualty. The work of these U. S. A. Medical Officers deserves special recognition. They have been invaluable and have worked under the most trying conditions and with great gallantry.'

"I thought you would like to know this, and I should be much obliged if you would show it to the Director-General. You are, of course, entirely at liberty to make it known in whatever way you wish, in fact, I should be glad if you would do so for I feel strongly how much we owe to your country, and I should like your people to know how well your Medical Officers are doing. . . . ."

General—then Colonel—Goodwin, it will be remembered, was in this country for over a year, and a large number of our readers will have personal remembrance of him.

It is gratifying to read the message General Goodwin sends. It must be borne in mind that the letter from which General Goodwin sends the quotation was not written with the idea that it would be presented to American readers, but for "home consumption."—*Journal A. M. A.*, June 8, 1918.

THE EARLY DIAGNOSIS OF CANCER OF THE STOMACH.

By C. J. FISHMAN, B. S., M. D.

Assistant Professor Internal Medicine, Medical Department, University of Oklahoma, Oklahoma City.

The early diagnosis of cancer of the stomach based only upon older clinical text-book symptoms may now be considered as an early autopsy diagnosis rather than clinical evidence of the disease.

The newer laboratory and X-ray methods have largely come to the front so that with a carefully obtained history, a thorough physical and laboratory examination, together with accurate X-ray technique, we may find early cancers of the stomach that are amenable to treatment and change materially the prognosis in a diagnosis of this disease. We must, however, never wait for the development of marked symptoms of cancer *per se*. The coffee-ground vomit with obstruction, absence of free hydrochloric acid and emaciation with a palpable tumor spells an absolutely hopeless case. I believe that the development in the diagnosis of cancer of the stomach will reach the point of perfection that the development in the diagnosis of acute appendicitis has reached in offering to the patient a decidedly favorable prognosis in early cases. Many cases will not be typical cancer cases but may be considered precancerous conditions of the stomach which are surgical in nature and operable from a prophylactic point of view. I look forward to the time when the finding of an inoperable carcinoma will reflect upon the diagnostic ability of the examining physician to some degree, as it reflects upon the diagnostic ability of a physician who has watched a case of acute appendicitis from the very beginning and ultimately brings the patient to the surgeon with a large abscess, insisting that such a case is still an acute appendicitis.

The diagnosis depends upon the most thorough painstaking investigation of each individual case. Nothing should be neglected in patients at or past middle life who have irregular and indefinite gastric symptoms which have not been precisely diagnosed. The investigation of these cases should be taken up under the following groups:

I. History Taking.

According to Smithies, this part of the investigation is considered most important as leading to a probable diagnosis, for he says, "There is no proved clinical procedure other than history taking which enables one to make an early diagnosis of gastric cancer." There should be one exception to this statement and that is the careful X-ray investigation of the upper gastro-intestinal canal.

There are in general, two clinical types of symptoms that are obtained in the history of most cancer cases.

Type I, in which there is a fairly definite and regularly accepted history of chronic recurrent gastric ulcer which has undergone degenerative malignant changes. This group is said to comprise two-thirds of the stomach cancer cases. The symptoms are present for a period varying from a few to many years (average about twelve) with periods of remissions and comparative good health.

There is usually pain or discomfort which is definitely related to the time, quality and quantity of food-taking. Large, heavy, coarse meals induce severe discomfort after a long period of freedom, while light, non-irritating foods induce severe discomfort after a long period of freedom, while light, non-irritating foods induce less pain and distress after a shorter period of freedom, The pain is often relieved by further food-taking, vomiting or the use of alkalies. The patients will usually have the "soda habit". Vomiting may occur at the height of the discomfort and hematemesis is also sometimes seen. The history of the beginning of the malignant degeneration often changes the above story decidedly. During the course of an attack the pain may become less severe but more continuous.

Epigastric distress may be more constantly noticed but the symptoms are all aggravated by food taking. There is a less tendency to an interval of complete freedom, as in uncomplicated ulcer. The symptoms are progressive. Blood is found in the stools in 93 per cent. of the cases if examined with sufficient frequency.

Type II, may be considered as "primary gastric carcinoma" cases in which a previous ulcer history is practically, if not entirely, absent. This group comprises approximately one-third of the cases studied. Nasuea, eructations, loss of appetite with occasional mucous vomiting, which is the text-book of chronic gastritis, should always be considered suspicious in patients over forty years of age who have previously never had stomach trouble. These patients usually say that they "never knew they had a stomach" and when complaint is made by such individuals the onset of a gastric cancer of primary type should be considered.

The absence of either of these symptom groups does not completely rule out cancer of the stomach. Cases are occasionally seen which have been diagnosed as primary pernicious anemia without stomach symptoms in which extensive cancer has been found either by operation or autopsy.

II. Physical Examination.

The local findings in early cases are frequently absent, but each patient should be thoroughly examined.

1. **Physical methods.** Palpation will rarely present any signs except a local point of tenderness with slight rigidity which are the principal signs in ulcers and may also be detected in most cases of early carcinoma and can therefore not be considered a differential point. The presence of a tumor, of course, rules out an early diagnosis, although some of these may be amenable to surgical treatment

2. **Stomach tube findings** are of value only when positive, particularly in the presence of a pyloric carcinoma, in which case obstruction symptoms in the form of retention are early present. In tumors of the lesser curvature or towards the fundus, there may frequently be no pathological signs until late in the disease. The presence, however, of microscopic food rests after an eight or ten hour fast is of aid in diagnosing a mild degree of retention, which together with other pathological findings will lead to valuable conclusions.

The stomach tube offers the only means of testing gastric secretion. Properly carried out methods with the Rehfuss tube gives evidence of the emptying power as well as of the latent bleeding.

At this point it may be well to mention a pharmacological-clinical method for the study of gastric function that should be used more extensively, both in connection with the chemical as well as the X-ray study of stomach conditions. I refer to the use of atropine in full doses to decide whether gastric retention is due to spasm associated with chemical changes or to actual tissue narrowing. In the latter case, gastric retention usually signifies a surgical condition, whether due to hyperplastic ulcer or to carcinoma.

III. Laboratory Examinations.

Laboratory tests should be carried out in all cases. There is not at this time any single method which has been proved to be reliable, but when used in connection with other methods of diagnosis often prove a valuable aid in drawing conclusions.

The tests for hydrochloric acid show no important changes in early cancer. The method of Gluzinski may be of service. According to him, ulcer is always accompanied by an active catarrh while cancer never develops without an associated mucous gastritis. He has found that the practical utilization of this fact has enabled him to develop a test which is of definite value. After an Ewald test breakfast there may be a normal amount af HCl. However, after giving a meal of two grated, hard-boiled eggs with a glass of water, the aspiration after one hour shows a reduced amount of free HCl. After a meal consisting of soup, a portion of steak, some potato and bread, the gastric examination after three hours shows a still further reduction in free HCl. Normally, there should be a progressively increased production after each test meal of this type.

The demonstration of the so-called cancer ferments and of protein content in test meals has not proved sufficiently reliable to depend much upon the use of these reactions. However, the Neubauer-Fischer Reaction and the Wolff-Junghans Test have been used sufficiently so that they are to be recommended in a complete examination.

In the serum reaction lies the best hope of a positive specific diagnosis of gastric cancer. However, as in all serological methods dependent upon the production of specific antibodies or ferments, it is doubtful whether a sufficiently early diagnosis will be available to offer a favorable prognosis intervention. These methods up to the present time have not been sufficiently perfected to be considered reliable.

Occult blood in the stool is present in 93 per cent of gastric cancers and is a valuable aid in diagnosis together with other signs. The patient should be kept upon a meat-free diet and the stools frequently examined.

Ultimately, the diagnosis of a malignant process depends upon the microscopic examination of the tissue and this should be carried out in all excisions of stomach ulcers in order to verify or exclude the presence of cancer. Ulcers yield promptly to skillful medical treatment and if no improvement is noted in three to four weeks, operative interference is indicated and the lesion under the microsope will frequently show early cancerous change.

IV. X-Ray Examination.

Roentgenologists as well as clinicians are of the opinion at the present time that X-ray examinations in the detection of cancer of the stomach take precedence over all other methods of diagnosis. In the Mayo Clinic, 95 per cent of gastric cancers have been given distinct roentgenologic signs of their presence. In view of these figures every patient of cancer age with indefinite stomach symptoms should be submitted to a thorough X-ray examination. The signs of the presence of a cancer depends upon the type which is developing as well as upon the basis upon which the tumor grows. The location of the cancer as well as the skill of the examiner will determine the percentage of early diagnoses that can be made.

A constantly found filling-defect with clinical signs is sufficient to make a positive diagnosis. Cancers developing upon an ulcer basis will show in many cases evidence differing very little from that of a chronic ulcer. In tumors of the pyloric region, there will be signs of obstruction and retention with irregularity of the pyloric ring.

Ideal results in diagnosing early cancer of the stomach will correlate X-ray and clinical evidence to perfect an early opinion of a suspicious case.

THE UREA INDEX.

Reginald Fitz (New York), France (*Journal A. M. A.*, June 8, 1918), reports the urea index as a test for kidney function in the war hospital. McLean's directions were followed exactly and Marshall's urease method was found most satisfactory, using the permanent preparation of urease described by Van Slyke and Cullen. Cases showing the prognostic value of the test are reported, and also the possibility of its application in a tent hospital with few laboratory facilities. It has the advantage over the phenolsulphonephthalein test in not requiring injections, which may possibly be a source of sepsis, and in being more agreeable to the average patient. As McLean claims, it gives results of practical value in the recognition, prognosis and treatment in certain conditions of impairment of renal function.

PROCEEDINGS OF CLINICAL SOCIETY—ST. ANTHONY'S HOSPITAL, OKLAHOMA CITY.

January 21, 1918

DR. A. A. WILL, President ·   DR. LEILA E. ANDREWS, Secretary

The Society elected the following officers for the ensuing year: President—Dr. Lea A. Riley; Vice-President—Dr. O. J. Walker; Secretary—Dr. Leila E. Andrews.

Dr. Leila Andrews presented a case of Hodgkin's disease that had been under observation for several months. The patient, Mrs.; M., age 29, married 8 1-2 years; father living and well; mother died few months ago, result of cardio-renal-vascular disease; four sisters living—one had an arrested pulmonary tuberculosis; others well; one sister died of puerperal asepsis.

Patient always well as child, except had colds. She was a mouth breather and had adenoids removed when 21. Never had tonsilitis or diphtheria. Had mild typhoid at 16, and arthritis of shoulder at 17. Her first menstrual period was at 11. She has always been regular. Had ·dysmenorrhea until after her first child. She was married at 20, became pregnant one year afterward. Her pregnancy was quite stormy—nausea, vomiting and stomatitis during the whole period. She had a normal delivery with laceration of her perineum. About one week after her confinement she developed a high temperature which lasted a few days, and then disappeared. After she was able to be up her mouth and gums gave her so much trouble that she was under the dentist's care for several weeks. She had during this time conjunctivitis and later was fitted with glasses. Her menstrual periods began when the baby was 1 1-2 months old and continued regularly. After the baby was 1 1-2 years old she began to gain weight and at the end of six months was in quite her usual health. I saw her first, three years ago, when she had a beginning cystocele and rectocele and was quite nervous. She had a repair of cervix and perineum, and the removal of some hemorrhoids. She recovered promptly, and again seemed in normal health. A year afterward she became pregnant and was delivered 2 1-2 years ago of twin boys, one weighing 7 1-2 and the other 5 1-2 pounds. This pregnancy was most miserable. She was toxic—nausea, vomiting and exaggerated stomatitis marked the whole period. Her gums were so swollen that they required attention during the whole time. The stools were lighter in color than normal and occasionally there was bile in the urine. The conjunctivae were slightly tinged with yellow and the skin itched. Blood pressure was never above 140-80. Her confinement was short, altho both babies were breech presentations. A few days after the delivery an anterior cervical gland appeared in the rt. supra clavicular space. This was very tender and painful. When the babies were a week old she began having afternoon temperature and at ten days it was present all day, rising to 103-4 in afternoons. One day she had a hard chill, temperature rising to 10o, followed by profuse sweat, and a fall below normal, at which it stayed for two weeks. She had no abnormal discharge, but smears from discharge from cervix showed the Neisser diplococcus. The gland in her neck remained the size of a hazelnut, and was very tender and painful. Her convalesence was rapid. Menstruation began when babies were seven weeks old. At six months she began to feel tired and easily exhausted. This isolated gland had persisted and under it there seemed to be another. In three months these had grown in size, and a cervical gland appeared in the left side. An X-ray was made of her chest and the mediastinum showed a marked enlargement of glands. The one cervical gland was removed under local anesthesia by Dr. Reed, and a culture was made from the inside of it. The gland was then sectioned and stained and showed the typical picture of Hodgkin's disease.

The patient had many blood examinations made during the three months she was under observation. She had a very moderate leukocytosis—usually ranging from 9000 to 1300². Her Wassermann was negative. She had her tonsils removed, some infected teeth extracted, and a most thorough treatment given the gums. She was placed upon X-ray therapy at a laboratory accustomed to treating this class of cases. She was given a vaccine made from the culture from the diphtheroid bacilli found in the tissue of the gland that was removed. She has been on active treatment for 1 1-2 years, and by the X-ray pictures presented at this meeting the mediastinum shows a marked decrease in glandular enlargement. There are only one or two palpable glands of the neck. None of the axilla. The blood count shows in fact, a leukopenia. She has greatly improved clinically, although the prognosis should be guarded.

WAR FRACTURES.

According to W. S. Baer (Baltimore), France (*Journal A. M. A.*, May 25, 1918), the treatment of fractures from battle causalties is for the most part the treatment of wounds of the soft parts, plus the added difficulities of injuries to bony tissue. Hence the importance of understanding the changes made in the treatment of the soft parts. The essential principles of war surgery are stated by him as follows: "1. All battle wounds are to be considered as infected. 2. It is necessary to remove all projectiles, clothing and devitalized tissue as early as possible, at least before the twelfth hour after injury. 3. These wounds can then be considered as aseptic in character and a primary suture made, thus converting compound fractures into simple fractures, and appropriate treatment for these simple fractures thereupon instituted." The advance in surgery which these imply and which he considers marvelous, is due to the combination and harmonious working together of the surgeon, the roentgenologist and the bacteriologist. The primary suture is the method of selection, when possible, for the beginning of the operation. And it is possible, he says, in 80 to 95 per cent. of the cases, this excluding such minor infections as stitch abscesses. The time in which sutures may be considered primary is the first twelve hours after the reception of the wound; slightly less in cases of face wounds. Its advantages are: lessened mortality from absence of infection; less suffering to the patient; absence or diminution of scar tissue; decreased period of hospitalization; saving of dressings, and often change of compound infected fractures into simple aseptic fractures that may be treated as such. The great enemy to success that is responsible for failure in 5 to 10 per cent. of the primary sutures is the streptococcus. The bacteriologic and roentgen reports are most useful in preventing this complication, and certain virulent streptococci, by themselves or associated with other organisms, may demand the immediate reopening of the primary suture. The delayed primary suture is the method adopted where primary closing of the wound is impossible, as when the patients must be removed at once from the hospital at the front. The tenchic is the same excepting that the skin is not closed and a dry sterile dressing is placed over the wound, and the skin edges brought together in three to ten days afterward. Baer's principal object in his article is to emphasize the necessity of early treatment of bone injuries by primary or delayed primary suture, for this is he, says, the keynote to the successful handling of war fractures. Bone infection is generally secondary to that of the soft parts, and it is in the handling of such cases that the combination of surgeon, bacteriologist and roentgenologist comes into play. The problem of the compound fracture is that of the simple one, and it should be operated on with the same principles, within eight or ten hours of the casualty. Hospitals of sufficient size must be located near enough the zone of advance, to enable the transportation of such cases early enough and should have a sufficient staff of specialists, constantly cooperating.

JOURNAL OF THE OKLAHOMA STATE MEDICAL ASSOCIATION

VOLUME XI	MUSKOGEE, OKLA., JULY, 1918	NUMBER 7

PUBLISHED MONTHLY AT MUSKOGEE, OKLA., UNDER DIRECTION OF THE COUNCIL

DR. CLAUDE A. THOMPSON, Editor-in-Chief

ENTERED AT THE POST OFFICE AT MUSKOGEE, OKLAHOMA, AS SECOND CLASS MAIL MATTER, JULY 28, 1912

THIS IS THE OFFICIAL JOURNAL OF THE OKLAHOMA STATE MEDICAL ASSOCIATION. ALL COMMUNICATIONS SHOULD BE ADDRESSED TO THE JOURNAL OF THE OKLAHOMA STATE MEDICAL ASSOCIATION, 308 SURETY BUILDING, MUSKOGEE, OKLAHOMA.

The editorial department is not responsible for the opinions expressed in the original articles of contributors.

Reprints of original articles will be supplied at actual cost, provided request for them s attached to manuscript or made in sufficient time before publication.

Articles sent this Journal for publication and all those read at the annual meetings of the State Association are the sole property of this Journal. The Journal relies on each individual contributor's strict adherence to this well-known rule of medical journalism In the event an article sent this Journal for publication is published before appearance in the Journal, the manuscript will be returned to the writer

Failure to receive the Journal should call for immediate notification of the editor, 307-8 Surety Building, Muskogee, Okla.

Local news of possible interest to the medical profession, notes on removals, changes in address, deaths and weddings will be gratefully received.

Advertising of articles, drugs or compounds unapproved by the Council on Pharmacy of the A. M. A. will not be accepted.

Advertising rates will be supplied on application. It is suggested that wherever possible members of the State Association should patronize our advertisers in preference to others as a matter of fair reciprocity.

EDITORIAL

CANCER INCREASE.

From statistics alone there would appear to be a marked increase of cancer in the civilized world, and while it is a generally accepted fact that figures do not lie, it is an open question as to whether the increase is real or apparent. There can be no doubt that improvements in diagnosis must account for at least a portion of the reported increase.

Many deaths now recognized to be from certain forms of cancer were earlier not diagnosed as such, but were reported as death from senility or some unknown cause.

When the statistician attempts to determine the relative value of this factor, difficulties are met that cause a divergence of opinion. One holds that cancer is increasing more or less rapidly, another will hold that the increase is only apparent, not real.

Cancer mortality is reported lower but appears to be increasing more rapidly in men than women. This may be apparent also and may be explained by the better methods of diagnosis and that the organs most commonly affected by cancer in men are less accessible than in women.

A parallel to the above is that the reported cancer mortality is lower in the negro than in the white, but is increasing more rapidly; here again this may be explained by the relative correctness of diagnosis.

The increase in reported appendicitis in the United States is parallel with the increase in the reported cancer mortality, which would seem to back up the presumption that the increase is due in large part, if not entirely, to improvements in diagnosis.

PERSONAL AND GENERAL NEWS

Dr. L. B. Sutherland, Ringling, is attending clinics in Chicago.

Alfalfa County General Hospital, Cherokee, was opened June 4th.

Dr. A. W. Harris, Muskogee, has been commissioned Lieutenant M. R. C.

Dr. Phil. F. Herod, Lieutetnant M. R. C., ElReno, has arrived safely in France.

Dr. T. A. Hartgraves, Lieutetnant M. R. C., Soper, is stationed at Camp Travis.

Dr. A. B. Montgomery, Lieutenant M. R. C., Checotah, has arrived safely in France.

Dr. H. B. Spaulding, Ralston, has been appointed Assistant Surgeon in the U. S. Navy.

Dr. J. M. Byrum, Shawnee, attended clinics in Chicago and Rochester, Minn., during June.

Dr. G. A. Wall, Captain M. R. C., Tulsa, has reported for active service at Camp McArthur.

Dr. W. G. Lemon, Lieutenant M. R. C., Tulsa, has been ordered to Fort Bliss for active service.

Dr. E. C. Wilson, Alva, and Miss Marie McManus of Knoxville, Tenn., were married May 11th.

Dr. R. L. Mitchell, Lieutenant M. R. C., Vinita, has been ordered to Camp Sheridan for duty.

Dr. J. H. White, Captain M. R. C., Muskogee, is at Rockefeller Institute for special instruction.

Dr. R. E. Thacker, Lieutenant M. R. C., Lexington, has been ordered to report to Washington, D. C.

Dr. Horace Reed, Captain M. R. C., Oklahoma City, was ordered to report June 22nd for active service.

Dr. W. Forest Dutton, Captain M. R. C., Tulsa, has received orders to report at Camp Mc-Arthur.

Dr. C. A. Thompson, Muskogee, Secretary of the State Association, is ill at Michael Reese Hospital, Chicago.

Dr. E. N. McKee, Lieutenant M. R. C., Enid, has received orders to report for active service at Columbia, S. C.

Dr. Wallace Aitken, Lieutenant M. R. C., Enid, has been ordered to report to Rochester, Minn., for intensive training.

Dr. W. P. Fite, Captain M. C. N. G., Muskogee, stationed at Camp Bowie, and Miss Maurine Mitchell of Fort Worth were married at Fort Worth June 1st.

The Haskell County Medical Society met June 6th and elected the following officers: President, A. B. Callaway, Stigler; Vice-President, J. E. Billington, Brooken; Secretary Treasurer, R. F. Terrell, Stigler; After the county meeting a Haskell County Medical Section of the Council of Defense was organized with the following officers: Chairman, R. F. Terrell; Secretary, T. B. Turner, Stigler.

CORRESPONDENCE

LIEUTENANT MARKS WRITES.

Pittsburg, Pa., April 28, 1918.

Dr. Claude A.. Thompson,
Muskogee, Oklahoma.

Dear Doctor:

I received the certificate of membership in the Oklahoma State Medical Society, today, for which I thank you.

I have just finished the course of special instruction given here and thought that you would be interested in the work.

Dr. William O. Sherman, the Surgeon-in-Chief for the Carnegie Steel Corporation, is giving this work to the Government, gratis. This month we have had thirteen Medical Officers detailed here for the instruction; a similar number is detailed here every month for this work. We have an immense amount of material to work with.

During the first part of the work we have lectuers and clinics, demonstrating the standard treatment of fractures and the use of ambrine in the treatment of burns and the Carrel-Dakin treatment of infected wounds. During the rest of the time we do the work ourselves under his supervision, and have lectures on the recent development of bacteriology, pathology and laboratory work under very competent men.

When we came here we were all very skeptical about what we supposed was the extravagant claims for these new treatments. As we had all read their condemnations both in the A. M. A. Journal and our respective State Journals, we were somewhat biased in our opinions. But after spending one month here and working with them we have been thoroughly convinced that they are a distinct advance in medicine and that where the confusion and adverse reports on them were made, it was probably from the lack of knowledge in the application of the proper technic.   Unless the instructions are followed out minutely, the value of the treatment would be modified or altogether worthless.

The very rapid recovery, the lack of pain and the general condition of the patients under these treatments are remarkable and are more than enough to convince us that in being so slow in adopting these new methods we are neglecting a very valuable aid in keeping up the high standard that we strive for in the profession.   These new treatments should be approached with a more open mind than we are accustomed to giving anything new in the medical line.

Dr. Sherman has accumulated a large volume of statistics supporting the value of these new principles when carefully carried out.   And has also thoroughly convinced us as to their value by actual demonstration.

I beg your pardon for taking up so much of your valuable time but thought that you would be interested in this work.

I am reporting the first of the month to the Base Hospital, Camp Sherman, Chillicothe, Ohio.
Yours very respectfully
Lieutenant W. R. Marks, M. R. C.
(Vinita, Oklahoma)

PROCAINE AND NOVOCAINE IDENTICAL.
To the Editor:

It appears that in certain quarters the attitude is taken that the local anesthetic sold as procaine is not identical with that marketed as Novocaine.   The Subcommittee on Synthetic Drugs of the National Research Council believes it important that this misunderstanding should be corrected and hence offers the following explanation:

The monohydrochloride of para-amino-benzoyldiethyl-amino-ethanol, which was formerly made in Germany by the Ferbwerke-vorm. Meister, Lucius and Bruening, Hoechst A. M., and sold under the trade marked name Novocaine, is now manufactured in the United States.   Under the provisions of the Trading with the Enemy Act, the Federal Trade Commission has taken over the patent that gave monopoly for the manufacture and sale of the local anesthetic to the German corporation, and has issued licenses to American concerns for the manufacture of the product.   This license makes it a condition that the product first introduced under the proprietary name "Novocaine" shall be called Procaine, and that it shall in every way be the same as the article formerly obtained from Germany.   To insure this identity with the German Novocaine, the federal Trade Commission has submitted the product of each licensed firm to the A. M. A. Chemical Laboratory to establish its chemical identity and purity, and to the Cornell pharmacologist, Dr. R. A. Hatcher, to determine that it was not unduly toxic.

So far, the following firms have been licensed to manufacture and sell Procaine:

The Abbott Laboratories, Ravenswood, Chicago.
Ferbwerke-Hoechst Company, New York, N. Y.
Rector Chemical Co., Inc., New York, N. Y.
Calco Chemical Company, Bound Brook, N. J.

Of these, the first three firms are offering their products for sale at this time, and have secured their admission to New and Nonofficial Remedies as brands of Procaine which comply with the New and Nonofficial Remedies standards.

While all firms are required to sell their product under the official name "Procaine", The Farbwerke-Hoechst Company is permitted to use the trade designation "Novocaine" in addition, since it holds the right to this designation by virtue of trademark registration.

In conclusion: Procaine is identical with the substance first introduced es Novocaine.   In the interest of rational nomenclature, the first term should be used in prescriptions and scientific contributions.   If it is deemed necessary to designate the product of a particular firm, this may be done by writing Procaine-Abbott, Procaine-Rector, or Procaine-Ferbwerke (or Procaine (Novocaine) brand)).

Yours truly, .
Julius Stieglitz, Chairman
Subcommittee on Synthetic Drugs,
National Research Council.

MISCELLANEOUS

GREAT DEMONSTRATION BY ARMOUR EMPLOYEES.

Fifteen thousand employees of Armour and Company, more than 75 per cent. of them of foreign birth, got a close up of "the Big Boss," at the Flag Day Exercises June 14 at the Chicago plant. They liked the personal touch and "the Boss" liked it.

When J. Ogden Armour appeared on the speaker's platform with Maclay Hoyne, the principal speaker of the day, and A. Watson Armour, F. Edison White, R. J. Dunham and G. B. Robbins, vice-presidents of the company, he was acclaimed in more than thirty tongues. Every foreign tongue spoken in the United States can be heard in a tour of the Armour plant and the "Viva, Vive, Evviva, Atzye, Niech zyje, Zivio, Eljen, Da, Zdravstvuet and Benzai," were given as lustily as were the typical " 'Ray's" of the Americans.

The real feeling of the crowd was expressed in the muttered comment of one member of the great throng when he spoke aloud to himself, "Gad, this is true Democracy."

Preceding the principal program which included the raising of the flag, a parade was formed which marched through the stock yards and through the streets between the plant buildings.

The Flag Raising Program was held in front of the Armour Wholesale Market and after the singing of the Star Spangled Banner, in which Mr. Armour led, the flag was raised while a bugler played "the salute to the Colors.' Then Mr. Hoyne was introduced and after a few words he gave way to Mr. Armour. When the chief of the great industry arose the stoch yards rocked with the cheers of the thousands. So affected was Mr. Armour that he could not speak and after a "Thank you, thank you, this is great," he called for a cheer for the flag. It was given as a cheer never before has been given in the stock yards. Then the crowd sang America.

During the program the crowd spoke in unison an "American's Creed," which follows:

"I believe in the United States of America as a government of the people, by the people, for the people; whose broad powers are derived from the consent of the governed; a demoracy in a republic; a sovereign nation of many sovereign states; a perfect union, one and inseparable, established upon these principles of freedom, equolity, justice and humanity for which American patriots sacrificed their lives and fortunes. I therefore, believe it is my duty to my country to love it; to support its constitution; to obey its laws; to respect its flag, and to defend it against all enemies."

THE HAY-FEVER PROBLEM.

Notwithstanding the many "specifics" and "near-specifics" for hay-fever that have been brought forward in recent years, the disease, if not precisely enigmatical, continues to baffle and perplex. It is evident that no single therapeutic agent has arisen that can eliminate, or even modify, the symptoms in all cases, individual sufferers presenting problems that are peculiar to themselves. The suprarenal substance, in the form of its isolated active principle, Adrenalin, is undoubtedly one of the most reliable alleviants. One feels justified in saying this in view of the long, efficient service it has rendered in the treatment of hay fever. Not infallible in a strict sense of the word, it affords grateful relief in a vast majority of cases. A powerful astringent, Adrenalin, topically applied, constricts the capillaries, arrests the nasal discharge, minimizes cough, headaches and other reflex symptoms, and hastens the resumption of natural breathing. Adrenalin Chloride Solution and Adrenalin Inhalant are the preparations commonly used, being sprayed into the nose and pharynx. The former should be diluted with four to five times its volume of physiologic salt solution, the latter with three to four times its volume of olive oil.

FROM THE STATE BOARD OF HEALTH, OKLAHOMA CITY.

Dr. John W. Duke, Commissioner.

SUMMER DISEASES.

While certain diseases are more prevalent at one season of the year than at another, it should be kept in mind that this is not so much due to climatic changes, as causes over which we have no control, as it is to our habits which to a large extent vary accordinz to the seeaons. In winter most of us spend a very large proportion of our time indoors and when it is cold we are apt to resort to all sorts of expedients to keep warm. The result is that quite often we subject our bodies to extremes of temperature or try to stay in rooms too "stuffy" for health, Consequently we are apt to suffer from "house diseases" in winter—diseases of the respiratory system, pneumonia, consumption, bad colds, grippe and the like. In addition, we have in winter those special diseases which come from close contact with others. Whooping cough is an example. Diphtheria is to a certain extent another, although this is more common in the fall than the winter.

In summer our habits change. Instead of staying indoors to keep warm, we get out-of-doors much of the time to keep cool. Our work, for a large part of the population, is more apt to take us out doors. The result is just what would be expected—a great decline in the number of respiratory diseases. Pneumonia, except under unusual conditions, seldom comes in summer. The same is true of grippe. Persons suffering from tuberculosis, if not cured, at least improve in condition when spring comes and they spend more time in the open

But if summer saves us from one group of diseases, it exposes us to another set, which might be called outdoor diseases. These are, as stated, essentially the result of our habits and our environments. Take typhoid fever for instance. The germ itself, the primary cause of this disease, is little affected by cold. It can be frozen and when thawed is as active and virulent as ever. Yet as a matter of fact there is less typhoid in winter than in summer. The reason is that our habits do not so much expose us to it and because the season is not so suitable for the carriage of germs from the sick to the well.

In summer, on the other hand, flies are bound to be almost everywhere. They are responsible to a considersble degree for the spread of typhoid. We work more in the open and therefore are more apt to get our hands soiled with the germs of typhoid. Thus it often happens that during August there is more typhoid than during the three coldest months of the year combined. Our diseases are as our habits—and this is the sum and substance of the principle upon which we must base our preventative measure.

Four habits which are largely responsible for the spread of diseases in summer are:

Carelessness in disposinz of the wastes from the human body.

Carelessness in protecting ourselves against summer insects.

Carlessness in our food and drink.

Carelessness in handling soiled articles of all sorts.

By the exercise of a comparatively small amount of care in these four directions the amount of summer disease could be greatly reduced.

PROTECTION AGAINST FLIES.

Everybody knows that flies are a pest and nuisance, but if people realized that they are also dangerous sources of disease stronger effort wculd be made for their elimination. The first practical step toward protection against flies is to have the house well screened. Flypaper, "swatters" and fly poison are also effective against those which get past the screens.   The best poison consists of a mixture of two tablespoonfuls of formalin to a pint of milk and water in equal proportions. This can be placed in saucers or shallow bowls, being more effective if a sponge or crust of bread is also placed in the saucer for the flies to light on. .

It should be remembered, however, that the fly is a tremendous breeder and that getting rid of manure piles and other breeding places is the most thorough and effective method of attacking this dangerous nuisance.

DEAD MEN THREE.

There were three of them trapped in an old chateau—Black Wolf and Terry and Dale.
And round them clamored the surging Huns, with weapons that would not fail.
So they held, each man, to his vantage point, and sent the steel in a storm
That broke the force of the frantic rush and scythe mowed the gray-green swarm.
Black Wolf, the son of a Shawnee chief, and a bad buck Indian, too,
Grinned as he ground at his Lewis gun while its "tac-tac" drilled them through.
Gone were the ways that the white man taught, and the polish of old Carlisle—
The Indian shouted his death song high, then bent to his work with a smile;
A volley shattered the Lewis gun—then he tore from the ancient wall
A battle ax of the olden days, and met the assault in the hall.
His was a death that the greatest chiefs might seek in a masterly pride,
For hand to hand, with a pale face foe, he went out as Tecumseh died!

Terry, the gunman, Bowery boy, fresh from a stretch in the pen,
Fired through the smoke till a stricken mass piled up in that devil's den— .
He smashed his rifle over a head—then his automatic gun
Answered his hand like a living thing as each shot sent death to a Hun.
He had broken his word to the Warden, yes—and under a new coined name
The honor man of the prison squad had plunged in the mightiest game.
His hand was red and his heart was black—at least so the records said—
But the ledger balanced and all was square as the boy pitched forward dead!

Then the citified and handsome Dale, at bay on a winding stair,
Drove back the press of the foremost foes and fought like a grizzly bear;
They rushed in a pellmell fury up, and his bullets dropped them back
Till the stairway's length was filled and choked with a red and hideous wrack;
They grappled him and dragged him down—as he strove beneath their feet
His dulling ears hear distant shouts—and a bugle called retreat!
The Huns gave way—they staggered out—they fled from the iron will
Of the Dead Men Three who had held them hard, till the Flag came over the hill!

—By W. A. Phelon.

COUNCIL ON PHARMACY AND CHEMISTRY.

Partial list of articles accepted in May, 1918.

Parke, Davis & Company: Antipneumococcic Serum, Type 1.

E. R. Squibb and Sons: Antipneumococcic Serum, Type 1.

NEW AND NONOFFICIAL REMEDIES.

Chlorcosane. A liquid, chlorinated paraffin, containing its chlorine in stable (non-active) combination. It is used as a solvent for dichloramine-T and is itself without therapeutic action.

Chlorcosane-Calco: A brand of chlorocosane containing from 31 to 35 per cent. of combined chlorine. The Calco Chemical Co., Bound Brook, N. J.

Chlorcosane-Monsanto: A brand of chlorcosane containing from 27 to 30 per cent. of combined chlorine. Monsanto Chemical Co., St. Louis, Mo. (*Journal A. M. A.*, May 18, 1918, p. 1459).

PROPAGANDA FOR REFORM.

Mayr's Wonderful Stomach Remedy. This is a "patent medicine" adaptation of the old "fake gallstone" trick, which consists of selling large doses of olive or other oil and a saline cathartic. The result of taking this combination is the passage of a number of soapy concretions which the victim is persuaded to believe are gallstones. In 1915 Mayr was convicted under the federal Food and Drugs Act for making false and fraudulent claims for his "remedy". As the Food and Drugs Act applies only to the packages of a preparation and not to store window displays and newspaper advertising, Mayr has revised the labels, etc., for his "patent medicine", but still makes misleading claims elsewhere (*Journal A. M. A.*, May 11, 1918, p. 1393).

Cotarnin. Cotarnin is an artificial alkaloid derived by oxidation from narcotin, by a process analogous to the derivation of hydrastinin from hydrastin (which again differs from narcotin only by an additional OCH₃ group). Cotarnin hydrochlorid is marketed as stypticin, and cotarnin phthalate as styptol. Cotarnin is used systemically mainly against uterine hemorrhage, especially in menstrual hemorrhage, endometritis and congestive conditions. It is ineffective against postpartum hemorrhage or bleeding from gross anatomic lesions, and probably also against hemorrhage in other internal organs. Local application of cotarnin in substance or concentrated solution has a direct vasoconstricting effect and is used in tooth extractions, epistaxis, etc. (*Journal A. M. A.*, May 11, 1918, p. 1396).

Syphilodol. According to the French Medicinal Company, New York, Syphilodol is a "synthetic chemical product of silver, arsenic and antimony", the effects of which are very similar to those of salvarsan and neosalvarsan, with the advantage that, in addition to being available in ampules for intramuscular or intravenous use, it is also furnished in the form of tablets for oral administration. The A. M. A. Chemical Laboratory reports that each Syphilodol tablet contained approximately 3-4 grain yellow mercurous iodid with minute traces of arsenic, silver and antimony. The laboratory further reports that a Syphilodol ampule contained a liquid having the characteristics of water, in which the presence of less than 1-6000 grain of arsenic could be demonstrated. Shorn of its mystery, Syphilodol therefore is essentially the old, well-known "protoiodid of mercury" (*Journal A. M. A.*, May 18, 1918, p. 1485).

Pyocyaneus Bacillus Vaccine. When this vaccine was admitted to New and Nonofficial Remedies in 1910 it gave promise of having therapeutic value. Now the firms whose products are described in New and Nonofficial Remedies advise the Council on Pharmacy and Chemistry that they have ceased to make the vaccine because of lack of demand. Holding the lack of demand as evidence that the vaccine had proved without value, the Council directed its omission from New and Nonofficial Remedies. (*Journal A. M. A.*, May 18, 1918, p. 1496).

The Dr. Chase Company. A fraud order prohibiting the use of mails has been issued by the post office department against the Dr. Chase Company. This patent medicine concern sold three remedies—pills—which, before the Food and Drugs Act made lying on the label irksome if not expensive, were known, respectively, as "Dr. Chase's Blood and Nerve Food", "Dr. Chase's Kidney Food" and "Dr. Chase's Liver Food". Since the enactment of the Food and Drugs Act, however, the term "food" in the name of the nostrums has been changed to "tablets" for obvious reasons. In 1917 K. E. Hafer, the proprietor of the Dr. Chase Company, was fined under the Food and Drugs Act for misbranding. (*Journal A. M. A.*, May 25, 1918, p. 1557).

Capsules of Bismuth Resorcinol Compound. According to the label, each capsule of Bismuth Resorcinol Compound (Gross Drug Co., Inc., New York City) contains bismuth subgallate, 2 grs.; resorcinol, 1 gr.; betanaphthol, 1-2 gr., and creosote (beechwood) 1m. The preparation was declared inadmissible to New and Nonofficial Remedies because unwarranted therapeutic claims were made for it; because the name is not descriptive of its composition, and because the combination of the stated drugs in fixed proportions is irrational (Reports Council Pharmacy and Chemistry, 1917, p. 139).

Elixir Novo-Hexamine. The A. M. A. Chemical Laboratory reports that Exilir Novo-Hexamine (Upsher Smith, St. Paul, Minn.) is not a "stable, palatable, potent preparation of Novo-Hexamine, an acid compound of hexamethylenamine", as claimed, but a flavored and colored solution of sodium acid phosphate and hexamethylenamine in diluted glycerol. The Council on Pharmacy and Chemistry considered the report of the laboratory and the advertising claims, and declared Exilir Novo-Hexamine inadmissible to New and Nonofficial Remedies because its composition is secret; because the ill-advised use by the public is invited; because unwarranted therapeutic claims are made for it; because the name is misleading, and because it is irrational to prescribe hexamethylenamine and sodium acid phosphate in fixed proportions (Reports Council Pharmacy and Chemistry, 1917, p. 142).

Formosol. Sunshine's Formosol (The Formosol Chemical Co., Cleveland, Ohio) is claimed to contain 18 per cent. formaldhyd in a solution of soap. The preparation was refused recognition by the Council on Pharmacy and Chemistry because it was advertised indirectly to the public and because unwarranted therapeutic claims were made for it (Reports Council Prarmacy and Chemistry, 1917, p. 145).

Kalak Water. Kalak Water (The Kalak Water Co., Inc., New York) is a carbonated, artifical mineral water, said to contain in one million parts sodium carbonate, 4,049.0; sodium phosphate, 238.5; sodium chlorid, 806.3; calcium carbonate, 578.2; magnesium carbonate, 48.9, and potassium chlorid, 47.9. In view of the false and absurd claims made, the Council on Pharmacy and Chemistry declared Kalak Water inadmissible to New and Nonofficial Remedies (Reports Council Pharmacy and Chemistry, 1917, p. 148).

Neurosine and the Original Package Evil. Neurosine advertisements ask that only original bottles of Neurosine be dispensed when physicians prescribe the nostrum. The reason is obvious: the bottle has the name blown in the glass and thus is an invitation to the patient to purchase more on his own initiative and also recommend the preparation to his friends. The danger to the public from the self-administration of mixtures of bromides, such as Neurosine, is obvious. Neurosine is said to contain potassium bromid, sodium bromid, ammonium bromid, zinc bromid, extract of lupulin, fluid extract cascara sagrada, extract of henbane, extract of belladonna, extract of cannabis indica, oil of bitter almond and aromatic elixir. This chemical blunderbuss has been advertised for use in insomnia, hysteria, neuresthenia, migraine, etc. It has also been recommended for children suffering from chorea. In all the years that Neurosine has been exploited to physicians with such remarkable claims, we have never seen a report of a careful clinical study in which the product has been used under the conditions which scientific investigation demands. (Journal A. M. A., April 27, 1918, p. 1251).

The Toxicity of Arsphenamin (Salvarsan). James C. Sargent, Milwaukee, Wis., and J. D. Willis, Roanoke, Va., report untoward effects from the intravenous administration of American-made salvarsan (arsphenamin). Such experiences are not unusual, but should be reported. Untoward results followed the use of the German salvarsan. Such reactions may be due to faulty preparation, to deterioration of certain ampules of a batch, to idiosyncrasy of the patient or to faulty technic or preparation or injection. There is no reason to believe that arsphenamin made in this country is more toxic or less satisfactory than that formerly imported from abroad (Journal A. M. A., April 27, 1918, p. 1254).

Misbranded Nostrums. The following are some "patent medicines" which the federal authorities held to be sold under false claims: Ascatco, containing over 13 percent. alcohol and some opium. Mexican Oil, containing over 57 per cent. alcohol, together with essential oils, glycerin ,red pepper, emodin, menthol and a small amount of opium alkaloids. Persil, containing 40 percent. alcohol. Though claimed to contain in addition, asparagus, parsley, celery, buchu, juniper berries, it contained no appreciable quantities of celery, buchu, juniper, asparagus or parsley Dr. D. Kennedy's Favorite Remedy, containing 18 per cent. alcohol, nearly 50 per cent sugar, and over 4 per cent. potassium acetate, with methyl salicylate, aloes, licorice and oil of sassafras. Our Standard Remedy, tablets containing rhubarb, senna,scoparius, licorice, red pepper and some ammonia compound with indications of aloes. Dr. King's Throat and Lung Balsam, claimed to relieve coughs and colds and consumptive patients in the last stages of the disease. "White Pine Expectorant" and "White Pine Balsam" (Allan-Pfeiffer Chemical Co.), a syrup containing alkaloid (probably morphine), chloroform, alcohol, benzoic acid and plant extract, but no extract or tar of white pine. California Tuna Tonic Tablets, pills containing iron carbonate and a small quanity of nux vomica alkaloids (strychnin, etc.). Alorine Antiseptic Suppository, containing quinin sulphate, boric acid and tannic acid. St. Joseph's Quick Relief, containing 32 per cent. alcohol with Peru balsam, camphor and red pepper. "Andrew's Wine of Life Root or Female Regulator", containing over 14 per cent. alcohol, sugar, methyl salicylate and tannin. "Andrews' Wine of Life Root Annex Powders", composed of sodium chloride and sodium bicarbonate, with a small amount of sodium carbonate. Clark Stanley's Snake Oil Liniment, a light mineral oil mixed with about 1 per cent. of fatty oil, red pepper and possibly a trace of camphor and turpentine (Journal A. M. A. April 20, 1918, p. 1183).

NEW BOOKS

Under this heading books received by the Journal will be acknowledged. Publishers are advised that this shall constitute return for such publications as they may submit. Obviously all publications sent us cannot be given space for review, but from time to time books received, of possible interest to Oklahoma physicians, will be reviewed.

MEDICAL WAR MANUAL, NUMBERS FIVE AND SIX.

(Authorized by the Secretary of War and Under the Supervision of the Surgeon General and the Council of National Defense)

Number Five. Lessons From the Enemy. How Germany Cares for Her War Disabled. By John R. McDill, M. D., F. A. C. S., Major, Medical Reserve Corps, U. S. Army. Illustrated. Price $1.50. Lea and Febiger, Philadelphia and New York.

We believe we have seen nothing approaching this little volume in the meatiness of its contents. The illustrations are good, practically all originals and the work contains so much that is new, every medical reserve corps man should have a copy.

Number Six. Laboratory methods of the United States Army. Compiled by the Division of Infectious Diseases and Laboratories, office of the Surgeon General, War Department, Washington, D. C. Illustrated. Price, $1.50.

A TEXT-BOOK OF OBSTETRICS. By Barton Cooke Hirst, M. D., Professor of Obstetrics in the University of Pennsylvaina. Eighth edition, revised and reset. Octavo of 863 pages, with 715 illustrations, 38 of them in colors. Philadelphia and London: W. B. Saunders Company, 1918. Cloth, $5.00 net.

THE PRACTICE OF PEDIATRICS. By Charles Gilmore Kerley, M. D., Professor of Diseases of Children, New York Polyclinic Medical School and Hospital. Second edition, revised and reset. Octavo of 913 pages, 136 illustrations. Philadelphia and London: W. B. Saunders Company, 1918. Cloth, $6.50 net.

PRINCIPLES OF SURGICAL NURSING. A guide to Modern Surgical Technjc. By Frederick C. Warnshuis, M. D., F. A. C. S., Visiting Surgeon, Butterworth Hospital, Grand Rapids, Michigan., Chief Surgeon, Pere Marquette Railway. Octavo of 277 pages with 255 illustrations. Philadelphia and London: W. B. Saunders Company, 1918. Cloth, $2.50 net.

THE NERVOUS SYSTEM AND ITS CONSERVATION. By Percy G. Styles, Assistant Professor of Physiology in Harvard University; instructor in Boston, School of Physical Education. Second edition revised. 12mo of 240 pages, illustrated. Philadelphia and London: W. B. Saunders Company, 1917. Cloth, $1.50 net.

DIFFERENTIAL DIAGNOSIS. Presented through an Analysis of 317 cases. By Richard C. Cabot, M. D., Assistant Professor of Clinical Medicine, Harvard University Medical School, Volume 2, Second Edition. Octavo of 709 pages, 254 illustrations. Philadelphia and London: W. B. Saunders Company, 1918. Cloth, $6.00 net.

OFFICERS OF COUNTY SOCIETIES, 1918

County	President	Secretary
Adair	A. J. Sands, Watts	A. J. Patton, Stilwell
Alfalfa	H. A. Lile, Aline	W. H. Dersch, Carmen
Atoka-Coal		A. Cates, Tupelo
Beaver		
Beckham		V. C. Tisdal, Elk City
Blaine	J. B. Leisure, Watonga	J. A. Norris, Okeene
Bryan	J. L. Reynolds, Durant	D. Armstrong, Durant
Caddo	A. H. Taylor, Anadarko	Chas. B. Hume, Anadarko
Canadian	P. F. Herod, El Reno	W. J. Muzzy, El Reno
Choctaw	V. L. McPherson, Boswell	E. R. Askew, Hugo
Carter	F. W. Boadway, Ardmore	Robt. H. Henry, Ardmore
Cleveland	J. J. Gable, Norman	Gayfree Ellison, Norman
Cherokee	W. G. Blake, Tahlequah	C. A. Peterson, Tahlequah
Custer	J. Matt Gordon, Weatherford	C. H. McBurney, Clinton
Comanche	E. R. Dunlap, Lawton	General Pinnell, Lawton
Coal-Atoka		A. Cates, Tupelo
Cotton		G. O. Webb, Temple
Craig		R. L. Mitchell, Vinita
Creek		H. S. Garland, Sapulpa
Dewey		E. J. Hughes, Vici
Ellis		
Garfield	*H. B. McKenzie, Enid	A. Boutrous, Enid
Garvin	H. P. Markham, Pauls Valley	N. H. Lindsay, Pauls Valley
Grady	D. S. Downey, Chickasha	Martha Bledsoe, Chickasha
Grant		C. H. Lockwood, Medford
Greer	Nay Neel, Mangum	Thos. J. Horsley, Mangum
Harmon	W. T. Ray, Gould	R. L. Pendergraft, Hollis
Haskell		R. F. Terrell, Stigler
Hughes		
Jackson	T. H. Hardin, Olustee	W. H. Rutland, Altus
Jefferson		L. B. Sutherland, Ringling
Johnson		H. B. Kniseley, Tishomingo
Kay		A. S. Risser, Blackwell
Kingfisher		C. W. Fisk, Kingfisher
Kiowa		A. L. Wagoner, Hobart
Latimer	E. B. Hamilton, Wilburton	E. L. Evins, Wilburton
Le Flore	E. E. Shippey, Wister	Harrell Hardy, Bokoshe
Lincoln	A. M. Marshall, Chandler	C. M. Morgan, Chandler
Logan		E. O. Barker, Guthrie
Love		
Mayes	J. L. Adams, Pryor	L. C. White, Adair
Major		
Marshall		
McClain	J. W. West, Purcell	O. O. Dawson, Wayne
McCurtain		R. H. Sherrill, Broken Bow
McIntosh	B. J. Vance, Checotah	W. A. Tolleson, Eufaula
Murray		W. H. Powell, Sulphur
Muskogee	J. G. Noble, Muskogee	A. L. Stocks, Muskogee
Noble	L. D. Stewart, Perry	B. A. Owen, Perry
Nowata	J. E. Brookshire, Nowata	J. R. Collins, Nowata
Okfuskee	J. S. Rollins, Paden	A. O. Meredith, Bearden
Oklahoma	John A. Reck, Oklahoma City	H. H. Cloudman, Oklahoma City
Okmulgee	W. C. Mitchner, Okmulgee	Harry E. Breese, Henryetta
Ottawa	A. M. Cooter, Miami	Blair Points, Miami
Osage	G. W. Goss, Pawhuska	Benj. Skinner, Pawhuska
Pawnee		E. T. Robinson, Cleveland
Payne	E. M. Harris, Cushing	J. B. Murphy, Stillwater
Pittsburg	T. H. McCarley, McAlester	J. A. Smith, McAlester
Pottawatomie	R. M. Anderson, Shawnee	G. S. Baxter, Shawnee
Pontotoc	B. F. Sullivan, Ada	Catherine Threlkeld, Ada
Pushmataha	H. C. Johnson, Antlers	Edw. Guinn, Antlers
Rogers	W. E. Smith, Collinsville	W. A. Howard, Chelsea
Roger Mills		Lee Dorrah, Hammon
Seminole		
Sequoyah	W. M. Hunter, Vian	Sam A. McKeel, Sallisaw
Stephens	D. M. Montgomery, Marlow	H. C. Frie, Duncan
Texas	W. H. Langston, Guymon	R. B. Hays, Guymon
Tulsa	H. D. Murdock, Tulsa	W. J. Trainor, Tulsa
Tillman		
Wagoner	C. E. Hayward, Wagoner	S. R. Bates, Wagoner
Washita	D. W. Bennett, Sentinel	A. S. Neal, Cordell
Washington	G. F. Woodring, Bartlesville	J. G. Smith, Bartlesville
Woodward	R. A. Workman, Woodward	C. W. Tedrowe, Woodward
Woods	G. M. Bilby, Alva	D. B. Ensor, Hopeton

*Deceased

OFFICERS OF OKLAHOMA STATE MEDICAL ASSOCIATION.

President—Dr. L. J. Moorman, Oklahoma City.
1st Vice-President,—Dr. E. D. James, Miami.
2nd Vice- President—Dr. H. M. Williams, Wellston.
3rd Vice-President,—Walter Hardy, Ardmore.
Delegate to A. M. A., 1919-1920—LeRoy Long, Oklahoma City.
Meeting place, Muskogee—May, 1919.

CHAIRMEN OF SCIENTIFIC SECTIONS.

Surgery and Gynecology—A. A. Will, Oklahoma City.
Pediatrics and Obstetrics—
Eye, Ear, Nose and Throat—
General Medicine, Nervous and Mental Diseases—F. W. Ewing, Muskogee.
Genitourinary, Skin and Radiology—
Legislative Committee—Dr. Millington Smith, Oklahoma City; Dr. J. M. Byrum, Shawnee; Dr. W. T. Salmon, Oklahoma City.
For the Study and Control of Cancer—Drs. LeRoy Long, Oklahoma City; Gayfree Ellison, Norman; D. A. Myers, Lawton.
For the Study and Control of Pellagra—Drs. A. A. Thurlow, Norman; L. A. Mitchell, Frederick; J. C. Watkins, Checotah.
For the Study of Venereal Diseases—Drs. Wm. J. Wallace, Oklahoma City; Ross Grosshart, Tulsa; J. E. Bercaw, Okmulgee.
Necrology—Drs. Martha Bledsoe, Chickasha; J. W. Pollard, Bartlesville.
Tuberculosis—Drs. L. J. Moorman, Oklahoma City; C. W. Heitzman, Muskogee; Leila E. Andrews, Oklahoma City.
Conservation of Vision—Drs. L. A. Newton, Oklanoma City; L. Haynes Buxton, Oklahoma City; G. E. Hartshorne, Shawnee.
First Aid Committee—Drs. G. S. Baxter, Shawnee; Jas. C. Johnston, McAlester.
Committee on Medical Education—Drs. A. L. Blesh; A. K. West; A. W. White, Oklahoma City.
State Commissioner of Health—Dr. John W. Duke, Guthrie, Oklahoma

COUNCILOR DISTRICTS.

District No 1. Texas, Beaver, Cimarron, Harper, Ellis, Woods, Woodward, Alfalfa, Major, Grant, Garfield, Noble and Kay.
District No. 2. Dewey, Roger Mills, Custer, Beckham, Washita, Greer, Kiowa, Harmon, Jackson and Tillman.
District No. 3. Blaine, Kingfisher, Canadian, Logan, Payne, Lincoln, Oklahoma, Cleveland, Pottawatomie, Seminole, and McLain.
District No. 4. Caddo, Grady, Comanche, Cotton, Stephens, Jefferson, Garvin, Murray, Carter and Love.
District No. 5. Pontotoc, Coal, Johnston, Atoka, Marshall, Bryan, Choctaw, Pushmataha and McCurtain.
District No. 6. Okfuskee, Hughes, Pittsburg, Latimer, LeFlore, Haskell and Sequoyah.
District No. 7. Pawnee, Osage, Washington, Tulsa, Creek, Nowata, and Rogers.
District No. 8. Craig, Ottawa, Delaware, Mayes, Wagoner, Cherokee, Adair, Okmulgee, Muskogee, and McIntosh.

STATE BOARD OF MEDICAL EXAMINERS.

Melvin Gray, M. D., Durant, President; B. L. Denison, M. D., Garvin, Vice-President; J. J. Williams, M. D., Weatherford, Secretary; O. R. Gregg, M. D., Waynoka, Treasurer; E. B. Dunlap, M. D., Lawton; Ralph V. Smith, M. D., Tulsa; W. LeRoy Bonnell, M. D., Chickasha; Wm. T. Ray, M. D., Gould; H. C. Montague, D. O., Muskogee.
Reciprocity with Georgia, Kentucky, Mississippi, Nevada, North Carolina, Wisconsin, Kansas, Arkansas, Virginia, West Virginia, Nebraska, New Mexico, Tennessee, Iowa, Ohio, California, Colorado, Indiana, Missouri, New Jersey, Vermont, Texas, Michigan.
Meetings held second Tuesday of January, April, July and October, Oklahoma City.
Address all communications to the Secretary, Dr. J. J. Williams, Weatherford.

IN WRITING ADVERTISERS, PLEASE MENTION THIS JOURNAL

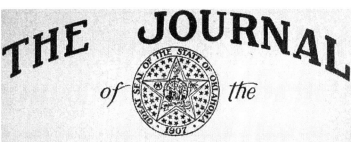

THE JOURNAL

of *the*

Oklahoma State Medical Association

| VOLUME XI | MUSKOGEE, OKLA., AUGUST, 1918 | NUMBER 8 |

RECTAL EXAMINATION IN LABOR.*

By C. V. RICE, M. D., Muskogee, Oklahoma

Every obstetrical case should be treated as a surgical case and have the same protection. The fact is now well known that childbed fever is in reality a wound infection similar to an infection after an accident or an operation, and it can be prevented by the same measure of cleanliness and asepsis which is used so universally in modern surgery. No surgeon of today would think of entering the abdomen without sterile gloves. Yet such is being done in obstetrics. The most frequent cause of infection in labor is by the vaginal examination and for all practical purposes one can gain the necessary information rectally. Experience has shown that the major part of all serious cases of infection at child-birth may be prevented by the application of such principles of hygiene and strict surgical cleanliness.

Dr. Grace L. Meigs of the Children's Bureau, Department of Labor, Washington, D. C., states that in the last thirteen years there has been no improvement in puerperal infection, while there has been a striking decrease of the mortality rates for typhoid, diphtheria, and tuberculosis. Typhoid has been cut in half, diphtheria reduced by more than fifty per cent., and tuberculosis about twenty-five per cent. There are eight thousand women who die annually in this country from this preventable infection, and in the child-bearing woman between the ages of fifteen and forty-four the death rate is second to tuberculosis. Where one woman dies of this infection, five get well. If this is so, then forty thousand cases of childbed fever occur each year in the United States.

Dr. De Lee states that in these mild cases of infection, the woman has slight rise of temperature, often lasting but a day or two. There may be only a slight pelvic pain, but anatomic traces of the infection are bound to be left. Later, we find peritoneal bands, occluded tubes, distorted and displaced uterus, rectum, bladder and ureters, and hundreds of thousands of women date life-long invalidism from an infectious process in the puerperium. He also states that obstetrical asepsis and antisepsis have not yet penetrated the body of the medical profession and in some instances they have hardly touched the surface.

While at the Chicago Lying-In Hospital, I made two thousand rectal examinations and those on about seven hundred women. Not one ever protested. Of course, there would be some who would remark that it was the first time they were ever examined by this method and would express their appreciation when told the object.

*Read at the 26th Annual Meeting, Tulsa, Okla., May 15, 1918.

251

If a vaginal was thought to be necessary, the patient was taken to the birth room, prepared and draped as for a delivery. The attending man would scrub, put on a cap, mouth-piece, sterile gown and gloves. This is the precaution that is taken at that institution and for this reason they can boast of a mortality of sixteen out of 30,000 cases.

After the external examination, what information is to be gotten, that cannot be obtained rectally? Per rectum, you can make out the dilatation, effacement, presentation, and engagement—membrane and bulging of same if intact and also sutures.

Rectal, as a substitute for vaginal examination, was suggested by Kroenig, before the Obstetrical Society of Liepzig, November 20th, 1893. Emil Reis, now of Chicago, began an investigation of the possibilities of rectal examinations and published his results a few weeks after Kroenig. De Lee and Edwards, then of Cook County Hospital, took it up in this country, not confining it to obstetrics alone. They abandoned the method, due to the fact that they had no rubber gloves at that time. The last few years, De Lee has been teaching rectal examination and the internes have been teaching same to the students during their dispensary service.

It has been seventy-five years since Oliver Wendell Holmes published his paper on the contagiousness of childbed fever, seventy-two years since Semmelweiss made his startling observations in the Vienna Hospital, and about forty years since Pasteur so positively declared that childbed fever was of bacterial origin and was carried by doctors and nurses. Still in this day of advanced medicine and surgery, the second greatest mortality in the child-bearing woman is childbed fever. Is this not sufficient proof that vaginal examination should be abandoned and replaced by the rectal?

Vaginal examination should not be made near term and if abortion is in progress. The rectal touch will furnish us with the desired information up to the point of operative intervention. In all cases of suspected cesarean section, the rectal should be practiced, as we know that the contamination produced by one or more vaginal examinations during the test of labor, influence the outcome of the end results more than anything else unless it is exhaustion or attempts at delivery with forceps or otherwise. Yet we hear of surgeons doing sections who have attempted version. We also hear of surgeons who have had the assistant place his hand in the vagina and push the engaged head out of the pelvis. This technique is very poor including the art and this kind of obstetrical practice adds to our high mortality list of twenty thousand mothers and over two hundred fifty thousand babies dying each year in child-birth in the United States.

The method of rectal examination is very simple. The woman during her antipartum treatment should be told that as soon as she feels pain, she must take an enema. The left index finger is used in the examination, as we should educate the left hand for sense of touch and the right for strength. If you arrive when the patient is in the second stage of labor, it is easy to slip on a rubber glove, lysolize and lubricate same and pass through the anus slowly and carefully, as this method of examination can be done without any particular preparation of the patient. At the same time you can obtain all the information as to the progress of labor and can adjust the time necessary to make the set up.

In conclusion I wish to say:

Vaginal examination should be made subordinate to the rectal.

That the rectal is as definite as the vaginal.

That the rectal should be made in all tests of labor.

In normal labors, with ordinary care, it eliminates all possible chance of infection which is the most important thing to consider in child-birth.

Discussion.

Dr. H. M. Reeder, Shawnee: When I was first asked to discuss this subject, I really did not know much about it, and after reading up all the literature I could get on the subject, I knew less about it than before.

Some years ago I read an article on rectal examination in labor, and I tried out one or two cases but I could not learn anything from such an examination myself. Possibly with greater experience I could have. It seemed to me with proper asepsis there is not a great deal of necessity for continual examinations anyway. What one has to learn from examining internally he cannot learn from external examination; a vaginal examination with me would be highly imperative and with proper asepsis, the same asepsis you give to other surgical cases of abdominal laparotomies and things of that sort, the danger of infection is practically eliminated.

That is all I have to say on this subject.

Dr. W. A. Fowler, Oklahoma City: Mr. Chairman, I want to say that I most heartily approve this paper in toto. I have been making rectal examinations for about two years.

At first the making of a rectal examination, as Dr. Reeder says, is worthless. You remember the first vaginal examination you ever made; don't you remember how perfectly useless it was to you, that you could not detect anything at all about the parts you were feeling for? You have to become accustomed to a rectal the same as you have become accustomed to a vaginal examination.

It is the exception in my own practice for a multipara to have a vaginal examination during labor, or a primipara with a border-line pelvis after the antipartum examination is made at least a month or six weeks before term.

I had a case yesterday, for instance, with a slightly contracted outlet and I told the patient of the condition, and I will make no vaginal examinations during the labor. I also told them that this is a case in which this patient will probably be able to deliver herself, but it is what we call a border-line case, and if they want the judgment of another man, now is the time to have the consultation. I told them I would be very glad to have any other man see this patient in consultation, but that if they wanted someone else to see her it will be very much better to have the consultant see the patient a month before term than during labor.

As a matter of fact, the patient goes into labor and we repeatedly examine her; the people become anxious, and while we might know the condition they ask for a consultation. The consultant comes in and examines her and we are multiplying the chances for infection. Abortion is followed by a higher percentage of morbidity than full term labor; and the old rule that was laid down a long time ago was not to invade the threshold of the vagina until you are ready to go to the dome of the uterus.

We are too careless of abortions; we go in and examine without using the technique that we do for labor. The test of labor, as I suggested, is something that we have not appreciated the meaning of. By waiting for the test of labor we mean that we wait for the natural forces of labor without our interference.

If we repeatedly examine the patient, if we attempt forceps, if we attempt version, we are not waiting for the test of labor; we are meddling and we are destroying the patient's chances to receive the best results from whatever operative procedure may be indicated.

The diagnosis of position is sometimes uncertain and in these cases I think we ought to make a vaginal examination. In the beginning of our rectal examinations, we will probably need to make a vaginal examination in every case because our diagnosis will not be accurate; but as we go along there will be few cases in which we are not just as certain as we would be by the vaginal examination, and in those cases in which we are in doubt—for instance if we suspect an occipital posterior and are not sure—we should make a vaginal examination.

Dr. J. A. Hatchett, El Reno: We cannot emphasize this subject too deeply. I began the practice of medicine when we attributed childbed fever to the providence of God, to the rarity of the atmosphere or something else we did not know what. We went on as best we could. We did not believe what was said about it and we were not taught to believe it; in our lectures there was nothing said about aseptic precautions in labor, and probably a few that hear me will bear me out in that assertion. When the change did take place, it took place very rapidly.

You will remember that Meade Potts vituperated Oliver Wendell Holmes, even attacking him personally for that grand masterly speech he made, so vindictive were they. And the very next year Penrose, their student, took up aseptic obstetrics and practiced it from that on.

But when the change did take place, it took place tolerably rapidly in the minds of a few, but the many remained dormant and paid no attention to this judgment of great men.

Twenty years ago I read a paper before this Oklahoma Medical Association in which I emphasized the importance of aseptic obstetrics and they laughed at me; there are men here in this house who laughed at me. They said, "There is something wrong with Dr. Hatchett; he is crippled in the brain; we do not have any of these troubles at all, we get along all right. Dr. Hatchett has overdrawn this thing and has put emphasis on a thing that really has no intrinsic value."

That hardly seems like the truth; that seems like I am telling you a yarn from this floor. But it is a fact and can be substantiated by some of the old members.

But the change took place rapidly. Dr. Hatchett kept on writing his papers and reading them, and he kept on emphasizing these things, and Dr. Hatchett has seen many close their eyes in death just at the time when a new world of happiness was pressing upon a heart. He has seen many a one, and he has seen many a one that was the result of his own hands, but he was not to blame a bit more than other people were to blame at those times. But now we are to blame; we all know. We all know in regard to these vaginal examinations. I used to make ten times as many as I ought to make. I conduct many of my cases without making a vaginal examination at all. It is just foolishness; it is idle interference with the case and not necessary.

After you have examined your case thoroughly, you watch your labor, watch the bulging of the perineum, keep your hands out. If it is a multipara you have made an external examination; you know where the head is; you may not know whether it is occipital or not but you know where it is, and I do not make an examination in that case.

The rectal examination is all right; I have never practiced it but it is all right. I can see that it is all right because the rectal and vaginal walls are very thin. We are surprised how well we can mark out the vaginal condition through the rectum. I heartily agree with the gentleman who read that paper and I believe that henceforth, though I am old and gray, when I make an examination I will make a rectal examination. There are several things that militate against them, but the idea is not to make any of them without they are absolutely indicated. We make so many vaginal examinations that we should not make!

Dr. W. W. Wells, Oklahoma City: Obstetrics is classed as surgery. Surgical asepsis and antisepsis in our development of the tactile sense through the rubber glove in surgery has become a fact. We can feel just as well with a rubber glove on as we can without one, for we have developed that. We can develop the tactile sense so that a rectal examination will tell us everything that we can find out by a vaginal examination. That means that we are able to tell the presentation, possibly the position. I have not developed it to that extent myself, but the presentation can be easily told. You can tell if the head is engaged or not. You can tell the amount of dilatation of the os, and those are the only things that are

necessary unless there is some malposition or some other trouble that·we want to
rectify. Consequently the rectal examination is simply an improvement over the
vaginal examination and only needs development by every one of us.

Dr. Lee W. Cotton, Enid: Dr. Hatchett speaks of us old men. I am not in
that class, I assure you, though in years I am not far from Dr. Hatchett; otherwise
I am not in his class.

I just wanted to run over the ground hurriedly in about a minute and a half,
I do not want to take up any time.

I just want to recall twenty or twenty-five years ago when I had the honor
of being under, as a preceptor, one of the best men of our country, in southeast
Missouri. He warned me always to use a fountain syringe, plenty of carbolic
acid, all that could be borne, and hot water.

We know different. I have often thought of the success that old doctor had
and how many—notwithstanding the large practice he had—how many mothers
he lost in the time that I knew him. I could count several that were undoubtedly
uncalled for.

We recognize obstetrics as strictly surgical; we all agree on that point, and
asepsis is the key-note to its success. I remember when I first began to try to
practice medicine that about every thirty or forty or sixty minutes, especially
when I was so anxious, I would exxmine a patient. I do not know how it is that
I ever got by as well as I did; I cannot understand it now. Now if I spend ten
minutes, I am going to get my hands clean; at least I think so. And soap and water
and work are the essentials.

I do not hesitate after I have done that and used a good antiseptic wash, to
make a thorough examination; I want it thorough and I only want one. I do not
meddle; I do not want to continue those examinations but I do want to know exactly
where I am and then I am done.

I can see at once the necessity and the advantages of a rectal examination,
yet I still contend and I believe and I know that if we follow those rules of absolute asepsis it is rarely, if ever, we need to infect our patient. Those cases of puerperal sepsis usually we know are infected from the outside, not in themselves.
Now when such a thing does occur, we must condemn ourselves for the trouble,
hence we cannot be too cautious.

I expect to try now to take up this point of rectal examination, yet on the
other hand if I do not find out exactly the position and exactly the progress that
has been made, I will not hesitate to make the examination as I have done for
the last few years.   .

But as I said before, we are not careful enough in getting our hands clean,
that is the point; we need not infect if we thoroughly clean our hands, there is
the danger. .

Dr. F. R. Wheeler, Mannford: There is just one point I wanted to bring out.
I guess I am like the two brothers, I am not a spring chicken. I remember the
first case where I ever had made an examination. I tried to look wise, like I am
trying to act now. I assumed everything was all right, and it so happened that
it turned out that way.

I forgot to say that there was nobody there but that girl and me. Her husband
had gone across the river after her mother and the bridge had floated away and
they did not get back.

Once in a while she said, "I wish my husband was here," and so did I. "I wish
my mother was here," and so did I. And she says, "Doctor, these pains are awful,
these are after pains." I says, "They may be after pains, but I think they are
before." Pretty soon I had a child; you know what I found out. So much for
that.

I can say I always use soap and water. I do not fear much from my first examination. · After you get your child out, keep your hand out. I do not believe anybody brought that out, but keep it clean after the child is out; keep your hands out after that.

Dr. W. A. Tolleson, Eufaula: I want to thank Dr. Rice for this paper and I am glad that I am here to hear it this morning. To my mind the strongest point in this paper is the fact of cleanliness, or a removal of the average practitioner from meddlesome midwifery. Another point we must bear in mind is—but this method with a large number of us will be in a certain sense impractical for the reason that there is a class of physicians in this country which does not have the opportunity of getting or having access to their patients in this line of work and cannot keep their patients in a condition for this character of examination. Much more information can be obtained from the external examination than is taken advantage of by the average practitioner. Many times you can determine—and I daresay that I can say this without fear ·of contradiction by the testimony of men who specialize in this line of work—whether or not there is a proper engagement, and you are able to determine the character of engagement or the position that the child will be delivered.

A rectal examination, if you can do what you say you can do and if that is the movement on the part of obstetricians at this time, will do great good because I know that much harm is done by meddlesome midwifery. But those who practice in certain sections of the country must keep in mind this fact, that the doctor's "all's well" must be heard.

I was very much interested in Dr. Fowler's discussion when he mentioned the fact that we are often confused as to what we have. Many times a breech is delivered before the doctor has determined whether or not he had a head or a breech; we all suffer this confusion.

For a long time I have contended for a cleanly procedure in the management of an obstetrical case, but as I said a while ago, those of you who are on the pavement are in a different situation from country doctors. The city physicians have an opportunity and have an advantage over those of us in the country, as was wisely suggested by one of the other members of this audience a moment ago. What are you going to do with the patient when you do not get there until labor is practically finished? Many times you do not have an opportunity, and we probably are to blame because we have not disciplined them to this point. But with those of you who can see your patients fifteen minutes after you leave your office, you can probably do these things.

On the other hand there are some objections to a rectal examination, where you will find an acutely sensitive condition, particularly with a primipara. My experience is that a primipara is likely to have a sensitive rectum and hemorrhoids that accompany pregnancy. And the rectum must be clean if you are going to get anything out of the examination.

Personally I have had no experience with rectal examinations but if I have the pleasure of meeting you at the next annual session of the Oklahoma Medical Association, I will know something personally of a rectal examination. The strongest point and the best point with reference to this is the emphasis upon a clean surgical behavior in the management of the average case of labor.

Dr. J. S. Hibbard, Cherokee: Just about one minute. I will not stop to say anything about the excellent paper. We all know the purpose of our discussion is to avoid after-trouble.

The point I wanted to bring out is the personal equation of the physician. All infections are not caused by the physician. I have waited on many cases, and we all have, where the woman herself has made an examination before the physician arrived; and we have waited on other cases where the marital relationship has been practiced ten hours before labor, and maybe after that. All these things enter into consideration. One thing I have noticed in my own work is the personal equation of the physician. For instance, our excellent chairman who has come from a case of erysipelas while I come from a bath, with the same care, may be more apt to have trouble than I would. I have noticed that the surgeons who seem to take the greatest care always get pus cases. I have noticed sometimes a physician more prone to infection, and with the same care is more apt to have trouble than other men. I remember one physician who was a co-practitioner with me whose habit was to use his hands, and if he could find soap he used it, and if he didn't he didn't and he never had any infections.

I never practiced rectal examinations, but it is ideal undoubtedly. My usual custom is to sterilize my hands thoroughly before I put on my sterilized gloves. I shave the pubis and then apply petrogen, iodin and alcohol, and then keep a sterile pack, and I do not have near as many infections as I used to have.

The point I wanted to emphasize is the personality of the physician. I mean in cases where the physician is guilty of the infection, that one physician must practice more care in sterilizing himself than another.

Dr. Rice, closing: In closing this paper I wish to thank the doctors for the generous discussion. For the benefit of Dr. Reeder I wish to say that there is not a great deal written on rectal examination. I think perhaps that De Lee's is the only American text-book that even speaks of it, and then in only two or three lines. Dr. Holmes of Chicago, who I believe is associated with Rush, a year or so ago wrote a very nice article on rectal examinations. But in De Lee's new book, which will be out in September, I am satisfied there will be a chapter or more on rectal examinations.

I appreciate the fact of course that judgment must be used in rectal examinations the same as in all others. For instance, if you have a long drawn out case of labor and you are not satisfied with your rectal examination, and perhaps your membrane is bulging and you cannot make out the line of suture, then you are justified in making a cleanly vaginal examination. Then again ofttimes you are not careful, and I will admit perhaps you can go to the extreme in rectal examination.

For instance, there a case happened of a prolapsed cord. The interne on this particular case made a rectal diagnosis of a prolapsed cord. He sent in for help and the senior interne went out on the case and instead of confirming that diagnosis by a vaginal, he confirmed the diagnosis rectally in a negative way. The fact is, it was a prolapsed cord and the patient did not go to the hospital until several hours later, possibly eight or nine hours, and there was no pulsation in the cord and the baby was lost. You must consider all those things.

As for the external examination, every case should have of course a thorough external examination made; and you can tell as much, or you can practically make a diagnosis externally without any internally whatsoever until the head enters the pelvis, and then you can tell the way the head rides, whether you have an occipital, posterior, anterior, transverse, or what it is.

OBSTETRIC SUPERSTITIONS.

Paul Titus, Pittsburgh (*Journal A. M. A.*, May 18, 1918), calls attention to the prevalence of obstetric superstitions, and gives quite a number of them as he has heard them in his practice. Some of them, like that of marking the unborn baby, are so common and persistent as to be hopeless, and some of them may, perhaps, be unfamiliar to the average physician, who may know of still others, unmentioned. When it is considered, he says, that obstetrics forms one of the main topics of conversation at Red Cross meetings and bridge parties, it may be understood how such a multitude of fanciful ideas have sprung up, and have been kept in existence. The less the pregnant woman thinks about herself the better, so long as her condition is normal and her progress is being watched by a competent physician. Titus says that it is his opinion that the more familiar the physician is with these common notions, the better is he able to allay fears, and explain away the doubts that these old-wives' tales produce.

THE PREVENTION AND TREATMENT OF PUERPERAL LACERATION.*

By W. W. WELLS, M. D., Oklahoma City

You will not expect me to treat this subject in detail, as this would require too much of your valuable time.

First let me briefly review the anatomy of the uterus, the vagina, and the perineal body. The uterus, as you all know, is made up of three distinct layers: the serous, the muscular, and the mucous. I scarcely need say that the serous coat does not cover the anterior surface of the cervix, nor that part of the posterior surface which projects into the vagina. The cervix, as you know, has two layers: the muscular, and the mucous. The cervix, unlike the body of the uterus, contains more connective and elastic tissue; therefore it is more firm and consequently more rigid. It also renders it capable of a greater amount of stretching without injury. I need not say that all blood vessels of the cervix are in the muscular coat, which has but few fibers; therefore there is a very poor blood supply.

The mucous layer of the cervix, you know, is continuous with the mucous layer of the body of the uterus; and differs only in this respect, that it is more fibrous and contains a great many more glands.

The vagina, as you know, has two coats: the muscular and the mucous. The muscular coat contains a great many blood vessels, while the mucous coat has very few glands in comparison with the mucous coat of the cervix.

Unlike the cervix, which depends upon its elastic tissues for dilating, the walls of the vagina simply lay in folds, or rugae, which are smoothed out in dilating.

The perineal body is composed of, or is the union of the transverse perinei, bulbocavernosus, and sphincter ani. It is located posterior to the vaginal orifice and anterior to the anus. It is covered with mucous membrane and skin.

The causes of the cervical tears are, too rapid dilatation, as when some such drug as pituitary extract has been used; manual or instrumental dilatation; non-elasticity in old primipara; and scar tissue in multipara, which has been repaired.

The preventive treatment, I scarcely need say, is simple. Unless there is some cause for a rapid delivery, the patient should be given plenty of time for the cervix to soften and dilate. If we leave the patient who has only two, three, or four fingers dilation, with pains only moderate, alone, we shall have fewer cases to repair later; and if we give a drug to stimulate the contraction and see that we are going to have a rapid delivery, ether, chloroform, or nitrous-oxide should be given to retard it.

We do not repair the cervix at the time, unless there is a hemorrhage. And, here let me make this statement, that if we examine the cervix in our cases of post partum hemorrhage, we shall find that there is in a great number of these cases, a deep tear involving the circular artery of the cervix, and that this tear is the source of the hemorrhage. These as you know are the cases that respond slowly to treatment; but if we take two strong gauze forceps and put one on the posterior and one on the anterior lip of the cervix, we can easily bring it down into view and determine where the hemorrhage is coming from. If from a tear in the cervix, it is no trouble to take one or two interrupted sutures.

The only precaution is that we must not try to do too good work. Do not take more than two or three sutures. The most important suture, as you know, is the one high up on the cervix and includes the circular artery.

The best of authorities are agreed that the cervix should be immediately repaired when you are working in a well-equipped hospital or when the cervical artery has been torn. The suture material should be No. 2 chromic or No. 3 for-

---

*Read at the 26th Annual Meeting, Tulsa, Okla., May 15, 1918.

malized pyoktanin catgut, as this does not have to be removed and seems to give as good satisfaction as the old method of using silkworm gut.

In the prevention and repair of tears of the vagina and perineum, we again call your attention to the rapid delivery.

Dr. Ochsner once said, "Do not use insane haste, nor imbecilic deliberation in surgery." This can well be applied to obstetrical surgery. Tears of the vagina are caused by the same conditions as those of the cervix. Too rapid delivery and malposition. These tears are never very deep because the vaginal wall is made up of only mucous membrane and a longitudinal muscular layer; therefore the tear is usually longitudinal.

It is this class of cases that give the most trouble. On inspection, the perineum may look normal, and hence these vaginal tears are overlooked. The index finger should be placed in the rectum and turn the vaginal wall out. In this manner the tear will be brought plainly into view. If these tears are not repaired, they may become infected. The skin being intact, pus can not drain out and we have the usual signs of infection, chills, fever, etc. It was in this class of cases that the now discarded vaginal and uterine douche carried infection into the uterus and tubes, and caused a general puerperal infection, or childbed fever. If we are unfortunate enough to get one of these tears infected, the patient should be set up to get free drainage; then paint the wound with iodin or put in a gauze wick drainage, and use the usual supportive treatment. These tears should be repaired at delivery, if we can be surgically clean. No. 3 pyoktanin catgut, in a running half-lock suture, is used.

Lacerations of the perineum are usually median and are classified as: first degree, which is a laceration through the mucous membrane; or second degree, where the laceration extends through the perineum down to the sphincter ani muscle; and third degree, where the laceration extends through the sphincter ani into the rectum.

These lacerations usually occur when the head is being delivered. Occasionally the shoulders will be delivered in such a position and with such rapidity that a tear occurs. To prevent these tears we give the perineum plenty of time to dilate; and when the head is seen to be coming through the vulva, the patient is turned on the side, with the upper leg flexed, with the foot on the lower flexed knee. In this manner the head does not press directly on the perineum.

With one hand covered with a sterile towel, pressure is made just below the coccyx and just back of the anus. This pushes the head against the pubic arch. Now with the other hand, we can hold the head from coming too fast, and can deliver the head between pains and get the least possible laceration.

In case we have an infantile vulva, or one that has had a perineorrhaphy, when the head has stretched the levator ani, the anus opens out, the perineum is resistant, and is seen to be about to tear, then an episiotomy should be done.

The repairs of the perineum should be divided into three classes, the same as the classification of tears. In the repair of the first class, or first degree tears, we use formalized pyoktanin No. 3 of chromic No. 2 catgut, beginning at the upper angle of the tear, using a continuous half-lock suture. These sutures do not have to be removed.

In the repair of the second class, or second degree tears, we retract the vagina laterally, to bring the tears into full view; then with plain catgut No. 2, on a round full curved needle, we go well out into the lateral walls, and bring the muscles together using interrupted sutures. Now we close the fascia over the muscle with a few interrupted sutures, the skin and mucous membrane being closed as in the repair of the first class of tears.

In the repair of the third class, or the third degree tears, we begin by suturing the rectal tear at its upper angle, with No. 2 catgut. It is best to make the sutures interrupted, and be sure to suture the rectum down to the skin beyond the mucoskin anal margin. Then bring the sphincter together with No. 2 plain catgut, also the levators and fascia, and close the same as in cases of first or second degree tears. We seldom use silkworm gut; but if there seems to be much tension, it is best to put in one or two tension sutures.

Thus we can, if the patient be in good condition, by using the suture material mentioned, repair all tears immediately after delivery. The sutures do not need to be removed, thus benefitting the doctor who cannot return the eighth or tenth day to remove them. In our hands this method has given better results than the old method of using silkworm gut.

Discussion.

Dr. Lee W. Cotton, Enid: The great war has focused the attention of the public on the necessity of conservation of health, and our country (this nation) has accepted the challenge to do everything in its power to promote the health and conserve the vitality of our people.

This is the slogan or watchword in all of our cantonments or training camps, and while this splendid campaign was started as a war measure, it has become a part of the permanent community life; hence we must at once conclude that this paper is not only timely, but in urgent demand, as it deals with the health, longevity and happiness of motherhood, which is the foundation stone of the home.

The first section of the subject (prevention) furnishes us with the most fertile field for preventive medicine and surgery, and at once suggests a closer supervision of our patients during the full term of gestation.

The invalidism resulting from childbirth is appalling, and a panoramic view of the real conditions, which now exist, should make any thoughtful considerate physician pause occasionally, and ask himself if he has not often been guilty of inexcusable carelessness and gross neglect bordering on criminality.

Rather obscure vital statistics claim about 20,000 deaths of mothers and about 250,000 of babies annually in the United States from childbirth, to say nothing of the postponed mortality from injury received during labor.

Doctor De Lee, one of our best authors, claims that 50 per cent of women who have borne children bear marks of injury sooner or later, and yet we contend that labor is a normal function of the human female. These are fine monuments of our carelessness and ignorance.

In order to intelligently protect our patient and prevent possible approaching danger, many factors must be considered. We need to know something of her hygienic surroundings, mode of living, manner of dress, occupation, heredity, etc.; if she is suffering from urethritis, endometritis or a salpingitis, size of the child's cranium and the position of the foetus, if the kidneys are secreting properly, and if she has persistent or even periodical attacks of vomiting, especially in the latter states of gestation.

Only last week we buried in a little town near Enid the wife of one of our best physicians, a splendid young woman in fine health seemingly. Those who attended her and those who know something of the family in considering this at our meeting the other night thought that we had certainly overlooked things that we should not have overlooked. That woman seemingly had been rather strong and in rather good condition, but at the seventh month and bordering on the eighth she began to have quite frequent attacks of vomiting, not much appetite, tongue dry; the urine was examined and there was possibly a trace of albumen, no high line case, no cast of any description that should make it very alarming. Yet she was brought to the hospital a little later and in a few days from that time she went into coma and died.

We had good physicians that looked into the case carefully. But now what did we have? She had persistent vomiting, that is, at times, yet some days it would pass over. It is a toxin in her condition; I do not know how to explain it, possibly some of you may be able to. We were not able fully to understand it; we know occasionally we have those conditions. The woman died; there was no real reason, so far as we could see, except she had a toxin from pregnancy that she died from some way or another. That is one thing I think we ought to look into more carefully.

I have had one or two cases where they did not die, but I was alarmed. I could not find anything alarming in the urine, yet they were very sick women. Now that is a condition I hope some of you will not pass over. Personally I would like to have more light on it; I know I am in a way in the dark, but I mention this because it is a factor and an important factor and if we are going to prevent these things we want to look at every phase of our case and we want to have every symptom. This is a very important symptom in my mind.

At the Bedside. The first prerequisite is absolute cleanliness, not necessarily antisepsis, but asepsis, and soap and water are the essentials.

The physician at this time needs in store a good stock of patience. It is said that time, patience, and perseverence will overcome all things, and nowhere in a physician's career are these essentials more appropriate.

We fully agree with Dr. Wells that the principal cause for cervical tears is due to too rapid dilatation. We believe that almost without exception this can be averted. As a remedial agent the old true and tried, chloral hydrate, in thirty grain or even drachm doses, seldom fails to bring happy results. Nitrous oxide, chloroform, etc., have their places. Ext. pituitrin, except where dilatation is complete, is not only likely to harm but dangerous.

Small tears of the cervix usually care for themselves, and it is only where the hemorrhage is profuse and rupture of the circular artery that surgical interference is necessary.

The technique of repair of the cervix, when necessary, has been so ably described by the author of this paper, we do not wish to further comment.

Injury to the vagina and perineum is much more common than is that of the cervix, yet the causes for tears are practically the same and are usually due to too rapid delivery. As a rule tears of the perineum should be repaired at the time of delivery, unless it is very slight indeed.

Many times what seemingly is only a slight tear of the perineum elicits the fact in after years that the pelvic floor has been seriously damaged, with the result of subinvolution of the uterus and later prolapse or marked displacement.

Dr. W. R. Joblin, Porter: There is a question in my mind whether a doctor in country practice should attempt an early repair of these tears. I generally do unless the surroundings are very bad. And I find that, as did the doctor who read the paper, the old English side position is one of the best positions to prevent a tear of the perineum; and I also notice that we find very few tears in negro and Indian patients who assume the squatting position. I have quite a large practice among the full blood Indians and the negroes and they nearly always assume the squatting position.

I know that I am neglectful, I let tears get by me that are obscured by the skin not being broken; vaginal tears and muscular tears get by me, and I know that we let more cases of that kind go by us, to the detriment of the patients in after years, than we should. It is a very small thing, but we overlook it. A man will look at the perineum and he won't recognize a tear there when he has got a vaginal or muscular tear and the muscles are separated widely, and the next thing you know you have an invalid patient. It is very hard, though, for a doctor doing practice under the hygienic surroundings that a country doctor has to contend with to repair all of these lacerations. But we are coming to a day and time when a doctor will be held criminally liable when he does not repair a lacerated perineum when the condition exists.

Dr. W. A. Fowler, Oklahoma City: Dr. Wells' paper is so important and so interesting that I feel like we ought to have more discussion on it, and I think that the key-note of the paper is absolutely right, and that is that the prevention of lacerations is more important and is a more fruitful field for our interest than the cure, and that the best thing in the prevention is to give the tissues time to stretch.

There are two or three features of the paper that I thought of particularly that might be dangerous in some cases. One is the practice of introducing the finger in the rectum. I have seen this procedure done in the course of repair of the perineum. Of course Dr. Wells did not mean that should be done, but that is sometimes practiced. The finger is introduced into the rectum and the glove not changed or rinsed off in a lime salts solution before being introduced into the vagina. That is a source of infection, and in a case of infection I think we had better accept a failure in the repair of the laceration and remove the sutures for better drainage. I believe that in home practice particularly—and it is my practice in all cases—the use of the silkworm gut externally will be better than the use of the catgut. If we get a mild infection with the silkworm gut, not sufficient to make them feel really sick, we can just leave the silkworm gut in, and we will get a much better result than using chromic catgut. I believe with the average man— and I put myself in that class—that the silkworm gut will give us better results. The thing about introducing a silkworm gut is to start it far enough from the edge of the tear so that it will be easily removed and swing the needle out so as to make a circle with your suture and not to leave a dead space in the tear and to leave it in long enough before being taken out. Personally I leave the sutures in two weeks before I remove them.

The practice of episiotomy recommended by De Lee does not belong in my opinion to home practice. I feel it is a very wise man who can tell by looking at the perineum that it is going to be torn or that it is not going to be torn, and I would not care to wilfully make a tear in the perineum when I could not be sure it was going to be a tear. I know some of the best authorities recommend that, Dr. De Lee among them.

The paper as a whole is excellent and I think it is one of the best we have had.

Dr. F. R. Wheeler, Mannford: I certainly like the paper, and the prevention is the biggest thing. I am isolated, like Dr. Joblin over there, although I never waited on but very few people outside of our own. I hardly ever have a consultant in the practice. I do not know why I get along, but I seem to pretty well.

Dr. W. M. Taylor, Oklahoma City: We all agree with Dr. Wells that the preventing of tears is more important. Some time ago Dr. Cook advocated the plan, instead of repairing our lacerations immediately, especially where our surroundings are bad, of waiting for a week, as much as seven days and then putting in a suture, that we would get better results than where you got in where the tear is fresh, and that he uniformly would get better results by waiting seven days than he would from work of that kind done immediately.

Of course the objection offered to his plan at that time was that the lacerations and blood vessels are left exposed and there are more chances for infection. There is a good point, but I am sure that in certain cases we would be justified and would meet with much better results if we postpone these operations of repair work.

Dr. W. W. Wells, closing: I thank you for the general discussion. In regard to what Dr. Taylor suggests, waiting seven days to repair, I want to say that I looked up the different authorities on that subject and see that a great many of them believe in waiting. However, an equal number repair the cervix and perineum immediately, and in many cases they get union by first intention and consequently get good results.

Another thing is that the patient will usually permit one or two sutures to be taken at this time and then you are through with the case. If you are not practicing in that neighborhood you do not necessarily have to go right back and see how the patient is getting along or go back in six or seven days, as the doctor suggested, and put in these sutures. Then you have another week that you do not know whether you are going to have infection or not.

Dr. Fowler, in speaking of the introduction of the finger into the rectum in these cases, called our attention to that danger. The introduction of the finger into the rectum certainly might cause infection; but after every injury, whether it be from obstetrical cause or other trauma, we always make a thorough examination of the parts injured, and that is the object in this case. You put the finger into the rectum and turn the vaginal wall out, and you do that to inspect it, then you know whether to prepare to do your surgical work or not. In this paper I have not touched on antisepsis or asepsis because we feel that as obstetrical surgeons we should be sterile.

Now in regard to repairing the cervix. I went down to the instrument display and got one of these forceps. This is a sponge forceps; it is curved. I use two straight ones; they do not cut the cervix. Now put one on the posterior and one on the anterior lip of the cervix; pull the cervix down into view. You can easily see the tear, it is usually on the side; you can take as many sutures as is necessary. Do not repair these cases unless it is absolutely necessary.

The silkworm gut usually shows in my hands deep ulceration around the gut down into the tissue. In general surgery they have always used silkworm gut in closing their abdominal wounds. Today there are very few men using silk worm gut in abdominal surgery. only where they think that they might have some infection or too much tension for catgut.

We have found that by using the plain catgut for closing the muscle, and the tissue closed with chromic or pyoktanin catgut and then the skin with plain iodinized gut, we are able to get a suture that will not ulcerate from any other cause.

The material we use is pyoktanin catgut No. 3, it is put up so that any one can carry it, it is sterile, it is in three packages, and I have always found that it gives us better results than the silkworm gut on account of the fact that we do not have the tissue with an unabsorbable suture material extending out through the skin along which infection can go down into the deeper tissues.

This pyoktanin gut will swell and fill the cavity, consequently it will not allow germs to pass down along the gut to the deeper tissues. The silkworm gut as the skin retracts from it leaves an opening that the germs can pass through.

THE EYES OF THE ARMY.

Allen Greenwood, Boston (*Journal A. M. A.*, June 29, 1918), describes what has been done for correction of eye defects in the army. Some criticisms have been made on the standard frame adopted, but it seemed to have more advantages than any other, with its three variations of bridge. The most frequent criticism, however, is of the round eye piece, and the disadvantage that the cylindric lenses may be turned in the frame. This is best answered by calling attention to the fact that all cylindric lenses when in place are marked on the side, at a point close to the middle of the temple attachment, and the soldier's attention is called to this, so that he can watch for any possible shifting. Other methods of meeting the difficulty are noticed, and a list of lenses supplied in the equipments of the various units. Steps were taken to have a first class optician in each of the cantonments. For the central optical unit, a full equipment of machinery for the surfacing and edging of lenses, and a plentiful supply of glass and blanks was provided to be used by skilled workers on the spot.

SOME SURGICAL ASPECTS OF OBSTETRICS.

By E. FORREST HAYDEN, M. D., Tulsa, Okla. .

The fact that I have been asked to write a paper, and that it has come in this important section and also has lined up under this particular part of this section, viz., obstetrics, and has furthermore partaken of a surgical nature, is a matter of evolution.

My first contribution in the way of a paper to the Oklahoma State Medical Association was on the subject of "Pneumonia in the Young." The second, "Pre-natal Influences," and today, because of the course of events and the nature of the greater part of my work, I am endeavoring to present an obstetrical subject from the standpoint of its surgical aspects. This, however, will be brief, for I think it is the tendency of modern times to make papers and addresses, and especially papers to be read before bodies of this sort, as concise as is in keeping with a good sense and a fair presentation of the subject in hand.

The main object in a medical meeting when its members assemble themselves is to give a fair opportunity to standardize medical thought, and to establish a mean and in a measure harmonize the extremes existing between the viewpoints of the very enthusiastic and those who are more than conservative. It is from the various discussions of the topic that we probably derive the most benefit. Men coming from different parts of the state who have been daily wrestling with problems peculiar to their communities and work, hold pent up in their experiences material which is wonderfully beneficial to the whole of us. This they produce on the spur of the moment, delivering their systems of some rich experiences that, though extreme or conservative, are very helpful to all of us, and thus we progress.

Papers that are well paragraphed outlining the fundamental features of the subject so as to readily merit discussion should meet with universal approval.

Papers that contain long lists of statistics or too many case reports with much irrelevant matter do not conserve time properly, and at once become tiresome and inefficient, oftentimes leaving the better part of a program unfinished. Things that are purely historic or academic in character have no part or place in a medical program such as we are now handling except under very rare conditions, consequently without padding or polishing, I pass to the essentials that have been the incentive for this production.

Obstetrics has its surgical aspects, and surgery sustains a relationship to the subject as a whole as much as does embryology, the physiology of the puerperium, the physiology and mechanism of labor, the pathology of labor, or any other of its subdivisions. In fact, it is the methods that are surgical in character that lend to the subject the results that are most positive in the alleviation of suffering, robbing birth of its pangs and giving promise of less mortality to both mother and infant. As the management of labor cases has passed from the control of the ignorant and untutored into the hands of the scientific and those who know how to be surgically clean, so have gone septicemia, infection, and death resulting from lack of knowledge and the neglect of rational and radical surgical procedure.

The responsibility of being clean begins at the bedside when we first approach a patient in labor, and we should begin after this manner: If a patient has not been long in labor and the cervix is dilated not larger than a silver dollar or the top of an ordinary tea cup, or if the membranes are not as yet ruptured, to be exactly right, give a vaginal douche of one-half gallon of warm bi-chloride solution 1-2000. Give an S. S. enema of the same amount. Place a pad underneath patient made of several thicknesses of newspaper and covered on both sides with thin cloth or canvas, otherwise use a Kelly pad. I use and prefer the Kelly pad, notwithstanding that it is condemned by a few, because I can boil it in a few minutes a nd be certain it is thoroughly sterile. Distribute a few more newspapers on the

---

*Read at the 26th Annual Meeting, Tulsa, Okla., May 15, 1918.

floor at the bedside, upon which set a slop jar with sleeve of the pad dipping into it. Drape a clean sheet about the legs of the patient, not being too afraid to expose her, and you are all ready to go, so far as the patient is concerned. While the Kelly pad is being boiled in a pan of water on a nearby stove, have a pair of rubber gloves in preparation at the same time. In the same pan above mentioned, place two Dudley ligament forceps, a needle holder and one pair of scissors, unless you prepare the scissors and a fish hook needle together with some few silkworm gut sutures on the side, in a separate dish of alcohol or phenol, anyway, have them ready and clean. Don one glove at least, at the first examination, which has been preceded by a bi-chloride 1-2000 vaginal douche. Lubricate two fingers with sterile white vaseline, using it from a flexible tube so that it cannot become contaminated. It is not necessary to put glove No. 2 on until the second stage of labor is practically over. Such preparation having been made, proceed to examine the patient. The first examination usually enables an experienced accoucher to predict the outcome of the whole labor. Every time the hand is removed from the birth canal it should be dropped into a bowl, close at hand, of 1-2000 bi-chloride of mercury before being re-introduced into the birth canal. With this surgical technique no such a calamity as puerperal septicemia need befall anyone, and I have not had such an accident to happen to me in a period of five or six years, and I have delivered many women under every variety of trying circumstances.

The different methods of all difficult labors are necessarily surgical, after a primary surgical preparation, then all labors which are natural are purely obstetrical, and remain so as long as nature affords a spontaneous process, which within itself is indeed marvelous.

The proper dress of the umbilical cord, though simple, is a surgical proposition. First we tie with sterile tape, or should do so, then dress with an aseptic powder and cover with sterile gauze, and if later the cord becomes too dry, we recommend a dressing of sterile vaseline. If too soft, on the other hand, we apply an aseptic powder again, boracic acid or bismuth formic iodide, etc.

I might go on enumerating the surgical aspects in obstetrical work indefinitely, but I will not do so, however, I will take the liberty to mention, concisely, just two or three more evidences. The one is the formidable placenta praevia, a problem that is not easily solved by the most skilled and one that should be approached with fear and trembling by anyone half prepared to cope with its enormous possibilities of danger.

Apart from surgical knowledge and technique, obstetrical practice resolves itself into a very crude and inadequate branch of medicine, and carries us back to the days when the process of labor and birth were handled by ignorant midwives; when it was no uncommon thing for women to die of what was then known as childbed fever.

Previous to the advent of Dr. Oliver Wendell Holmes, puerperal septicemia was not recognized as such, and its exact causes were not clearly and definitely known, but about this time a revolution in the science of obstetrics was begun which has continued to develop into our present day perfection.

In referring to placenta praevia, I do not propose to enter into its classification, it is of no particular concern as to whether it is divided into three or four different varieties, neither do I need, in this, instance to consider its diagnosis, etiology or prognosis, but we must remember that it requires strict and accurate surgical treatment.

In the early cases of three or four months the best thing to do is to tampon the vagina tightly after having thoroughly cleaned the vagina and put the patient strictly to bed, keep her quiet on a liquid diet. If nothing develops after a period of twenty-four hours, repeat the process in exactly the same manner, and wait another period of hours, during this time, however, pituitrin cautiously administered acts admirably, and as a rule when the tampon is removed the third time the cervix will have been well dilated, and most likely the foetus will immediately follow up the removal of the tampon or it can be readily removed with the fingers or a placenta forceps, and without any hemorrhage of consequence.

In the more advanced stages of pregnancy, say six or eight months, the process is somewhat different, and I think the tampon unnecessary and of no benefit, perhaps dangerous. Wide dilation is required which is accomplished by means of a uterine dilator, a Ribes bag or the fingers, of course the membranes are ruptured as soon as can be conveniently done thereby permitting and encouraging the uterus to contract down on its lower and soft segment as soon as possible, which materially controls the hemorrhage. So soon as the cervix is sufficiently dilated to permit the introduction of the hand, a bipolar version is done and the whole affair is safely finished. I have a large four-pronged uterine dilator with which I can safely dilate any cervix that I have seen within the short interval of four or five minutes sufficiently to introduce my hand, and large enough to drag down and deliver the oncoming head without danger of lacerating the cervix.

I intended to mention briefly septic abortion and also cesarean section but I failed to get to them. Of course we are pro and con as to the treatment of septic abortion, some believing in going in and cleaning out the uterus, and others believing in staying out.

As to the cesarean section I am highly in favor of doing cesareans whenever it is apparent that the mother is incapable of delivering her child in a reasonable time. There was a case of mine I had ten days ago. Three years ago the mother, who was thirty-eight years old, went into labor on Thursday evening and remained until Saturday with one physician in attendance when the second one was called, and then continued until Monday, when a third was called, and somehow they hitched on with forceps and delivered the baby dead and the mother half dead.

On this occasion she came to me very much alarmed, pregnant again. I explained to her what cesarean meant and if it came up again we would do the cesarean, which we did. When I went out I found that the bag of water had ruptured, the head had no tendency to engage in the pelvis, and knowing the history I sent her out to the hospital and up to the operating room and did the cesarean. Consequently they have a fine boy, and the mother is in good condition. Of course we have the pros and cons on this subject; some say it is bad and some good. I will leave it up to you.

Discussion.

Dr. L. J. Moorman, Oklahoma City: Mr. Chairman, I am sorry I have been called upon instead of someone else. I appreciate the paper very much but this subject is one to which I have given but very little attention and really am not capable of discussing it.

I feel very keenly the necessity of having such a subject thoroughly discussed in such a meeting as this. We all know that even with our modern ideas of asepsis and antisepsis, puerperal sepsis is still quite common in the hands of the average practitioner, and I believe that it is not due to lack of knowledge but due to lack of caution, due to carelessness chiefly. While I am not doing obstetrics at all and never do surgery, I feel like since you called upon me to make these remarks I want to say that I think that is true. I think if we had the statistics we would find that the mortality from childbirth has not been reduced as it deserves to be reduced, with our present understanding of labor, which really is a major surgical, it seems to me.

Dr. J. A. Hatchett, El Reno: Mr. Chairman, I will say that I enjoyed that paper very much. Of course the subject of the surgery of obstetrics is broad.

He spoke of the cesarean section, and there has been a revolution taking place in that regard in the last few years. We would be better off, much better off if we would do a great many more cesarean sections than we do, if we have favorable surroundings. If we have a hospital to take our patients to, and competent surgeons, we will find it greatly to our advantage to have more of that work done. We lose too many children by running the risk of using forceps in cases that produce the death of the child. Many times we lament the fact; we make our measurements and we examine thoroughly, and we say we can save this child by a forceps operation, and we apply our forceps and the child is lost. I remember in the New York Maternity, the last day I was there, I saw two fine children lost by high forceps, both of them died from high forceps. I thought at the time how much better it would have been if they had had a cesarean than to have tried the high forceps. I also think in our home practice many times we ought to use the cesarean when we do not.

I had a case not long ago where the mother was getting along in years, and the father was getting along in years; they had lost the previous child, and they were very anxious. The mother was approaching that period of life when she would cease to bear children; the father was beyond fifty. They were exceedingly anxious to have an offspring. Their first child was a breech and the pelvis was somewhat contracted; the measurements were short and they lost the child. Well, they came to me and told me that they were very anxious to have a living child. I examined the case thoroughly, found that the measurements were somewhat short, not very much so but somewhat short; enough to make a person anxious of the consequences. The woman could have gotten through all right with another breech. Jsut as soon as I found it was another breech, that ended it, I was not going to run any risk at all. Here were these people that wanted an offspring, and I might have brought that child alive but I might not, we do not know. The best calculations, the finest discriminations as were made in these two children that were lost by high forceps went wrong. That was carefully considered, and they decided that high forceps were better than the cesarean section in those two cases, but they made a mistake, in all probability, and they would have been better off if they had had a cesarean section. In this case I had a cesarean section and the parents had the much desired child.

We have many such cases, and you and I have often been chagrined and our heads have been bowed in humility and weakness when we bring forth a large child and it has cerebral hemorrhage and dies. We have all done that. It makes us sad; it makes us feel like we had better have done something else.

Dr. C. V. Rice, Muskogee: Speaking of the cesarean: The mortality of the Chicago Lying-In Hospital—pardon me for referirng to that institution, but it is a very good example—the low mortality of that institution is due to judgment. Now De Lee would not think of doing a cesarean where there had been a hand in the vagina; he would not think of doing a cesarean where there was complete dilatation or a rupture of the membranes. He would not think of doing a cesarean where there had been forceps applied.

After excluding the cesarean, there are two operations that he considers. He never does a high forceps in this way (indicating), that is, he never puts on the forceps and pulls. He makes eight or nine tractions, and if the head does not come he gives that up as not a forceps case. He either does a pubiotomy or a craniotomy, and that depends upon the conditions. If the baby's heart tones are good and the mother is in good condition, he does a pubiotomy, and with all success; but he absolutely would not think of doing a cesarean where there had been manipulation with forceps and examination and ruptured membranes.

I saw a very sad case there, due to a cesarean, that was performed where they had complete dilatation, the head was engaged, but an outside man did the work. In this particular case he had opened a Bartholin abscess perhaps a month or so before she went to term, before she went to labor, and she developed infection, the worst case De Lee ever saw, and she died. When he pulled the head up, it just drew the infection up into the uterus.

Dr. W. W. Wells, Oklahoma City: This just simply goes to show that obstetrics is surgery. Every man who attempts to do obstetrics is a surgeon or must know the principles of surgery; he must know what to do and when to do it. I say what to do, I mean by that to know not to do a whole lot of things that we do; to leave the patient alone just as much as possible if you know that everything is going well.

Last summer I had the pleasure of being in the New York Lying-In, and went there specially to get a lot of work on cesarean sections and I found out there was very little of it being done. They had lost some mothers, and it seems that it is a great deal worse to lose mothers than it is to lose babies. If you notice in these papers, they tell the mortality of mothers and then the mortality of the babies, and the babies reach into the thousands or hundreds of thousands in the United States in the last year.

Now our business is that of obstetricians and pediatricians in this land at the present time—which I may say is the greatest profession in medicine because we have to do with the coming generation, we have to do with the preservation of life in the United States at the present. There is more responsibility on us than there is in general medicine or in surgery. Surgery, which has taken the lead previous to this, has now gone to war and it is up to the obstetricians and the pediatricians to take care of the world and our future generation in the United States.

Dr. Roberts, Nash, Oklahoma: Most of these papers that have been written and the discussion is all for the city physician who has access to a hospital. It is the man who goes out into the country all the way from three to fourteen miles from a railroad who recognizes these conditions ought to be in a hospital.

I find that the high forceps delivery in my hands has been a failure. I find if you do the podalic version you get along better and you will deliver more children alive than you do with the high forceps delivery.

One great mistake made by we men out in the country is that we have not equipped our obstetrical bags sufficiently. I know I have been guilty of that error, and it is only in the last week that I feel I have begun to get my obstetrical bag equipped. When you go into a country home and try to do any surgery whatever, the first thing you are up against is to find something in which to sterilize your instruments. We should have a bag equipped with a sterilizer; we can get one very easily at most instrument houses with a sterilizer in the bottom of it which you can carry with you most anywhere, and that objection is removed. The only thing you will generally find in most homes is a little bit of a round sauce pan about big enough to hold a teaspoon, or the dishpan. You know how the dishpan is, Dr. Moorman; I graduated up there in your country from obstetrics. You will find maybe a little ring of grease around the top of it where the ladies have failed to wipe it out.

These are the things that the country practitioner comes up against. So I advise all of you to get your obstetrical bags equipped with a sterilizer, one that is long enough for your forceps, and you will get along a great deal better, since you cannot have the hospital.

Dr. W. A. Fowler, Oklahoma City: The point which I think is deserving of emphasis is that the cesarean operation ought to be a selective operation. Just as far as we are able, we ought to select the cases beforehand that are going to need the cesarean. It is dangerous to do cesarean operations after examination or other methods have been attempted, and probably the better procedure in these cases would be to sacrifice the child and save the mother and give her an opportunity for another pregnancy.

The second thing that I think should be unqualifiedly condemned is the antipartum vaginal douche. I think it has been abandoned and I am sure that though it is dangerous it is very often practiced. In the first place, it robs the vagina of the very useful lubricants, and I think we ought to condemn that procedure.

Dr. E. Forrest Hayden, closing: There is not much more I wanted to say because after I read my paper I always feel like apologizing for not having done it better.

It seems to me that the cesarean feature has been the one that has received the most attention. Of course it is spectacular, more spectacular than it is difficult to do. Being clean is the first essential, of course; and some doctor said it should be selective, that is good. It should have a little examination before we attempt an operation, but what examinations have been done should have been cleanly done. Of course we do not expect much harm to come to the mouth from an examination that has been carefully and cleanly performed.

As to the rupture of the membranes, the doctor said that they should not be ruptured before the operation. I am at a loss to know just why that is; I do know in my experience with cesareans, about three—and I haven't lost any of them, thank the Lord—that when the membrane is ruptured and all the contents of the uterus emptied, then you have less material to overflow into the belly. In the case which I mentioned a while ago, I ruptured the membrane before I sent her to the hospital and when I opened the belly I didn't have any overflow into the belly and I had no sepsis of any sort, and the mother is a living example at the Oklahoma Hospital, unless she went home yesterday.

As to the pubiotomy and craniotomy: I have never done but one craniotomy and I never will do another one; I think it is absolute murder and unnecessary. Some doctor suggested the podalic version; I think that is preferable to any forceps operation whatever. Some have delivered the placenta in the third stage, allowing it to pass out through the uterus after dilatation, of course. I have taken the placenta out through the belly with the child, stripped the uterus of all of its membranes and left it clean.

RUPTURE OF THE UTERUS.

After noticing the comparative infrequency of rupture of the uterus after and because of previous cesarean section Emil Novak, Baltimore (*Journal A. M. A.,* July 13, 1918), reports a case occurring about six weeks after the usual duration of pregnancy operated on by subtotal hysterectomy with recovery. The rupture was unaccompanied with internal hemorrhage or shock. This observation was not unique, a similar case having been reported before by Neill. The uterine scar seems to have been separated without producing any hemorrhage, perhaps because of the tampon-like action of the fetal head, as it was delivered through the gap. The most important feature of the case, however, is the history of an infected abdominal incision after the previous cesarean section, as it seems to have been demonstrated that a perfectly normal recovery from cesarean section is not followed by danger of subsequent rupture. The invasion of the uterine scar by decidual elements in subsequent pregnancy is probably much less important. In Novak's opinion the occurrence of stitch infection in the abdominal incision after the prior section may be taken as prima facie evidence of infection and poor healing of the uterine incision. As held by most obstetricians, the management of cesarea patients in subsequent pregnancies should not be too strongly influenced by the fact that rupture of the uterus occurs in a very small proportion of cases, probably not exceeding 2 or 3 per cent.

TYPHOID FEVER.*

By T. W. BREWER, M. D., Miami, Oklahoma

It is not the purpose of this paper to go into an exhaustive discussion of this subject, but merely to bring out some of the most important points, which are already well known to the profession, and to open the way for a full discussion, by the members of the profession. And to this end, a review of the prevention, nursing, treatment, contagion, and a short discussion of the pathological conditions, and a review of the phenomena, as it presents itself at the bedside is, I think, in order.

It has long been known that typhoid is a general infection and ulceration of the lymph follicles of the gut, swelling of the mesenteric glands and spleen, and parenchymatous changes in other organs, especially effecting the lungs, spleen, kidneys, and cerebrospinal system. The fever is accompanied by a rose colored eruption, appearing from the seventh to the eleventh day of its inception. Such symptoms as the pea soup stool, abdominal tenderness, and tympanics, are all too well known in this disease to receive special attention.

These symptoms, as well as others, even the fever itself, are inconstant, and no one of them is to be entirely relied upon, and one or more may be absent altogether. It has been well said that typhoid is an index to the sanitation of the community, and often to that of the family or individual. It is seldom met with in young children, is badly borne by patients over forty-five years of age, and it may, I think, be generally said to reach its height of severity between the ages of eighteen and forty-five. The bacillus is killed with carbolic acid, one to two hundred, or bichloride of mercury, one to twenty-five hundred, and it is said that a single bacillus will, with proper incubation, produce a billion in ten days.

In its ravages on the gut, hyperesthesia involves the glands of Peyer, in the jejunum, and ilium, and those of the large intestines The follicles are swollen and of a grayish white in color, resolution and necrosis takes place prior to the eleventh day, and the enlarged cells are destroyed and absorbed, leaving little pits, not unlike the pits of an eruptive fever. Superficial hemorrhage, sloughing, with ulceration, follow or may occur at this time, from the edema blocking the blood vessels. The ulcer may penetrate the peritoneum, especially in the region of the iliocecal valve. The entire Peyer's patch may slough away, in from six to eight inches of the ilium. Perforation takes place in about 5 per cent of all typhoid cases and may occur at any time from the seventh day of the attack to two weeks after the temperature becomes normal. The sigmoid probably being the most liable to attack. Rupture of the spleen, gangrenous abscesses, parenchymatous degeneration of the liver, acute nephritis, catarrh of the bladder, diphtheritic inflammation of the viscus, orchitis, ulceration of the larynx, edema of the glottis, lobar pneumonia, fibrous pleurisy, emphysema, typhoid gangrene from thrombosis, embolism in the veins and arteries, optic neuritis, aphasia, and muscular abscesses, especially in the body of the psoas, are all common complications, and in a disease so complex there can be no hard and fast lines of treatment, but the physician at the bedside must be the judge on the lines of treatment to pursue.

The period of incubation is from eight to twenty-three days. The prodromes are marked by a feeling of lassitude, headache, chills, anorexia, constipation or diarrhoea, abdominal pain and tenderness, and at last the patient takes to his bed, and from this date the attack is supposed to start. The evening record gradually grows higher and higher each day, advancing about one and one-half degrees daily until it reaches 103 to 105 degrees   The pulse will show a low tension, and will beat from 100 to 110, and often dicrotic. The tongue is coated, often red at the point, and sometimes with a red and angry looking center; cough and bronchial symptoms are marked; the rose colored spots appear at about the end of the first

*Read before the Ottawa County Medical Society, June, 1918.

week. The second week is an aggravated picture of the first, the face looks heavy
and mental dullness is marked, pronounced nervous symptoms, hemorrhage and
perforation may occur. The third week is marked by morning remissions of fever,
heart feebleness, pulmonary complications, delirium, muscular tremor. The
fourth week is an aggravated picture of the third, unless the fever leaves at the end
of the third week. After the second week, the tongue is likely to become dry and
cracked, pulse irregular and feeble, abdomen distended, and the patient lay in a
profound stupor, with eyes partially open, and defecation, and incontinence invol-
untary. Heart failure is liable to occur at any time and the friends and relatives
should be aware of the dangers that are likely to arise. The onset may show
cerebrospinal symptoms, facial neuralgia, headache, convulsions, pulmonary
symptoms, bronchial catarrh, chills, pleurisy, severe vomiting, smoky or bloody
urine with albumen.

In the ambulatory form, where the patient is up and around, with a temperature of 104 or 105, and as they say fighting the fever off, I have at once resorted
to powdered opium and constipation, and the application of cold, but in spite
of my best efforts, a death certificate is the rule, as death generally ensues from
hemorrhage. Post-typhoid will be recognized by a normal temperature for several
days, and then a sudden rise to 104 or 105. This phenomena is generally caused
from indiscretion in diet, and will pass off in a few days and the patient go on to
recovery. Relapsing typhoid will be recognized by the step-like rise after the
fever has run its course and become normal.

A subnormal temperature is of no special consequence, while a sudden drop
in the temperature indicates a hemorrhage. Chills, fever and sweats are often
encountered after the second week, and generally indicate pus somewhere in the
body. Bed sores should be avoided, but if present, see that all pressure and irritation is removed from them, use the air or water pad, and keep clean from infection. Sudden death may occur from embolism or uremia, either at the height
of the fever or during convalescence, and it is well to keep the old axiom that a
case of typhoid is never too light to prove fatal, nor too hopeless for recovery,
constantly before our own minds as well as before the minds of the relatives and
friends of the patient. In case of typhoid dementia, separate the patient from
sympathizing friends, for a month or two will generally result in a recovery. Hydro-
therapy, massage, and the wet pack are invaluable in typhoid; use cold water,—
externally, internally, and eternally. Careful nursing, restricted diet, and ventilation should receive proper attention, and the attending physician must be resource-
ful and meet conditions and complications as they arise from time to time.

All persons coming in contact with the infected individual or who have been
subjected to the same environments, should be immunized. The excretions from
the sick room should be properly disinfected, and the sick room kept quiet and
cool, with special attention to the relative humidity of the air in the room. The
physician should always write all directions plainly, and have the nurse check
as the directions are followed. I consider it good practice to thoroughly cinchonize
the patient at the onset, and caster oil is a most valuable remedy. Calomel is
valuable as symptoms demand, and a high enema and a mild intestinal antiseptic
do no harm; give lots of cold water, watch the stool, watch the temperature,
watch the pulse, watch the bladder, watch the tympanitic condition of the bowel,
watch the base of the brain and the spine; examine the stool for curds, and if
found, weaken the diet. If the bowel moves too often, and application of cold
fails to control them, use starch and opium. In case of hemorrhage, give full
doses of opium, or acetate of lead and opium, cold and adrenalin; use stimulants,
and if need be, use normal salt solution subcutaneously. In severe nerve symptoms,
use Dover's powder. Bandage in case of phlebitis, typhoid spine drags for months,
and massage is probably the most effective treatment; allow no solid food for ten
days after the fever becomes normal, always remember that one-half drachm of guaiacol, painted on the flank, will cause a prompt fall in temperature. Typhoid in
pregnancy should be carefully watched, and in case of a dead foetus, void the

uterus. In intercurrent typhoid, the temperature will drop to about 100 and in a few days the patient will become normal. Spurious typhoid generally lasts from five to seven days.

Typhoid fever is most variable in its manifestations, and typhoid malaria does not exist. The physician, who claims to be a dead shot on typhoid, either displays his ignorance, or is preying on the ignorance of the laity. It is always well to look out for malaria, pyemia, and miliary tuberculosis, in making the diagnosis. A good test is the best, and the best test is with the microscope. The prognosis should be most guarded, especially in high fever at the onset, toxic manifestations, early hemorrhage, or early involvement of the brain and nervous system. In conclusion, I would say, the prognosis should always be guarded, and that the resourcefulness of the attending physician, and careful nursing are the cardinal points to the life of the patient.

DUTIES OF THE DERMATOLOGIST.

H. H. Hazen, Washington, D. C. (*Journal A. M. A.*, June 29, 1918), calls attention to certain matters having special reference to the medical duties of the dermatologists as regards the profession and the public. The meeting of specialists' societies and of sections of the larger association have not done, he thinks, all that might be expected of them. Their meetings have been pleasant social occasions with some good papers and valuable discussions, but more might be asked. Would it not be fair to ask such societies to give out general authoritative information for the benefit of the practitioner, the lay citizen, and governmental guidance. A standard publication committee might occasionally publish cretiques, answer proper questions, and assign definite problems to members to be reported on. These are only suggestions for the future. As regards duties to patients, one important thing must be emphasized; the duty to recognize serious ailments that may be developing, such as early cancer and first or obscure symptoms of constitutional disease. Reference to skilled specialists is also a duty as well as consultation in such cases. There has, Hazen thinks, been too much deference given to Teutonic authority in dermatologic matters, and if the students who have gone to Germany had realized that frequently their provat-docent or professor was too ignorant or conceited to recognize work done in America, it would have been better for them. To some of us it has always been a marvel that more of us could not see through the folly of taking too seriously the work of a man who could publish a lengthy bibliography with no American references whatever, and scarcely any but German ones. We must prepare to train dermatologists and syphilologists, and have fewer and better clinics, so as to spare us the necessity of going abroad. The arsphenamin situation is also discussed, and we should see that we are not crippled by a renewal of the monopolies that existed before the war. The duties of a dermatologist to his government and country are referred to at length by Hazen, and he gives a list of some of those who have given all their services to the Government and a few who have even given their lives in active service. There are others, however, who, without giving their all, could give services of greatest value, as consultants and visitors to hospitals and camps in the same capacity in which they now act for the civil hospitals. Army physicians would thus secure additional aid and training, and be freer to fulfill their multifarious military obligations unhampered. At the same time we must appreciate the tremendous difficulties that have attended the sudden expansion of the medical corps of the Army. These are offered as suggestions worthy of consideration.

JOURNAL OF THE OKLAHOMA STATE MEDICAL ASSOCIATION

VOLUME XI   MUSKOGEE, OKLA., AUGUST, 1918   NUMBER 8

PUBLISHED MONTHLY AT MUSKOGEE, OKLA., UNDER DIRECTION OF THE COUNCIL

DR. CLAUDE A. THOMPSON, EDITOR-IN-CHIEF

ENTERED AT THE POST OFFICE AT MUSKOGEE, OKLAHOMA, AS SECOND CLASS MAIL MATTER, JULY 28, 1912

THIS IS THE OFFICIAL JOURNAL OF THE OKLAHOMA STATE MEDICAL ASSOCIATION. ALL COMMUNICATIONS SHOULD BE ADDRESSED TO THE JOURNAL OF THE OKLAHOMA STATE MEDICAL ASSSOCIATION, 308 SURETY BUILDING, MUSKOGEE, OKLAHOMA.

The editorial department is not responsible for the opinions expressed in the original articles of contributors.

Reprints of original articles will be supplied at actual cost, provided request for them is attached to manuscript or made in sufficient time before publication.

Articles sent this Journal for publication and all those read at the annual meetings of the State Association are the sole property of this Journal. The Journal relies on each individual contributor's strict adherence to this well-known rule of medical journalism. In the event an article sent this Journal for publication is published before appearance in the Journal, the manuscript will be returned to the writer.

Failure to receive the Journal should call for immediate notification of the editor, 307-8 Surety Building, Muskogee, Okla.

Local news of possible interest to the medical profession, notes on removals, changes in address, deaths and weddings will be gratefully received.

Advertising of articles, drugs or compounds unapproved by the Council on Pharmacy of the A. M. A. will not be accepted.

Advertising rates will be supplied on application. It is suggested that wherever possible members of the State Association should patronize our advertisers in preference to others as a matter of fair reciprocity.

EDITORIAL

NEW ARMY NEEDS FROM OUR PROFESSION.

Four months ago the Surgeon General's office indicated there would be needed immediately 8,000 physicians to equalize the needs of the 800,000 registrants to be called in 1918. This estimate was shortly thereafter reduced to 5,000. Almost immediately the country was electrified by the statement that we "now have more than half a million men in France." Soon the mark reached a million. Every great railway line running across the country bore evidence that there was a constant stream of trained men going to the seaboard for embarkation and coincidentally with the superactivity the Provost Marshal General began his insistent calls for thousands of new men to take the places of those who were leaving the cantonments; these calls came in such rapid succession as to amaize people who had not noticed the work particularly before. In many places Class 1 was exhausted by them.

This preliminary statement is made to show the impossibility of anyone trying to gauge the demands of the Medical Department for medical men. We thought we needed the 8,000, but as a matter of fact that 800,000 that we were to have have called out leisurely in 1918 has probably long since been sucked into the rapidly expanding and hungry maw of our training camps and when we have cast up our figures at the end of the year we will likely find that 3,000,000 for all Army branches will be nearer the number than the first estimate.

To meet this demand we must place more medical men in the field than we ever thought would be needed. Already the number runs far above twenty thousand (estimate) and the American Medical Association, which has completed an exhaustive, grass-roots survey of the situation, believes that we will be called to furnish approximately 40,000 men before we are through with the war if the ratio of men to the number of soldiers in service is maintained as heretofore.

They are now formulating the suggestion to all county organizations to secure at least 20 per cent. of their registered practitioners for the service.

A survey has already been made of our State's resources in this respect or is being made, and we should soon know approximately how many men have gone from each county, how many are left and of those how many probably can be spared.

It is suggested that no locality should, unless clearly oversupplied, send more than 50 per cent. of its practitioners, for it must not be overlooked that the civilian population at home, after we have an army of five million men in France, will approximate more than one hundred million people and they must necessarily have medical attention or the suffering will be incalculable. We have some localities heretofore oversupplied with physicians, but as a rule the rural districts have had localities where there·were not enough. Obviously such districts as the latter should be very carefully approached and the committees having charge of the consideration of ways and means should make their suggestions square with the facts and needs of each community. It has been said that some one with supposed authority has promised to send physicians to localities needing them. It must be said right here now that is a practical impossibility and was a promise made with little knowledge or study of the situation. The rural community now deprived of its physicians will remain in that state until the war ends, for the attractive lure of the cities will take those who can move, so it follows that the first and severe demands should be made on the cities where hospitals and centralized population makes it easier for physicians to centralize and systematize their work in such manner that they may, in the aggregate, do twice or thrice the work they formerly did. We have remaining in Oklahoma many men who by a little stretch of management could arrange their affairs to make the sacrifice entailed on entering the service of their country. These men should now prepare to answer the call soon to be made on them. We should not forget that the most important thing confronting the free peoples of the world today is winning the war and the efforts toward building up private practices and furthering selfish and personal ends must be relegated until the most important work is finished. Unless we win the war physicians may well look forward to conditions of impoverishment, taxation rates undreamed of and possibly such impossible interference with the intimate and personal affairs of the American family life as to make our lives unbearable.

The only thing we have to suggest in this matter is that each physician must be the sole judge of whether he should go or not, but the man who can go and trumps up this and that trivial excuse for not going is soon likely to become a mark for derision from his fellow man.

PERSONAL AND GENERAL NEWS

Dr. R. Keyes, Castle, has moved to Okemah.

Dr. and Mrs. W. S. Larrabee, Henryetta, are touring Colorado by automobile.

Dr. G. H. Wetzel, Sapulpa, has been commissioned in the Medical Reserve Corps.

Dr. Lea A. Riely, Oklahoma City, has been made a Captain in the Medical Reserve.

Dr. E. W. King, Bristow, has received a commission as first lieutenant in the Medical Reserve.

Dr. H. T. Ballantine, 1st Lieutenant, M. R. C., Muskogee, was ordered to report for duty Aug. 5.

Dr. A. B. Fair, located for many years at Frederick, will move to his old home, Ottumwa, Iowa.

Dr. Edwin F. Davis, Oklahoma City, has been commissioned a Captain in the Medical Reserve Corps.

Dr. R. J. Shull, Hugo, has been commissioned and received orders to report for Medical Reserve Corps duty.

Dr. C. E. Calhoun, Sand Springs, has moved his family to Springtown, Ark. He will soon enter the Medical Reserve.

Drs. A. B. Fair and J. Angus Gillis, Frederick, have dissolved their partnership. Dr. Fair will seek a new location.

Pauls Valley physicians have announced a substantial raise in their professional charges on account of the H. C. L.

Dr. C. C. Shaw, McAlester, who has been penitentiary physician for several years, has been commissioned in the Medical Reserve.

Dr. McLain Rogers, Clinton, is preparing to enter active service in the Medical Reserve and is visiting his old home in North Carolina.

Okmulgee physicians and civic societies are putting in execution a plan for the securing of free ice and milk for sick children in that city.

Okfuskee County organized a medical council of defense recently. Dr. B. Watts was made Chairman and Dr. H. A. May, Secretary.

Muskogee City is preparing to erect a tuberculosis pavilion. It will be located near the city hospital. and be managed by the organization of that institution.

Capt. William P. Fite, M. R. C., Muskogee, received orders July 17 to report on the Atlantic seaboard. He had been stationed at Camp Bowie for a year as Sanitary Inspector.

Oklahoma City's Maternity Hospital will not be closed, according to a statement from Mark Kessler, Commissioner, who announces there will be sufficient funds to operate during the coming fiscal year.

Dr. Claude Thompson, Muskogee, holds this as permanent announcement place of continued illness. Attempts to resume his work late in July resulted in a relapse. He was sent home from Oklahoma City.

Dr. B. F. McClure, McCurtain, despondent over failure to enter army, committed suicide July 22. Dr. McClure was 44 years of age and was considered a good practitioner and a good man by all who knew him

Dr. A. C. Hirshfield, Oklahoma City, has been commissioned in the Medical Reserve Corps. He has already seen service, having been attached to surgical units in both the Russian Navy and Army earlier in the war.

Drs. S. W. Aiken and L. D. Bruton, Muskogee, were bound over without bail July 29th charged with the murder of a Miss Malone of Stigler due to the alleged performance of an illegal operation, the girl dying the day after. Bail was granted later.

Creek County has organized a medical section of the defense council by electing Drs. H. S. Garland, Sapulpa, J. M. Wells, Bristow, and A. W. Holland, Drumright, a committee to act for the body. Lieutenant Justice, M. R. C., Sapulpa, presided at the meeting.

Pushmataha County Medical Society organized a county council of defense, medical section, June 27th. Drs. H. C. Johnson was elected president and Edw. Guinn, secretary. Drs. E. P. Wright of Albion and Guinn of Antlers volunteered their services to the Medical Reserve Corps.

Dr. Harry Walker, Pawhuska, died July 26. Dr. Walker was formerly of Oklahoma City, was appointed Osage physician during the McKinley administration and has resided in the Osage since that time. He leaves three sons, Dr. Roscoe of Pawhuska and two others who are officers in the army.

University Hospital, Oklahoma City, had a narrow escape from destruction by fire June 26. The nurses on duty, directed by Miss Holland, Superintendent, prevented a panic among the patients and handled the situation in a masterly manner. The damage was slight, amounting to only $150.00, according to reports.

Dr. S. P. Rawls, one of Jackson County's oldest physicians, who had resided at Altus for many years, died in that city June 20th. His death was due to intracranial hemorrhage ten days prior to the fatal outcome. He was for many years health officer of his county and was held in high esteem by his fellow practitioners.

Carter County Medical Society held a patriotic meeting June 9th. Drs. M. S. Alexander, Wirt; N. R. Barker, Healdton; T. H. Ware, New Wilson; J. F. Son, J. C. Best, G. W. Denham and A. G. Cowles, Ardmore, and two negro physicians, D. B. Scott and G. W. Hill, of that city, volunteered their services to the War Department.

Dr. Leroy Long, Dean of the Medical Department, Oklahoma University, made a plea before the medical section, State Council of Defense, for the retention at home of several physicians who had been slated to enter service. The plea was based on the greater need of the medical school which would have been stripped of valuable men and severely crippled. The idea that the school should not be crippled prevailed and the men were released to the faculty.

Dr. J. B. Gilbert, City Superintendent of Health for Tulsa, announces that there will be a radical change in the sanitary conditions of that city's restaurants or at least one-third of them will be closed. He is to be congratulated. The traveling public who have to patronize the alleged eating places in that city will raise a protest on the mildness of his figures. It is admitted that a good mop and hot water and soap might improve the condition of their best hotel.

CORRESPONDENCE

THE OKLAHOMA ASSOCIATION FOR THE PREVENTION OF TUBERCULOSIS.

Oklahoma City, Okla., July 25, 1918.

Dr. Claud A. Thompson, Sec.,
  State Medical Association,
    Muskogee, Oklahoma.

Dear Dr. Thompson:

I am giving you a brief account of the conference of the state medical examiners held in this city July 16, 1918.

At a recent conference held in Saint Louis between the State Tuberculosis Association and the Southwestern Division Headquarters of the American Red Cross, the following plan for the care of soldiers discharged and returned on account of tuberculosis was proposed and accepted. As soon as notification is received of a soldier's discharge, the Home Service Section of his locality is required to advise with the man and obtain for us information called for in the following questionaire:

1. Exact location of the discharged soldier, including his nearest railway station.
2. His apparent physical condition, whether in apparent normal health, debilitated, or actually sick.
3. His financial condition, or his ability to meet all or part of the cost of care, approximately from $18.00 per week.
4. His educational standards and those of his family, rated as excellent, good, fair, or poor.
5. His home conditions, rated as excellent, good, fair, or poor.
6. The name of the family physician, and his willingness to co-operate in this program, indicated by "yes," or "no" or "doubtful."
7. The desire of the discharged soldier and his family for expert diagnosis and treatment, indicated as "willing," "uninterested," or "opposed."

One copy is sent to our office, one to the Division Headquarters of the American Red Cross, and the third copy remains on file with the local chapter.

With this information at hand, we notify the Home Service Section to send this man to our special medical examiner in that district, who has been appointed for the purpose of examining discharged soldiers. The medical examiner is notified in advance of the patient's coming, and performs the examination without any fee. It is agreed that if the patient cannot afford to make this trip that the Home Service Section shall pay all costs of transportation.

The physician records the results of his examination upon a special card prepared by the Association and a duplicate copy of this report is sent to the state office.

After the physician has outlined a course of treatment, we send a special field nurse to confer with the local Home Service Section, and visit the patient to see that the instructions of the physician are carried out. It is our plan to educate the Red Cross worker so that she may be of help to the patient. It is also our plan, wherever possible, to arrange for sanatorium care for these men. If necessary, the local Home Service Section will pay part of the patient's maintenance during his stay at the sanatorium.

At the conference held July 16, there were present the following examiners, appointed by the State Association: Dr. Bitting, Enid; Dr. Campbell, Mangum; Dr. A. S. Risser, Blackwell; Dr. D. A. Myers, Lawton; Dr. H. T. Price, Tulsa; Dr. Wilkiemeyer, Muskogee; and Dr. L. J. Moorman, State Medical Director. Others appointed, but who could not attend the meeting, are Dr. T. S. McCarley, McAlester; Dr. Walter Hardy, Ardmore; Dr. Lamb, Clinton; Dr. Blair Points, Miami.

The meeting was held with the co-operation of The Tuberculosis Committee of the State Medical Society, The State Council of Defense, and The Southwestern Division of the American Red Cross.

The morning was spent in the Tuberculosis Dispensary, conducted by the Oklahoma Anti-Tuberculosis Society with Drs. L. D. Moorman and C. J. Fishman in charge. The clinic was unusually interesting and instructive, because of the great variety of clinical material and the very complete social, medical, and laboratory data. At a short conference in the office of the State Association held in the afternoon, I presented the problem of the returned and discharged soldiers as it confronts Oklahoma. A very fruitful discussion followed. From here the meeting adjourned to the Oklahoma Cottage Sanatorium where Dr. Moorman outlined standard methods for diagnosis and management of cases. A very interesting case of a patient receiving artificial pneumothorax treatment was discussed and introduction of gas was witnessed by those present.

Altogether the day was very profitably spent, and the men who attended the meetings felt well repaid for their coming and were very enthusiastic about helping in the solving of the problem of reconstruction, even before the closing of the war.

I have had to describe this meeting at great length, because I wanted to be sure you understood our general plan. You may use such of this material as you see fit.

With kindest regards, I am,

Very sincerely yours,

OKLAHOMA ASSOCIATION FOR THE PREVENTION
OF TUBERCULOSIS.

Jules Schevitz, General Secretary.

MISCELLANEOUS

NEW MEDICAL RESERVISTS.

Supplementary List, April 1 to 30, Inclusive.

George Norton Bilby_____Alva
James La Salle Miner_____Beggs
Frank Thomason_____Drumright
Edward Nelson McKee_____Enid
Lawrence Henry Hill_____Idabel
John Hutchings White_____Muskogee
Samuel Robert Cunningham ___Oklahoma City
Robert Lord Hull_____Oklahoma City
Joseph M. Postelle_____Oklahoma City
Charles Benjamin Taylor_____Oklahoma City
Walter William Wells_____Oklahoma City

Antonio DeBord Young_____Oklahoma City
Elmer Clarence Byram_____Okumlgee
Benjamin Franklin Newlon_____Ponca City
Thomas Spencer Williams_____Stilwell
William Albert Cook_____Tulsa
Hardin Davenport Irvan_____Tulsa
William Gladstone Lemon_____Tulsa
William Bliss Newlon_____Tulsa
Edward Frank Stroud_____Tulsa
William Joseph Trainor_____Tulsa
Robert Lee Mitchell_____Vinita

Supplementary List, May 1 to 31, Inclusive.

Charles Judson Brunson_____Adamson
Arthur Ernest Hale_____Alva
William Bertram Berninger_____Atwood
James Theodore Lowe_____Blair
Emery Wilbur King_____Bristow
Onis Franklin_____Broken Arrow
Walter Alonzo Howard_____Chelsea
Victor Clifford Tisdal_____Elk City
Henry Selwyn Drummond_____Haileyville
Edwin Davis_____Haskell
Harry Elwood Breese_____Henryetta
Arthur Fletcher Hobbs_____Hinton
William Reed Leverton_____Hobart
Roy Lewis Pendergraft_____Hollis
Daniel Boy Ensor_____Hopeton

Emmett Johnson_____Kinta
Virgil Henry Barton_____McAlester
Charles Cicero Shaw_____McAlester
Will Curd Wait_____McAlester
Clyde Oscar Williams_____McAlester
P. R. Davis_____Noble
Robert Dow Lowther_____Norman
Horace Reed_____Oklahoma City
Harold Blake Justice_____Sapulpa
Carl Lorraine McCallum_____Sapulpa
John David Leonard_____Strang
Victor Maurice Gore_____Taloga
Roy Wilton Dunlap_____Tulsa
W. Forest Dutton _____Tulsa
Gregory A. Wall_____Tulsa

"THE LABORATORY THAT KNOWS HOW."

The Cutter Laboratory, of Berkeley, Calif., has for twenty years been serving the physicians of the country; but in order to better meet the requirements of the profession, they have re-organized and enlarged their Chicago office, and are better prepared than ever before to serve the interests of our readers. Accordingly this Journal has accepted their page announcement, and is printing that announcement in this issue. If you find their service available for your practice, we bespeak for the Cutter Laboratory a share of your patronage.

TO CLASSIFY DOCTORS.

Council of National Defense, Medical Section.

Washington, July 16, 1918.

To State anp County Committees, Medical Section:

1. By authority of Surgeon General Gorgas of the Army, Surgeon General Braisted of the Navy and Surgeon General Blue of the Public Health Service, the Chairman of the General Medical Board of the Council of National Defense has appointed the following committee on classification of the medical profession of the United States for military and civil purposes to aid in enrollment in the Army, Navy, Public Health Service and the Volunteer Medical Service Corps:

Colonel R. B. Miller, M. C., U. S. A.; Colonel V. C. Vaughan, M. C., N. A.; Lieut. Colonel H. D. Arnold, M. C., N. A.; Surgeon R. C. Ramsdell, U. S. N.; Surgeon J. R. Phelps, U. S. N.; Dr. Joseph Schereschewsky, U. S. P. H. S.; Dr. Otto P. Geier, Dr. John D. McLean, Dr. C. E. Sawyer.

Ex-Officio: Surgeon General W. C. Gorgas, U. S. A.; Surgeon General W. C. Braisted, U. S. N.; Surgeon General Rupert Blue, U. S. P. H. S.; Lieut. Colonel F. F. Simpson, Dr. Franklin Martin.

2. This committee is authorized to meet at regular intervals and to cooperate with the Committee on States Activities, the State and County Committees and other agencies and societies engaged in advisory or executive functions dealing with classifications and enrollment for military, industrial and home needs.

Franklin Martin,
Member of the Advisory Commission.

TRAINING CAMP AT FORT RILEY.

W. M. Bispham, Fort Riley, Kansas, says (*Journal A. M. A.*, July 20, 1918), that it is not necessary to show the reasons for the establishments of training camps for the Medical Department. The view was held from the beginning the proper principal to go on was to make medical officers 100 per cent military men, and in this way they would be of more value to their government in whatever position they were placed. There has been nothing in the course of months of experience to change this view. In the beginning, therefore, the course as outlined was distinctly military, with, of course, a considerable amount of professional instruction along the medico-military lines. The keynote has always been discipline, not servile, but it was impressed on the physician from his arrival that in doing any work with the army in the field ready and willing obedience to regulations was a first essential. It is well understood that the physical condition of the soldier of today, whether in the line or the medical department, must be as perfect as it can be made. The physical instruction is progressively more strenuous, and the results have shown that a three months' intensive course makes the officer leaving the camp capable of performing all his duties. The medical officer in the army comes in very close contact with the enlisted man, and unless he understands the point of view of the latter, he is incapable of performing his duties as the government requires. Therefore, at the training camp he is put practically in the potion of the enlisted man, in barracks, in which his rank of lieutenant, captain or major is ignored. This basic course is continued for there months, and he further receives instruction in Army Regulations, the manual of the Medical Department, and all the medico-military work which he ought to know. The last half of the course is taken up with actual field instruction, giving the officer maneuvers and field services in which he takes an active part. It was soon found, also, that something more than the mere military instruction could be profitably given. Certain special branches of medicine require more attention in military work that in civil life, and separate training schools were established to meet the need, one of these at Fort Riley. Some of the most important men, in their lines, were sent as instructors and the clinical material at the base hospital at Fort Riley permitted a very high class of instruction to be given. In the army the preventive side of medicine properly receives more attention than in civil life, hence special schools were established for instruction in sanitation and prophylaxis, and attached to this department a sanitary laboratory to enable the medical officer to study under practical demonstration the sanitary applicances used in the field and experiment with new ones. The enlisted men of the medical department were trained both generally and in special organizations, such as ambulance companies, field and base hospitals, etc., and the officer in training comes in close contact with these units. The results have been excellent. The effect on the individual as regards *esprit de corps* and general character and conduct is striking.

ARMOUR AND COMPANY ANNOUNCE NEW PRODUCT.

www.ingramcontent.com/pod-product-compliance
Lightning Source LLC
Chambersburg PA
CBHW071411050326
40689CB00010B/1826